# Notes for the MRCP

# Other Examination Preparation Books Published by Petroc Press

Obtainable from all good booksellers or, in case of difficulty, from Plymbridge Distributors Limited, Plymbridge House, Estover Road, PLYMOUTH, Devon, PL6 7PZ, Tel. 01752–202300, Fax 01752–202333.

# Notes for the MRCP

## N R BALCOMBE

*Consultant Physician/Geriatrician*
*St Cross Hospital, Rugby*
*Walsgrave Hospitals NHS Trust*

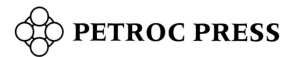 PETROC PRESS

*Petroc Press,* an imprint of LibraPharm Limited

**Distributors**
Plymbridge Distributors Limited, Plymbridge House, Estover Road, Plymouth PL6 7PZ, UK

Published in the United Kingdom by
LibraPharm Limited
Gemini House
162 Craven Road
NEWBURY
Berkshire
RG14 5NR
UK

A catalogue record for this book is available from the British Library

ISBN 1 900603 47 0

Typeset by WordSpace, Lewes, East Sussex
Printed and bound in the United Kingdom by Cromwell Press Ltd, Trowbridge, Wilts BA14 0XB

# Dedication

To my wife Sue – forever together

# Contents

# Preface

Welcome to the MRCP examination and to this book, which I hope will prove a valuable aid in your quest for success.

The book is aimed at candidates taking either the Part I or Part II examination, and as such should prove useful for a prolonged period of time. Furthermore, even after you have jumped the MRCP hurdle, I hope this book will prove to be a useful source of information in the future.

For the Part I examination a large amount of factual knowledge is required. A strong theme of the book, therefore, is to provide as much factual information as possible. Much of this is presented in the form of lists. The aim has been to make these as comprehensive and user-friendly as possible by indicating the common features by underlining. The extensive use of diagrams and flowcharts also allows information to be presented in a format that aids learning.

For the Part II examination little new knowledge is required over and above that needed for Part I, and so this book should be a useful revision aid. The book also contains features specific to Part II, such as common cases encountered in the clinical exam. The old Part II clinical examination has recently been replaced by a new format (PACES), and details of this examination are given in the first chapter.

Another important aspect of preparation for these exams is revision and exam techniques, and so handy hints for improving these are given in the first chapter.

The book covers all the major medical specialties and the basic medical sciences. It also contains a chapter on geriatric medicine. Although this has not been a popular area covered in past exams, in the near future it is likely to become an increasing feature of both Parts. This book represents one of the first to go into this specialty in any detail with the MRCP examinations in mind.

Finally, I would like to wish you all the best of luck.

*April, 2001*                                                                                            NB

# Acknowledgements

My sincere thanks go to everyone who has guided me through my professional career. In particular, I would like to thank Dr W M Saweirs (Consultant Physician/Geriatrician, Queens Hospital, Burton-upon-Trent) and Professor A J Sinclair (Professor of Medicine, University of Warwick), who have become valuable mentors and who continue to provide outstanding support in matters both professional and personal. Thanks also go to my wife and four wonderful children for their constant support and understanding. Particular thanks also go to my parents for all their efforts on my behalf, and especially to my mother for her help in the preparation of this manuscript.

# Section I

# Handy Hints for Passing the MRCP Examinations

# Introduction

In life there are seldom absolute certainties, but one thing that is certain is that to pursue a career in any branch of hospital medicine you will have to pass the MRCP examinations. To most candidates these appear a daunting and, at times, seemingly insurmountable hurdle. Their purpose is to test your knowledge of the principles and practice of medicine: there is therefore no substitute for thorough knowledge and competent clinical ability. However, as with any game, although good knowledge and ability are central to success, clever tactics and well planned strategies are also crucial elements of a winning package. Many candidates with excellent knowledge repeatedly fail because of poor exam technique. In the process of ploughing through the mountain of information required to attain a sufficient level of knowledge, while at the same time satisfying busy clinical demands, exam technique is an aspect of revision that is often overlooked. However, time spent on improving exam technique is vital and is often the difference between success and failure. This particularly applies to the Part I examination.

In this section I hope to be able to give you some useful guidance on how to improve your chances of success. Although certain principles apply to both parts of the examination, I will consider each part separately. I will also explain the format of the new Part II clinical examination (PACES) and illustrate how it differs from the old format.

# MRCP Part I

## Revision technique

*Time*

It is obvious to say that before you can begin your revision you must first create adequate time for it. This requires the production of a timetable. To produce a realistic and successful timetable you must plan to begin your revision well in advance of the exam (usually 3–6 months is adequate). A successful timetable should comprise mainly of a long-term plan taking you up to the exam itself, but it can also be useful to set short-term goals within this grander plan. It is important to try to stick to your timetable, but you will need to allow some flexibility. If you fall behind with your revision this may be because the timetable is unrealistic or because there have been unexpected events, or simply because you have not worked hard enough. Obviously it is important to identify what the problem is and to correct it. If you have allowed flexibility in your timetable, this will help you to catch up with your revision. A good way of incorporating such flexibility is to deliberately leave one or two revision sessions towards the end of the week empty. Thus if you have fallen behind at the beginning of the week you will be able to use these free sessions to catch up. If you have managed to keep to your timetable, these empty sessions are still not wasted and can be used either to revise an area of weakness again or to make a start on the next week's revision, allowing you to stay even further ahead of time. Staying on time is important in order to maintain confidence and prevent feelings of panic while revising, which undoubtedly impairs learning ability. Finally, remember to get your study leave requests in early.

## Learning strategies

### What to revise

Having developed a timetable it is now important to decide what you are going to revise and what sources of information you are going to use. At present the College does not produce a syllabus for its examinations, but past exams are useful pointers. Many mistakenly think the exam is a test of knowledge of rarities, and focus their revision accordingly. Although it is true that a great depth of knowledge is required, it is a mistake to skip over the common conditions. A natural behaviour during revision for any exam is to repeatedly cover areas in which your knowledge is already good. This has the effect of boosting your confidence by creating the feeling that you know what you need to know. However, it also leads to a false sense of security and, while confidence is important, it is essential that this cycle of revision does not develop because if it does, come the big day, even though you may be a world expert on a particular subject you will be doomed to failure when there are no questions on your specialised subject but a lot on topics you know less well. It is essential that your knowledge is equally good in all areas, and when you begin your revision programme it is important to ensure that you devote sufficient time to all topics on which you may be tested. Once you are into your revision programme, it is important to identify areas of weakness and to ensure that you devote more time to improving them rather than revising what you already know well. Flexibility in your timetable should allow you to follow this approach.

### Sources of information

The major medical textbooks remain the mainstay as information sources, but be realistic. It is not humanly possible to learn the *Oxford Textbook of Medicine* from cover to cover, and in trying to do so you will probably end up learning nothing. Although such definitive texts are undoubtedly valuable as reference books, you are much better choosing a smaller textbook as your main source of information. As I will discuss shortly, practice questions will also help to improve your knowledge.

### How often to repeat a topic

Some candidates seem to possess a photographic memory and are able to remember huge amounts of information after one sitting. If you are like this you are indeed fortunate, but if you are a mere mortal you will probably have to cover each topic several times (I would suggest at least two or three). Decide what you need to do, based on your previous experiences, and ensure that your timetable allows for whatever strategy you decide upon.

It is also important to get the timing of your revision correct. If you need to cover a topic two or three times it is no good revising it 6 months before the exam and again 2 weeks later. Although you will have covered the topic twice, in the intervening 5½ months you will undoubtedly forget some of what you have learned. It is better to cover all topics in a short period of time and then to duplicate your timetable. The number of times you will have to repeat topics will determine how much time you should allow to cover all areas. For example, if you begin your revision 6 months before the exam and you need to go through each topic three times, you will need to produce a timetable that allows you to cover all areas in 2 months. This 2-month timetable can then be repeated three times.

### To work alone or with others

Generally people fit into two categories. First there are those who prefer solitude when revising and find the involvement of others distracting or intimidating. Second there are those who derive a sense of wellbeing from being able to demonstrate in front of others what they know. These are the sort of candidate who often attempt to astonish others by their knowledge of rarities. This environment often creates a competitive atmosphere. For some this is beneficial, with such competition acting as a source of motivation. However, remember that in the exams you are not competing with your peers but with the Royal College of Physicians. For some candidates a competitive environment can be intimidating and lead to feelings of inferiority and reduced confidence and should be avoided. If you do find yourself in such an environment, for example on a course, do not allow yourself to be put off: remember, a knowledge of rarities does not equate to a knowledge of common conditions, and you will not pass unless you know the common things. If you are on a course and the atmosphere is intimidating, take yourself away from the environment as much as possible and steer clear of people who want to tell you how much they know. Don't worry if you appear as a loner and unfriendly: after all, you are there to prepare for your exam, not to make lifelong friends.

## Relaxation

One of the keys to successful revision is the ability to work smarter. Efficient revision equates to more successful revision. To achieve this, it is important to incorporate into your timetable time for relaxation. Assigning one night a week free from study is recommended. There are very few people who can revise effectively when tired, and late-night revision is a pitfall to be avoided. In contrast, early morning is often the time when the mind is at its clearest and best able to absorb knowledge. Tiredness can also seriously affect performance during the exam. Relaxation is particularly important in the week leading up to the exam itself. If an efficient and sensible revision programme has been pursued there should be little need for last-minute cramming, which usually increases stress levels and fails to add to your knowledge. Avoid revision on the night before the exam for similar reasons: what you do not know then you will not know the day after. All you will do by working the night before the exam is increase your anxiety and impair your performance on the day. It is far better to relax and remain calm. Going out, with friends who are not taking the exam with you, is a useful way of taking your mind off things. Do *not* go out with friends who are also taking the exam, because you will all undoubtedly talk shop and defeat the purpose of going out!

## Practice

A vital part of revision is MCQ practice. This is essential for two reasons. First it sharpens your skill in answering such questions, leading to improved exam technique, and second, if done properly, MCQs can be a valuable source of information, adding to the knowledge gained elsewhere. In particular, the past papers published by the College provide the best guide to the style of the exam and should be purchased at the earliest opportunity.

# Examination technique

It is important to remember that there is no fixed pass mark for the exam. Instead, a fixed number of candidates are passed (30%). This means that the pass mark does vary, although it does so within a small range (usually 50–60%). With the negative marking scheme used in the exam, to be successful it is important to have good technique. As previously mentioned, it is easy to fail because of poor technique despite good knowledge. When faced with a question in the exam, the first thing you must do is read it carefully and ensure you understand what it is asking. With regard to the answer, you will find that your degree of certainty falls into one of three categories: 1, absolutely 100% sure (convinced, no doubts); 2, moderately sure (fair idea but not absolutely sure); 3, totally unsure (no idea, pure guess). You may be tempted to think that if you are absolutely sure about 50–60% of the questions, then you will pass by answering only those. This would be a mistake, because in reality you will never get 100%: probably you will get around 90% right and 10% wrong. With negative marking, this will reduce your overall mark by 20%, making your mark 30–40% and leading to failure. Consequently you will need to answer more questions, but remember, of these questions of which you are moderately sure, you will get a higher percentage wrong than of those you are absolutely sure of. What you must determine before the exam is your degree of certainty when answering questions. This is done by doing three practice exams and in each one answering the questions in three different colours, according to your degree of certainty. Then calculate what percentage of each group you get right and wrong. You will find that your degree of certainty is consistent in each practice exam. This will then give you an idea of how many questions you will need to answer in the exam. Some candidates claim to answer every question. To pass by following this course of action you either have to have a tremendous depth of knowledge or a great deal of luck.

When sitting the exam it is advisable to first go through the paper fairly quickly, answering only the questions you are absolutely sure about. In particular do not be put off by the first few questions, which are often deliberately made harder to test a candidate's mettle. Start by finding an easy question that you can answer in full. This will get you off to a good start and help your confidence. Remember, there are no rules about the order in which you have to answer questions.. Add up the number you have answered and decide whether you need to answer more (you probably will). Then go through the paper again answering questions about which you are moderately sure. Make sure you do not guess at this stage. After you have calculated how many you have answered, try and work out, from your predetermined degree of certainty, what your mark will be. Then decide if you need to guess any more answers (if your knowledge is good this will not be necessary). Finally, the exam normally allows ample time to complete the paper and many candidates have half to one hour spare. This is a very dangerous time. Many candidates, during this time, review their answers and look at questions they have left out. This behaviour inevitably leads to changes of heart and to some answers being changed and others being guessed in a last-ditch attempt to improve your score. However, the result is usually a worsening of one's score. First impressions are usually more accurate than careful deliberations at the end of the exam, so do not fiddle with your previous answers and do not be tempted into guessing. If you have followed the above advice you should be able confidently to leave your paper and walk out of the exam room before time.

## Definitions

Many exam questions use key phrases and terminology that can confuse candidates as to their meaning, leading sometimes to an erroneous answer. It is important to understand what is meant by certain terms.

**Only, always, never** It is very rare for something to be as black and white as these words imply, and a question comprising them is usually false.

**Pathognomonic** This means it only occurs in one particular condition and its presence or absence immediately allows a diagnosis to be made or excluded. If it is truly pathognomonic you should know it. If you do not, the answer is likely to be false.

**Characteristic** This means that it is usually present in a particular condition and its absence might put doubt in your mind about the diagnosis. It may be characteristic for more than one condition. Again, if it is true you should know this; therefore, if you do not the answer is likely to be false.

**Typical** This means that you would expect it to be present. It is similar to 'characteristic'.

**Recognised** This means that it may be present in a particular condition but is not essential for a diagnosis to be made. To be able to answer these questions requires a good depth of knowledge.

**Associated with** This is similar in meaning to 'recognised'.

**Probably, frequent, often, likely** These are confusing terms but usually indicate a false answer.

**Possible, may, rarely, can** These are also confusing terms that usually indicate a true answer.

# After the examination

After the exam you will probably be wondering how you have done, and will find it difficult not to replay some of the questions and your answers over in your mind. This is best avoided if possible, as it usually leads to candidates believing they have done badly. What is probably worse is being in a group of people doing the same thing, particularly if some of them are the type that likes to air their opinions in front of an audience: remember that this behaviour is often a sign of insecurity and lack of knowledge. After the exam, forget it and steer clear of the mass hysteria that can develop outside. After all, you will have been working hard for some time and undoubtedly deserve a break. Enjoy it and look forward to receiving the letter 2 weeks later telling you that you have passed. Then you will have done it and will be able to look forward to taking Part II (but that's another day).

# MRCP Part II

## Written paper

After the gruelling encounter of Part I I am confident that you will find revising for Part II relatively enjoyable. This is mainly because it tests your ability to apply what has been learnt for Part I in a clinical setting. It therefore more closely reflects what you do daily as part of your clinical duties, and as a result is less of an unknown. Many of the principles I have already discussed with regard to revision and exam techniques apply just as much to this exam and should not be forgotten. However, there are some important differences in your approach that need to be mentioned.

There is no need to spend vast amounts of time ploughing through the major textbooks from cover to cover, as you did when revising for Part I. Instead, the emphasis for revision should now shift towards applying your knowledge to the questions posed in the written Part II paper. This can only be done by practising questions. Get your hands on every Part II question book that has ever been written and do the questions again and again and again, so that your mind becomes attuned to the style of this exam. You will begin to recognise topics and conditions that commonly crop up, and you will learn a tremendous amount of new and relevant information from the answers and explanations that are usually given. You may even enjoy your revision. Keep the major medical textbooks on the shelf, but within reach to enable you to use them for reference.

The exam is divided into three sections: picture slides, grey cases and data interpretation. Revision time should initially be divided equally between the three, but remember to allow flexibility in your timetable as before.

## Picture slides

This is often the most difficult section of the exam, simply because there is such a huge selection of pictures that could be shown. The only way to prepare for this is to see as many slides as you can (I would suggest somewhere in the region of 1000–2000). The most important thing to remember when faced with a picture slide is to look at it carefully and, more importantly, to look at all of the picture and to pick up clues that are sometimes given in the periphery. This is particularly important when faced with X-rays. Do not miss the absent breast shadow in an apparently normal-looking female CXR, and do not be fooled by an apparently normal but reversed CXR of a patient with Kartagener's syndrome. These points may be obvious, but they are often forgotten

when candidates enter the pressure-cooker atmosphere of the exam itself.

## Grey cases

Again, there is no substitute for endless question practice. After a while you will begin to see common topics and styles of questions emerging, which will help your preparations tremendously. Again, during the exam itself the most important thing to do is to read the question carefully and thoroughly. What you have to do is to put all the information together in a logical fashion to come up with an overall answer. In most of the questions a lot of information is given (including some red herrings to beware of). Sometimes it is useful to summarise the question by breaking it down into the main findings. If you have done enough practice questions in your build-up you should very quickly be able to get a feel for what the question is asking for, and this will help you formulate your answers accordingly. Remember that this exam is not a test of rarities but, rather, a test of your ability to apply your basic knowledge in a clinical situation that you may encounter in the future. Therefore, what the examiners want to see is that you have a solid grasp of the basic principles of clinical medicine and that, faced with the clinical situation given, you would perform logically, competently and safely. Remember that common conditions are common: if you are faced with a patient in Casualty with abnormal liver function tests, the examiners want to see that you would think of alcohol- or drug-induced liver disease rather than yellow fever.

Also, when answering the questions try and give as full an answer as possible. This is important because marks are awarded in a graded fashion and you can easily lose valuable marks if your answers are not thorough enough, even if they are essentially right. For example, if faced with a patient with a generalised purpuric rash, fever, neck stiffness and photophobia, the answers 'meningitis' or 'bacterial meningitis' would gain some marks, but to score full marks the answer should be 'meningococcal meningitis and septicaemia'.

## Data interpretation

This is probably the easiest section of the paper because there is obviously a limitation to the number of medical investigations that can be performed, and therefore that you can be asked about. Remember to read the questions carefully and give as full an answer as possible. Again, if you have prepared well, you will see common themes cropping up time and time again. If you are really lucky you may even get one or two questions in the exam that you have seen before. However, there is a note of caution to add to this statement, and that is that the question setters sometimes alter a question slightly so that the correct answer is altered. When candidates see questions they recognise, they are often tempted to proceed straight to the answer without reading the whole question properly. This may lead to an erroneous answer if the question has been changed from when they saw it. Hence, it bears repeating: read the questions thoroughly before committing to an answer.

# Clinical examination

Well, you are nearly there, having completed two-thirds of the exams you need to pass in order to enable you to put MRCP after your name. However, you still have one hurdle to go, and to many candidates this is the most daunting of all. Suddenly, sitting a multiple-choice paper or written theory paper, in solitude with no-one looking over your shoulder, seems

a pleasurable and preferred option. There is no doubt that having to perform in front of professors and eminent consultants seems to make clinical exams a very stressful experience. This is what they are all about: they are purely and simply a test of candidates' ability to perform in a stressful environment. The content of the exam is extremely straightforward for any candidate that has had good clinical experience, as most will have done during a busy SHO rotation. All the exam asks is that you do what you have been doing during the course of your clinical work, but what makes it a supreme test is the environment in which it asks you to do it. Some people say that the level of pressure makes it an unfair test, but in the real world, as an on-call SHO with five patients waiting to be seen, the ability to work under pressure is critical, and the exam therefore provides a perfect test of competence in such an environment.

## New exam format (see opposite)

### PACES (Practical Assessment of Clinical Examination Skills)

Until now, the clinical examination has been comprised of a long case (20 minutes), short cases (30 minutes) and a viva (20 minutes). As of June 2001, this format will change to become the new PACES examination. The new format is designed to provide the following advantages in comparison to its predecessor:

- A more standardised and objective assessment of examination skills
- A direct assessment of history taking and communication skills
- Assessment by ten examiners rather than six
- Increased throughput of candidates per host centre
- Improved patient efficiency
- Improved feedback to those who fail

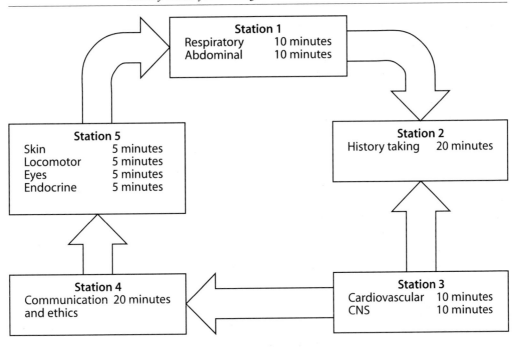

**The carousel of PACES stations**

The new examination will consist of five stations. Candidates will begin at any one of the stations and rotate around the carousel of stations at 20-minute intervals, until they have completed the cycle. At each station, candidates will be assessed by two examiners. In contrast to the old exam format, each pair of examiners will remain based at a particular station. This means that over the five stations, candidates will be assessed by a total of ten examiners. Each of the five stations will be of a standard design.

### Stations 1, 3, 5 (Clinical short cases)
These stations will be similar to the old short case section of the exam. The objective of these stations will be to assess candidates' ability to examine patients, interpret clinical findings and discuss cases. Although similar to the old exam format, two important differences in the new exam will be that candidates will be given written rather than verbal instruc-

tions for each case, and a time limit for each case will be set. In the three stations, various organ systems will be addressed in a standardised manner:

*Station 1*
• Respiratory system (10 mins)
• Abdominal system (10 mins)

*Station 3*
• Cardiovascular system (10 mins)
• Central nervous system (10 mins)

*Station 5*
• Skin (5 mins)
• Locomotor (5 mins)
• Eyes (5 mins)
• Endocrine system (5 mins)

### Station 2 (History taking)
This station will assess candidates' ability to gather information from patients, assimilate it and discuss the case. As such, this part of the new exam represents the

nearest thing to the old long case section. In the new format, candidates will be given written instructions five minutes before they start and only 15 minutes will be allowed for the history taking, leaving the last 5 minutes for questioning by the examiners.

### Station 4 (Communication and ethics)

While the other stations represent variations of the old exam format, this station represents a new topic for examination. It will assess candidates' ability to guide and organise an interview with a subject, to provide emotional support, and to discuss patient management strategies. The subjects may be patients, relatives or healthcare workers, who will be briefed before the candidate begins. Candidates will again receive written instructions at the start of the station and 15 minutes will be allowed for interaction between the candidate and subject, leaving 5 minutes for discussion between candidates and examiners at the end.

# Helpful hints for the PACES

## History taking

As I have already said, what you are asked to do in this section is what you will have been doing since you qualified from medical school. To pass the section requires an understanding of what the examiners want from you. They do not primarily want to see if you can examine the patient, because they know this will be tested at the other stations. What they do want is to test your ability to take a comprehensive history. What you must try to do is gather all the relevant information in as much detail as possible. For example, if you are presented with a patient with bronchiectasis, you don't just need to

know that the patient produces purulent sputum, but also how often and how much. In terms of patient management, you will need to mention drainage procedures, yearly flu jabs, prompt treatment of infection, giving the patient a supply of antibiotics at home, how will you monitor the condition etc.; if you remember what I said earlier about these exams being a 'game', you will see that what you have to do to be successful is learn to apply the information and your knowledge in a way that is adapted for the exam.

The first thing you will do in the long case is meet the patient. This is an important moment and it is critical that you get the patient on your side by being polite and introducing yourself. If you can put them in a comfortable frame of mind and make them feel safe in your hands, they will be much more inclined to help you, by telling you the diagnosis and other important points that you may have failed to pick up.

When taking the history, ensure that it is thorough and keep thinking about what the examiners are likely to ask about. For example, in a patient with rheumatoid arthritis the examiners will probably not be interested in their bowel habits, but more in their functional ability and social history. Conversely, in patients with inflammatory bowel disease the bowel symptoms are likely to be central to the case.

At the end of the 15 minutes of history taking, the examiners may take one of two approaches. They may ask you to present the case as you would normally do on your consultant ward rounds. Alternatively they may move directly to questions about the information you have gathered. If asked to present your findings, ensure that you speak slowly and clearly, maintaining eye contact with the person asking the questions. Make sure your presentation is smooth and well ordered. Present only the positive findings and relevant negative findings. Do not enter into a long monologue of irrelevant negative findings, as this irritates the examiners and demonstrates poor preparation and an inability to formulate your thoughts.

After some initial questions about the history, you will probably be asked more questions about the management of the patient and of the condition in general. Again, if you have prepared properly, you should be able to predict what you will be asked and be ready with some slick answers.

At the end of the time, make sure you thank the examiners and are polite and gracious in your departure, even if you have had a rough time. As you leave the room, clear your mind of any negative thoughts or mistakes you have made and begin to focus on the next section to come.

## Clinical short cases

Many candidates find this section of the exam the most gruelling and, again, this is almost certainly due to the intense scrutiny that candidates are put under. This section is designed to assess candidates' ability to examine a patient competently and professionally and to put together what is found in a logical order, leading to a sensible diagnosis. Again, what candidates are asked to do is the same as is done on a daily basis. Any reasonable SHO should be more than capable of examining patients, but, again, in order to pass the exam, candidates have to play the 'game'. For this section examination technique is all-important, and there is only one way to get it right: practise. It is obviously very useful to practise on patients with signs, but of paramount importance is your ability to perform a system examination smoothly and without hesitation.

In order to hone this skill it is often useful to practise your examinations on friends. If you imagine that there are six or seven systems that you might be asked to examine, with each taking 2–3 minutes, it should take no more than 30 minutes to run through every system, allowing time for appraisal. If you spend 30 minutes every day for 3 months doing this, your examination technique will improve dramatically. The key thing you must achieve is the ability to examine someone without needing to stop to think what you have done already and what you need to do next. If you fall into this trap, while you are examining the patient you will not be able to think about what signs you have found and how they fit together. Instead, you will have to assimilate this information when you have finished your examination, when what you should be doing is giving a slick presentation of your findings to the examiners. If you fall into these traps there will be long pauses during your case, and to the examiners, it is these pauses that indicate insufficient ability, leading to failure. It is terribly easy for an examiner to see what is going through candidates' minds while they are examining patients, and the poorly prepared candidate whose examination routines are not ingrained is rapidly spotted.

When you are preparing for the exam it is vital that you are taken round by someone who will push you hard, and at times make you feel uncomfortable without completely destroying your confidence. It is no good being taught by someone who smiles and tells you everything is fine, because unless you are really good, you will be misled into thinking your performance is good enough when it is not. My advice is that the best people to teach you are registrars and consultants who regularly examine for the exams. It is also important to practise in front of others to simulate exam conditions. You will be surprised how much more difficult it is to perform in front of an audience.

When you walk into the examination cubicle you will come face to face with a patient. Immediately, before you receive your instructions, take the opportunity to look at the patient to pick up any obvious visual clues. Also look around the cubicle for any other clues that might indicate a diagnosis, such as a hearing aid, diabetic chart, PEFR (peak expiratory flow rate) meter etc.

Pay close attention to the instructions you are given. For example, if you are asked to examine the cardiovascular system your examination will begin with a period of observation followed by examination of the hands. However, if you are asked to examine the praecordium you will irritate the examiners by examining the hands. Whatever you are asked to do there are some important things you must do before you even touch the patient. First, you must introduce yourself to the patient and ask them if you may examine them. Of course no patient will refuse your request, but by asking you are again demonstrating a professional approach. You must also ensure that the area you want to examine is fully exposed and that the patient is in the right position (e.g., at 45° to read the JVP – jugular venous pressure).

Once you have begun your examination, be thinking all the time of what you have found and how the findings fit together to form a diagnosis. It is also important to 'master the case'. This is done by thinking of associated conditions that may be found with the primary diagnosis, and to demonstrate to the examiners that you are thinking this way by proceeding to look for them. Also, try to demonstrate that you appreciate how the diagnosis relates to the patient as a whole. For example, if you are presented with a patient with rheumatoid hands, do not just examine the joints and note the

deformities, but go on and assess the patient's functional ability by asking them to hold a cup, pick up an object, unscrew a lid etc. Often items are deliberately put near the patient as a cue for you to use them. By the time you have finished examining the patient you should have formulated your thoughts and be ready to give a slick presentation. At the end of your examination you must perform the most important act in the whole process, and that is to thank the patient and cover them up. If you do not do this and leave the patient exposed as you turn away, you will fail immediately.

Pressure does funny things to people and one of the commonest effects it has is to make people say things they do not mean. Examiners look forward to the occasion when candidates make this mistake and manage to dig a hole as deep as the Atlantic ocean. There is one thing you can be sure of, and that is if you dig a hole the examiners will push you in. There is one certain way to avoid this, and that is to think before you speak. If you have followed the steps regarding a smooth examination, you should already have formulated your thoughts by the time you finish, and this will help. Once you have started to speak, be clear and to the point.

A good way to start your presentation is to tell the examiners that you have seen the patient and not just 'the chest'. Start with 'this is a [young, middle aged, elderly] [man, woman] who is [comfortable at rest, dyspnoeic etc.]. Once you have begun, do not then enter into a long monologue presenting the signs or lack of signs that you found in the order you found them. This demonstrates that the candidate has not thought through what he has done, and is taken as evidence of lack of examination skills. It is always best to start by pointing out the most obvious abnormality, and follow this with a statement of the other positive findings and important negative findings that support your diagnosis. While presenting the case, be clear, concise and confident, and do not be tempted to mention things you cannot justify. Also avoid using expressions such as 'I think' or 'possibly', which indicate uncertainty. Finish your presentation with a single diagnosis if it is clear, or two or three differential diagnoses if it is not, and when you have stated your diagnosis, shut up! At this point the examiners may pause, leading to a few moments of silence. Do not be tempted at this point to say anything else or you will probably begin digging the hole the examiners are waiting for. The examiners may then ask you some supplementary questions about the condition, direct you straight to your next case, or question your diagnosis. Without doubt, the best way for an examiner to determine a candidate's competence is to ask them 'Are you sure?', sometimes with a frown to add to the psychology. For a candidate who is not entirely sure of what they have said, this response is usually taken as a sign that they have made a mistake. They may then change their minds and backtrack on what they have said, and on many occasions this leads to a correct answer being changed to an incorrect one. Remember the hole that you will end up digging? In order to avoid this scenario you must concentrate and be clear about what you are doing, what you are finding and what you are saying. This comes back to adequate preparation. If you are confident that you are right you should not be put off if the examiners use this tactic. Simply and confidently restate your findings and conclusions. If, however, you realise that you have made a mistake, or the examiner tells you that you have made a mistake, admit it immediately and do not argue or try and bluff your way out of it. Remember that you are not expected to know everything, and you do not want to

waste valuable time being questioned on areas of weakness as this will reduce the amount of time when you can show the examiners what you do know.

Some people mistakenly think that to pass the short cases you have to get all the diagnoses correct. This is a mistake, and although you must get the obvious diagnoses you may be presented with some rare conditions, which you will not be expected to get right in a few minutes. What is more important is your ability to perform a competent and professional examination and make logical conclusions.

Another important point is that you should not be put off by the examiners' expressions or mannerisms. It is not uncommon for pairs of examiners to consist of a Dr Jekyll and Professor Hyde, with one appearing benign and pleasant and the other malignant and stern. However, you should remember the phrase 'Beware the smiling death', which tells you that it is often the pleasant half of the partnership that is busy failing you. Remain focused on what you are doing and do not let disgruntled expressions faze you or pleasant expressions relax you too much.

For you to be successful in this section there needs to be a lot of confidence around. You need to feel confident that you are doing well, and the examiners need to feel confident about your abilities. You will do wonders for everyone's confidence if you make a good first impression, and therefore it is helpful to do well in your first case. However, if you do badly in this or any other case, do not panic. As soon as you leave the cubicle, put it behind you and focus on the next case. Do not allow negative thoughts to impair your performance in the next case.

## Communication and ethics

While this station of the PACES represents a new facet of the MRCP clinical examination, many of the general principles that I have already discussed are relevant. Ensure that you behave in a professional manner at all times, be polite and courteous to patients and examiners, be sure to introduce yourself and thank your patients after you have finished the station. As this is a new assessment in the exam, it is difficult to advise on what you may be asked to do, but I suggest that the following scenarios may be quite likely:

- Breaking bad news
- Informing patients of a diagnosis of cancer
- Discussing resuscitation orders
- Discussing artificial enteral nutrition in older patients with stroke disease or dementia
- Giving prognosis in acute stroke
- Chronic disease management
- Discussing long term care placements
- Giving advice on post-MI rehabilitation

# Finally...

Remember that you are not alone in your quest for glory. As well as all the other candidates who will be feeling just like you (even if they do not show it), your consultants and professors will still remember what it was like for them and hence how you will be feeling. Your examiners may even be as nervous as you. It is obviously important to work hard, but pay attention to revision and exam techniques, particularly for Part I. Above all, stay relaxed and focused on your mission. Do not allow others to distract you or feelings of panic to overwhelm you. Do not allow your morale to slip. You will find success if you 'work hard and play hard'. Good Luck!

# Section II

# Basic Sciences

# 1  Pharmacology

## Contents

## Pharmacodynamics

This is the study of the biochemical and physiological effects of drugs and their mechanisms of action. There are three major ways by which drugs can produce a pharmacological effect: interaction with specific receptors; alteration of physiological enzyme processes; and direct physical or chemical action.

### Interaction with specific receptors

- Specific receptors are usually found on cell surfaces (Table 1.1)
  *Agonism*: binding of drug to receptor provokes a biological response
  *Partial agonism*: an antagonist which provokes some but not a full biological response
  *Antagonism*: binding of drug to receptor prevents other agents from producing maximal effect
  *Full (non-competitive) antagonism*: antagonist has no efficacy of its own and simply binds irreversibly to receptor to prevent action of agonist.
  Reduces number of receptors available for agonists

*Partial (competitive) antagonism*: binding of antagonist is reversible and can be overcome by increasing the proportion of agonist.
Full complement of receptors available to agonist

### Alteration of physiological enzyme processes

- Drugs acting this way most commonly inhibit enzyme processes.
- This inhibition may be competitive or non-competitive

### Direct physical or chemical action

- Osmotic laxatives
- Chelating agents
- Local and general anaesthetics

## Pharmacokinetics

Before a drug can exert a biological effect it must first reach its site of action; after exerting its effect it must be removed.

**Table 1.1: Receptor types**

| Receptor type | Receptor subtype | Agonists | Antagonists |
|---|---|---|---|
| Adrenergic | $\alpha_1$ | Noradrenaline Phenylephrine | Prazosin |
| | $\alpha_2$ | Noradrenaline Clonidine | Yohimbine |
| | $\beta_1$ | Adrenaline Dobutamine | Atenolol |
| | $\beta_2$ | Adrenaline Salbutamol | Propranolol |
| Cholinergic | Muscarinic | Acetylcholine Carbachol | Atropine |
| | Nicotinic | Acetylcholine Nicotine | Tubocurarine |
| Histaminergic | $H_1$ | Histamine | Chlorpheniramine |
| | $H_2$ | Histamine | Ranitidine |
| Dopaminergic | $D_1$ | Pergolide Apomorphine | |
| | $D_2$ | Bromocriptine Pergolide Apomorphine | Metoclopramide Domperidone Phenothiazines |
| Opioid | $\chi$ | Dynorphin | |
| | $\delta$ | Enkephalins | |
| | $\epsilon$ | $\beta$-endorphin | Naloxone |
| | $\mu$ | $\beta$-endorphin Morphine | Naloxone |

# Drug absorption and bioavailability

Bioavailability is the proportion of a drug reaching the systemic circulation. The intravenous route has 100% bioavailability.

## Oral route
• Both acidic and alkaline drugs are absorbed predominantly in the small bowel
• Acidic drugs may be absorbed in the stomach
• Absorption through bowel wall occurs in four ways:
*Passive diffusion*: drugs diffuse through bowel wall along a concentration gradient that depends on the lipid solubility of the drug

Most important mechanism of drug absorption
*Active transport*: drugs similar to natural substances use existing transport systems
*Filtration through pores*: only possible for small drugs
*Endocytosis*: drugs engulfed by cell in bowel wall
Of little importance to drug absorption

### Factors affecting gastrointestinal absorption
• *Gastrointestinal environment*
Some drugs cannot be administered orally as they are degraded by gastrointestinal enzymes (insulin) or by acidic environment in the

**Box 1.1: Drugs undergoing extensive first-pass metabolism**

**Analgesics**
Aspirin
Morphine
Paracetamol
Pethidine

**Cardiovascular drugs**
Isoprenaline
Lignocaine
Nifedipine
Propranolol
Verapamil
Isosorbide dinitrate
Glyceryl trinitrate
Labetalol
Metoprolol
Prazosin

**CNS drugs**
Chlormethiazole
Chlorpromazine
Levodopa
Nortriptyline

**Miscellaneous**
Salbutamol
Terbutaline
Oral contraceptives

stomach (benzylpenicillin)
The presence of food may increase or decrease absorption
• *Lipid solubility of drug*
Absorption dependent on lipid solubility
Some drugs remain ionised and not lipid soluble, and are therefore poorly absorbed
In acidic environment acidic drugs more lipid soluble
In alkaline environment alkaline drugs more lipid soluble
• *Formulation factors*
Important in determining rate and

extent of absorption
Diluents and other agents may be added to improve absorption
Sustained-release preparations delay absorption rate
• *Gastrointestinal motility*
Delayed gastric emptying delays absorption rate of most drugs, but may enhance absorption rate of acidic drugs in the stomach
Diarrhoea and malabsorption reduce amount of drug absorbed

***First-pass metabolism***
• Following absorption, drugs enter the hepatoportal system
• To reach the systemic circulation, they must survive exposure to liver enzymes
• If drug has extensive first-pass metabolism (Box 1.1), the amount reaching the site of pharmacological action may be drastically reduced

## Intramuscular
• Avoids presystemic metabolism and degradation by gastric acid
• Absorption rate varies with muscle group used (faster from deltoid than from gluteals)
• Dependent on adequate tissue perfusion

## Rectal
• Does not completely avoid presystemic metabolism
• May be poorly tolerated and give erratic absorption
• Small surface area may make absorption slow

## Buccal
• Avoids presystemic metabolism and degradation by gastric acid
• Not all drugs able to penetrate buccal mucosa

## Transdermal

- Avoids presystemic metabolism
- Absorption limited, therefore only useful for potent drugs

## Intrapulmonary

- Useful for drugs affecting lung function
- Reduced systemic absorption and side effects
- Allows lower doses to be used

# Drug distribution

Apparent volume of distribution is a measure of the proportion of drug present in the plasma relative to the rest of the body at any particular time.

- In plasma, drugs bind to plasma proteins
- Acidic drugs in plasma most commonly bound to albumin
- Alkaline drugs may also bind to $\alpha_1$ glycoprotein
- Bound drugs are unable to exert any pharmacological effect
- Only free unbound drug is active
- Tissues also contain proteins that bind certain drugs
- Active transport mechanisms also promote tissue uptake of drug
- Distribution enhanced by: high lipid solubility (reduced by ionisation)
  Hypoalbuminaemia
  Low plasma protein binding
  High tissue binding

# Drug clearance and excretion

The liver is the major site of metabolism for most drugs.

## Phase I reactions

- Cytochrome P450 enzymes lead to oxidation, reduction and hydrolysis, which produce water-soluble compounds
- End products may have some pharmacological activity

## Phase II reactions

- Conjugation most commonly with glucuronide
- May also occur with sulphate, amino acids (glutathione), acetyl CoA (acetylation)
- Acetylation genetically controlled
- Leads to pharmacologically inert products

## High-extraction drugs

- Metabolised at a high rate
- Clearance dependent on hepatic blood flow
- Lignocaine, propranolol, pethidine, morphine

## Low-extraction drugs

- Metabolised at a low rate
- Dependent on the concentration of drug at receptor site and, hence, free plasma concentration
- Theophylline, diazepam, warfarin, chlorpromazine, paracetamol
- Kidneys are the major site of excretion
- Lipid-soluble drugs must be metabolised to produce water-soluble compounds that can be excreted by the kidneys
- Water-soluble drugs can be excreted

---

**Box 1.2: Drugs to avoid in slow acetylators**

Hydralazine
Isoniazid
Procainamide
Dapsone
Nitrazepam
Sulphonamides
Phenelzine
Sulphasalazine

unchanged (digoxin, gentamicin)
- Some drugs are actively secreted into convuluted tubules (probenecid, penicillin, amphetamine, salicylates)
- Drugs may also be conjugated and excreted in the bile
- These drugs may be reabsorbed in the terminal ileum following deconjugation by intestinal flora
- This leads to the development of an enterohepatic circulation and reduced drug clearance
- Metabolism may be reduced at extremes of age
- Chronic liver disease is associated with impaired metabolism (particularly phase I reactions)
- Renal failure reduces renal excretion

# Steady-state pharmacokinetics

When a drug is introduced into the circulation its plasma concentration declines exponentially. The time taken for the drug concentration to fall to 50% of its original value is called the half-life (Fig. 1.1).

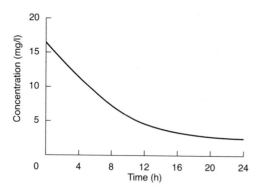

**Fig. 1.1: Plot of concentration against time after a bolus intravenous injection**

*The interception of the y (concentration) axis is the concentration resulting from the instantaneous injection of the bolus dose.*

## First-order kinetics (a)
- A fixed proportion of the drug is eliminated per unit time
- The rate of elimination is proportional to the amount of drug
- The amount of drug eliminated per unit time falls
- Steady state is reached when the rate of drug administration equals the rate of drug elimination
- Time taken to reach steady state equals 5 half-lives
- For drugs obeying first-order kinetics the concentration at steady state is proportional to the dose and inversely proportional to clearance

## Saturation kinetics (b)
- As the amount of drug increases, clearance falls
- Relationship between dose and steady state concentration is curvilinear
- Increases in dose lead to disproportionate increases in drug concentration, leading to an increased risk of drug toxicity

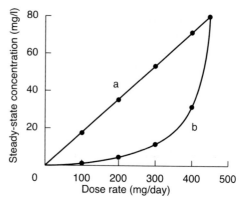
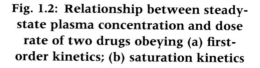

**Fig. 1.2: Relationship between steady-state plasma concentration and dose rate of two drugs obeying (a) first-order kinetics; (b) saturation kinetics**

**Box 1.3: Increased risk of adverse drug reaction**

Extremes of age
Polypharmacy
Previous history of adverse reactions
Pregnancy
High drug dose (type A reactions)

**Box 1.4: Drugs most commonly implicated as causes of adverse reactions**

Antibiotics
Aspirin
Digoxin
Diuretics
Heparin
Warfarin
Insulin
Prednisolone

# Adverse drug reactions

## Type A

- Dose-dependent and predictable
- Most common variety (75%)
- Often insidious onset
- Low mortality
- Commonest in renal and liver disease
- May be attenuated by dose reduction

## Type B

- Non-dose-dependent or idiosyncratic
- Unpredictable
- Usually acute onset
- May be high mortality
- Related to hereditary enzyme deficiencies or hypersensitivity reactions (all four types)
- Dose reduction unhelpful
- Immediate cessation and lifelong avoidance of drug required

# Drug interactions

## Pharmaceutical interactions

- Interactions occurring prior to entry of drug into body
- Occurs when drugs are mixed together, or when drug interacts with infusion fluid

## Pharmacodynamic interactions

- One drug alters the response to another
- This may result from interaction at receptor site or a different site
- Forms the basis for actions of antagonists and agonists

    *Synergy:* two drugs given together produce a pharmacological effect greater than would be expected from the combined effects of the two drugs alone
    *Potentiation:* one drug enhances the pharmacological effect of another

## Absorption

- Drugs may interact with each other to alter the rate or extent of absorption of a certain drug
- Some drugs may increase gastric emptying
- Chelating agents, ion exchange resins and antacids reduce absorption

**Table 1.2: Other important drug interactions**

| Drug | Interacts with | Effect of interaction | Mechanism |
|---|---|---|---|
| Warfarin | Salicylates<br>Fibrates<br>Thyroxine | Increased anticoagulant effect | Pharmacodynamic potentiation of anticoagulant effect |
| | Oral contraceptives | Reduced anticoagulant effect | Pharmacodynamic inhibition of anticoagulant effect |
| Oral contraceptives | Broad-spectrum antibiotics | Reduced contraceptive effect | Interruption of enterohepatic circulation |
| Digoxin | Amiodarone<br>Verapamil | Increased effect of digoxin | Reduced renal clearance |
| | Potassium-losing diuretics | Increased effect of digoxin | Pharmacodynamic potentiation by hypokalaemia |
| β-Blockers | Verapamil | Increased effect of β-Blocker | Pharmacodynamic potentiation |
| | NSAIDs | Reduced hypotensive effect | Salt retention |
| ACE inhibitors | NSAIDs | Reduced hypotensive effect | Sodium retention |
| | Potassium-sparing diuretics | Hyperkalaemia | Additive effects |
| Lithium | Thiazide diuretics | Increased effect of lithium | Increased renal tubular reabsorption of lithium |
| Iron | Antacids | Reduced effect of iron | Reduced absorption from gastrointestinal tract |

Box 1.5: Drugs affected by changes in liver enzymes

Warfarin
Phenytoin
Carbamazepine
Oral contraceptives
Theophyllines
Cyclosporin

## Distribution

- Drugs may compete for albumin-binding sites or active transport processes

## Metabolism

- Many drugs affect the activity of cytochrome enzymes found in the liver

### *Alteration of cytochrome enzymes*
*Enzyme inducers*
- Barbiturates
- Primidone
- Phenytoin
- Carbamazepine
- Rifampicin
- Cigarette smoking
- Griseofulvin
- Spironolactone

*Enzyme inhibitors*
- Antibiotics:
  Ciproxin
  Erythromycin
  Metronidazole
  Sulphonamides
  Chloramphenicol
  Isoniazid

*CNS drugs*
- SSRI antidepressants
- Monoamine oxidase inhibitors
- Chlorpromazine
- Sodium valproate

*Analgesics*
- Phenylbutazone
- Dextropropoxyphene

*Miscellaneous*
- Allopurinol
- Amiodarone
- Cimetidine
- Ketoconazole
- Fluconazole
- Warfarin

# Drug level monitoring

## Reasons for monitoring drug levels

- To ensure adequate therapeutic drug levels
- To detect overdose
- To assess compliance
- To reduce risk of toxicity (especially drugs with narrow therapeutic range)

## Therapeutic index (Fig 1.3)

- This is the ratio of the toxic dose to the therapeutic dose

Box 1.6: Common drugs monitored

Digoxin
Anticonvulsants
Aminoglycosides
Theophylline
Lithium
Paracetamol
Salicylates
Vancomycin
Cyclosporin

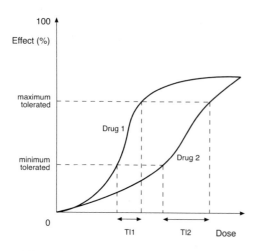

**Fig. 1.3: Dose–response relationship for two drugs with narrow (Drug 1) and wide (Drug 2) therapeutic indices (TI1 and TI2 respectively)**

*The minimum tolerated effect corresponds to the minimum dose of drug that is required to produce the desired pharmacological effect. The maximum tolerated effect represents the dose of drug that leads to intolerable side effects.*

- Dependent on the dose–response relationship
- Drugs with a steep dose–response curve have a narrow therapeutic index (Drug 1)
- Drugs with a flat dose–response curve have a wide therapeutic index (Drug 2)

# Drugs to avoid

The lists that follow are not comprehensive. For more comprehensive lists, consult the *British National Formulary* (BNF).

## Renal failure

Drugs that are hydrophilic and excreted unchanged via the kidneys.

### Drugs to avoid in renal failure
- Antibiotics (tetracyclines, nitrofurantoin, amphotericin B)
- Potassium-sparing diuretics
- Narcotics
- Non-steroidal anti-inflammatory drugs (NSAIDs)
- Lithium

### Drugs needing dose reduction in renal failure
#### Antibiotics
- Penicillin
- Ampicillin
- Aminoglycosides
- Cephalosporins
- Sulphonamides
- Vancomycin
- Metronidazole

#### Cardiovascular drugs
- Methyldopa
- Digoxin
- Procainamide
- Disopyramide
- Flecainide
- ACE inhibitors

#### Miscellaneous
- Chlorpropamide
- $H_2$ blockers
- Insulin

# Liver disease

### Drugs to avoid in liver disease
- Acarbose
- Anabolic steroids
- Androgens
- Chloramphenicol
- Dantrolene
- Gemfibrozil
- Ketoconazole
- Labetalol
- Lamotrigine
- Metformin

- Oestrogens
- Progestogens
- Terfenadine

# Pregnancy

## *Drugs that are teratogenic in the first trimester*
- Danazol
- Lithium
- ACE inhibitors
- Warfarin
- Metformin
- Quinine
- Tetracycline
- Trimethoprim
- Rifampicin
- Anticonvulsants
- Streptomycin
- Thalidomide
- Hydralazine
- Cytotoxics
- Radioiodine

## *Drugs to avoid in later pregnancy*
- Sulphonamides
- Chloramphenicol
- Aminoglycosides
- Amiodarone
- Carbamazepine
- Radioiodine
- Thrombolytics

# Breastfeeding

Most drugs pass into breast milk, but usually in low concentration without harmful effects.

## *Drugs to avoid during breastfeeding*
- Sulphonamides
- Chloramphenicol
- Isoniazid

> **Box 1.7: Substances not adsorbed to charcoal**
>
> Cyanide
> Ethanol
> Ethylene glycol
> Iron
> Lithium
> Methanol
> Petroleum
> Strong acids and alkalis

- Tetracycline
- Opiates
- Benzodiazepenes
- Amantadine
- Oestrogens
- Lithium
- Antithyroids
- Radioiodine
- Phenindione
- Cytotoxics
- Amphetamines
- Androgens
- Ciproxin

# Drug poisoning

## General management

### *History*
- If not available from the patient this should be obtained from relatives or friends
- Ask particularly:
  Has the patient taken an overdose?
  When was the overdose?
  What drug(s) has the patient taken?
  How many tablets has the patient taken?
  Is the patient on any other regular medication?
  Is there evidence of serious intent (suicide note, associated violence)?

## Examination

- Pay particular attention to:
  Level of consciousness
  Pupils (small in opiate overdose, large in tricyclic overdose)
  Blood pressure
  Respiratory depression (barbiturates, opiates, benzodiazepenes)
  Temperature (hypothermia worsens prognosis)
  Focal neurology (other cause for coma)
  ECG (arrhythmias in tricyclic overdose)

## Removal of drug from stomach

- Should be performed within 2 hours of ingestion for most drugs
- Can be performed up to 6 hours following ingestion of tricyclic antidepressants, aspirin, antihistamines
  *Gastric lavage*: contraindicated in young children and following ingestion of petroleum or corrosives
  Unconscious patients require intubation prior to procedure
  *Induced emesis*: contraindicated in unconscious patients, children and following ingestion of petroleum or corrosives

*Drug adsorption*: using activated charcoal
Repeated dosing usually required

## Enhanced drug elimination

- *Forced alkaline diuresis*: administration of sodium bicarbonate alkalinises urine
  Increases the ionisation of acidic drugs in alkaline urine, leading to reduced tubular reabsorption and increased excretion
  Can be used for aspirin, herbicides, barbiturates
  Complications: water intoxication, pulmonary/cerebral oedema, alkalosis, hypokalaemia
- *Forced acid diuresis*: acidifies urine using ammonium chloride, lysine or arginine hydrochloride
  Can be used for amphetamines, quinine
- *Haemodialysis*: useful for drugs with low plasma protein binding, poor lipid solubility and low volume of distribution
  Indicated in: lithium overdose with levels > 3 mmol/l
  severe alcohol overdose
  salicylate overdose with severe metabolic acidosis
  barbiturate overdose
  methanol, ethylene glycol overdose

### Table 1.3: Specific antidotes

| Drug | Antidote |
|------|----------|
| Paracetamol | N-acetylcysteine, methionine |
| β-blockers | Glucagon |
| Opiates | Naloxone |
| Benzodiazepines | Flumazenil |
| Digoxin | Specific antidigoxin antibody fragments (Fab) |
| Cyanide | Dicobalt edetate, sodium nitrite, sodium thiosulphate |
| Methanol and ethylene glycol | Alcohol |
| Iron | Desferrioxamine |
| Heavy metals | Dimercaprol |
| Copper | Penicillamine |
| Organophosphates | Atropine, pralidoxime mesylate |
| Paraquat | Fuller's earth |

- *Haemoperfusion*: can be used to remove drugs not removed by haemodialysis owing to high lipid solubility or high plasma protein binding
  Low volume of distribution still required
  Reserved for severe cases of overdose with: theophyllines
  short-acting barbiturates
  salicylates
  chloral hydrate

# Management of paracetamol overdose

## Recognition
- Patient may be asymptomatic and deny overdose, particularly if truly suicidal
- Always have a high index of suspicion
- Initial symptoms may consist of nausea, vomiting, abdominal pain
- Liver damage manifests after 3 days
- Severe overdose may lead to metabolic acidosis, hypoglycaemia, hypotension, cardiac arrhythmias, acute renal failure, pancreatitis

## Immediate management
- Gastric lavage within 2 hours of ingestion
- Baseline blood tests: FBC, renal function, liver function, clotting profile, blood sugar
- Paracetamol levels (unreliable < 4 h after ingestion)
- I.V. acetylcysteine if levels high (Fig. 1.4): (a) 150 mg/kg in 200 ml 5% dextrose over 15 min
  (b) 50 mg/kg in 500 ml 5% dextrose over 4 h
  (c) 100 mg/kg in 1000 ml 5% dextrose over 16 h
- Oral methionine may be given if < 8 h after ingestion or anaphylaxis to acetylcysteine
- High-risk patients: associated alcohol

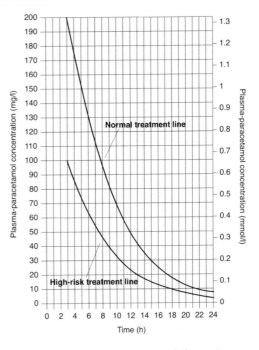

**Fig. 1.4: Treatment guidelines in paracetamol poisoning**
*All patients should receive acetylcysteine or methionine if paracetamol levels are above the 'normal treatment line'. High risk patients should be treated similarly if paracetamol levels are above the 'high risk treatment line'.*

ingestion or chronic alcohol abuse
already taking liver enzyme-inducing drugs
HIV-positive patients
malnourished patients
- Beware of errors in timing of overdose
- Always treat if in doubt

## Subacute management
- Daily renal and liver function, blood sugar, INR
- Observe for signs of encephalopathy
- Contact liver unit if:
  INR > 3
  renal failure
  raised aspartate amino-transferase (AST)
  encephalopathy
  pH < 7.3 after 24 h

# 2 Immunology

## Contents

# Anatomy of the immune system

## Cellular immunity

Cell-mediated (natural) immunity depends on the integrity of the following:

### Granulocytes
- Multi-lobed nuclear cells, 12–15 μm in diameter
- Cytoplasm contains two types of granule:
  *Primary*: contain myeloperoxidase, acid phosphatase, acid hydrolases
  *Secondary*: contain alkaline phosphatase, lysosyme
- Mature granulocytes circulate for 10 hours before migrating into tissues
- Main functions include chemotaxis, phagocytosis, killing of bacteria

### Monocytes
- Large mononuclear cells, 16–20 μm in diameter
- Cytoplasm contains granules similar to granulocytes
- Mature cells circulate for 20–40 hours before entering the tissues to mature as macrophages
- Macrophage lifespan may be as long as several months or years
- Main functions as for granulocytes
- Also act as antigen-presenting cells
- May adopt specific functions in different tissues

### T lymphocytes (Table 2.1)
- Represent 70% of circulating

### Table 2.1: T-Cell surface antigens

| Surface antigen | % of circulating T-cells | Recognition antigen | Function |
|---|---|---|---|
| T4 (CD4) | 65 | Class II HLA | $T_H$ and $T_{DH}$ cells |
| T8 (CD8) | 35 | Class I HLA | $T_S$ and $T_C$ cells |

*$T_H$: involved in antigen recognition and presentation; $T_{DH}$: involved in delayed hypersensitivity reactions; $T_S$: interfere with development of an immune response; $T_C$: involved in regulation of immune response and in cell lysis*

lymphocyte population
- Provide protection against intracellular organisms, protozoa and fungi
- Also involved in graft rejection, control of neoplasia and delayed hypersensitivity reactions

### Natural killer (NK) cells
These are cytotoxic lymphocytes involved in recognition and destruction of virus-infected cells and tumour cells.

### Killer (K) cells
These cytotoxic lymphocytes are involved in antibody-dependent cellular cytotoxicity.

# Humoral immunity

- Humoral (adaptive) immunity is based on B lymphocytes and the production of antibodies
- B lymphocytes represent 10% of the circulating lymphocyte population
- Provide protection against pyogenic bacteria, bloodborne infection and neutralisation of toxins

### Antibodies (Immunoglobulins)
- Each antibody is composed of two heavy and two light polypeptide chains
- The two chains are linked by disulphide covalent bonds (see Fig. 2.1)

  *Fab fragment*: antigen-binding site
  *Fc fragment*: complement fixation site
  *Light chains*: molecular weight 23 000 Daltons
  2 types (κ and λ)
  Each immunoglobulin (Ig) has either two κ or two λ light chains
  *Heavy chains*: molecular weight 50 000–75 000 Daltons
  Fc fragment of heavy chains

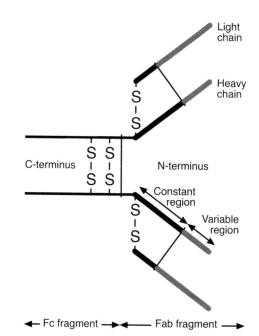

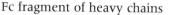

**Fig. 2.1: Structure of immunoglobulin**

determines antibody type (Table 2.2)
*Constant region*: amino acid sequences of immunoglobulins of the same class are identical
*Variable region*: amino acid sequences of immunoglobulins of the same class differ from molecule to molecule
*Isotype*: the class or subclass of immunoglobulin
*Allotype*: genetically determined variant of immunoglobulin class or subclass
*Idiotype*: specific immunoglobulin with uniquely shaped antigen-binding site

# Complement (Table 2.3)

- A second line of defence comprising 20 serum proteins
- Synthesised by macrophages and hepatocytes

**Table 2.2: Immunoglobulin classes**

| Class | Heavy chains | MW (Daltons) | % of Ig | Function |
|-------|-------------|--------------|---------|----------|
| IgG | γ | 150 000 (monomer) | 80 | Found in blood and interstitial fluids<br>Major Ig of the secondary immune response<br>Only Ig to cross the placenta<br>Opsonisation<br>Complement activation |
| IgA | α | 160 000 (dimer)<br>370 000 (secretory form) | 13 | Main Ig in secretions<br>Defence of mucosal surfaces<br>Activates complement |
| IgM | μ | 900 000 (pentamer) | 6 | Mainly intravascular<br>Major Ig of primary immune response<br>Opsonisation<br>Activates complement |
| IgD | δ | 170 000 (monomer) | 0.6 | May be involved in B-cell activation |
| IgE | ε | 185 000 (monomer) | 0.4 | Immediate hypersensitivity reactions<br>Control of parasitic infections |

- Circulate as inactive proenzymes
- Activated in sequence
- Two pathways: classical and alternative (Fig. 2.2)
  *Classical pathway*: activated by antigen-antibody complexes
  *Alternative pathway*: activated by bacteria, viruses, immune complexes, endotoxins

**Table 2.3: Functions of complement**

| Function | Main components implicated |
|----------|---------------------------|
| Chemotaxis | 5, 6, 7 |
| Opsonisation | 3b |
| Stimulate inflammation | 1, 2, 3a, 4a, 5a |
| Cell lysis | 5, 6, 7, 8, 9 |

## Major histocompatibility complex (MHC)

This constitutes a small cluster of genes on the short arm of chromosome 6 (HLA region). These genes determine the structure of HLA antigens.

- *Class I antigens*: HLA A, B, C, found on all nucleated cells
  Concerned with antigen recognition by $T_C$ cells
- *Class II antigens*: HLA DP, DQ, DR, found on antigen-presenting cells (APC)
  APC include B lymphocytes, dendritic cells of the spleen and lymph nodes, macrophages and Langerhans' cells in the skin
  Concerned with initiation and control of immune response (Table 2.4)

# Normal immune response (Fig. 2.3)

All immune responses have certain common features:
- Presentation of antigen (APC)
- Selection of antigen-specific lymphocytes (cell mediated or

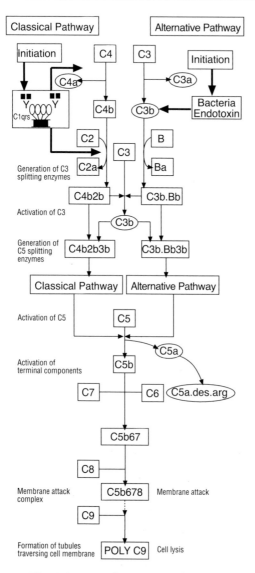

**Fig. 2.2: Complement pathways**

## Table 2.4: HLA-associated diseases

| Disease | HLA associations |
|---|---|
| Haemochromatosis | A3, B14 |
| Behçet's disease | B5, DR4 |
| Ankylosing spondylitis | B27 |
| Reiter's syndrome | B27 |
| Psoriatic arthritis | B27 |
| Multiple sclerosis | B7, DR2 |
| Pernicious anaemia | B7, DR2, DR5 |
| Dermatitis herpetiformis | DR3 |
| Coeliac disease | B8, DR3, DR7 |
| Sjögren's syndrome | B8, DR3 |
| Primary biliary cirrhosis | DR3 |
| Chronic active hepatitis | B8, DR3 |
| Addison's disease | B6, DR3 |
| Systemic lupus erythematosus (SLE) | DR3 |
| Graves' disease | B8, DR3 |
| Hashimoto's thyroiditis | DR3, DR5 |
| Insulin-dependent diabetes mellitus | B8, DR3, DR4 |
| Myasthenia gravis | B8, DR3 |
| Rheumatoid arthrtitis | DR4 |
| Ulcerative colitis | B5 |
| Pemphigus vulgaris | DR4 |
| Narcolepsy | DR2 |
| Goodpasture's syndrome | DR2 |

humoral response)
- Clone formation of appropriate lymphocytes
- Differentiation of lymphocytes into effector cells (T lymphocytes into $T_H$ or $T_C$, B lymphocytes into plasma cells)
- Generation of memory, required for secondary immune response
- Regulation and control of immune response (cytokines) (Table 2.5)

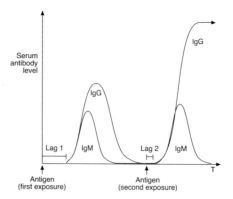

**Fig. 2.3: Primary and secondary antibody responses after repeated exposure to a common antigen**

**Table 2.5: Cytokines**

| Cytokine | Major source | Function |
|---|---|---|
| Interleukins (1–17) | APC<br>T lymphocytes<br>Bone marrow stromal cells | Stimulation of haemopoietic stem cells<br>Activation of T, B lymphocytes, NK cells, neutrophils |
| Interferon | Macrophages<br>Fibroblasts<br>T lymphocytes | Antiviral |
| Tumour necrosis factor | Macrophages | Antitumour, vascular damage<br>Antiviral |
| Colony-stimulating factors | Macrophages | Growth and maturation of neutrophils, eosinophils, monocytes |
| Tumour growth factor | T lymphocytes<br>Monocytes | Inhibition of T- and B-cell proliferation and NK activity |

# Immunodeficiency

## Defects of neutrophil function

Usually presents with recurrent bacterial and fungal infections.

### Defects of chemotaxis
- *Congenital*:
  Lazy leucocyte syndrome
  Complement abnormalities
- *Acquired*:
  Drugs (steroids, aspirin, tetracyclines)
  Alcohol
  Hypophosphataemia
  Raised plasma osmolarity
  Myeloid leukaemias
  Myelodysplasia
  Malnutrition
  Hodgkin's disease
  Renal failure
  Severe burns
  Systemic lupus eruthematosus (SLE)
  Rheumatoid arthritis
  Sarcoid
  Crohn's disease

### Defective phagocytosis
- Hypogammaglobulinaemia
- Complement deficiency (Table 2.6)
- Splenectomy
- Sickle cell disease
- SLE

### Defective killing
- Chronic granulomatous disease
- Myeloperoxidase deficiency
- Chediak–Higashi syndrome
- Acute myeloid leukaemia
- Chronic myeloid leukaemia
- Myelodysplasia
- Jobs's syndrome
- Severe G6PD deficiency
- Drugs: steroids, colchicine

**Table 2.6: Complement deficiencies**

| Deficient component | Clinical features |
|---|---|
| C1 esterase inhibitor | Hereditary angioneurotic oedema |
| C1–4 | Immune complex diseases |
| C3 | Recurrent bacterial infections |
| C5–9 | Recurrent *Neisseria* infections |

# T-Cell deficiencies

These usually present with viral, fungal, opportunistic or chronic bacterial infections.

## Primary
- DiGeorge syndrome (thymic aplasia)
- Isolated T-cell deficiency
- Chronic mucocutaneous candidiasis

## Secondary
- Lymphoproliferative disorders (lymphomas)
- Infections: measles, rubella, HIV, EBV, tuberculosis, brucellosis, leprosy, syphilis
- Drugs: steroids, cyclophosphamide, cyclosporin
- Miscellaneous: malnutrition, zinc deficiency, rheumatoid arthritis, sarcoid, pyoderma gangrenosum, diabetes mellitus, alcohol abuse

# B-Cell deficiencies

Usually present with bacterial infection.

## Primary
- Selective IgA deficiency
- X-linked agammaglobulinaemia
- Common variable immunodeficiency
- Acquired hypogammaglobulinaemia
- Transient hypogammaglobulinaemia of infancy
- Selective IgG subclass deficiency
- Functional antibody deficiency
- Transcobalamin II deficiency

## Secondary
- Artefactual due to haemodilution
- Decreased production:
    Lymphoproliferative disorders (CLL, myeloma)
    Splenectomy
    Malnutrition
    Marrow infiltration
    Drugs (cytotoxics, gold, phenytoin, penicillamine)
    Radiation
- Increased loss:
    Protein-losing enteropathy
    Nephrotic syndrome
    Malabsorption
    Erythroderma
    Burns
    Dystrophia myotonica

# Combined B- and T-cell deficiencies

- Severe combined immunodeficiency (SCID)
- Ataxia telangectasia
- Wiskott–Aldrich syndrome
- Bloom's syndrome
- Orotic aciduria

# Hypersensitivity

## Type I (immediate hypersensitivity, anaphylaxis)

- Precipitated by the formation of IgE antibodies
- IgE binds to mast cells
- Mast cells degranulate and release inflammatory mediators
- Inflammatory mediators include histamine, leukotrienes, prostaglandins, chemotactic factors, kinins, platelet-activating factor
- Inflammatory reaction may be localised or systemic, leading to shock and cardiovascular collapse
- Responsible for allergic conditions (hayfever, asthma, eczema, drug allergies)

## Type II (antibody-mediated)

- Antibody-mediated complement activation and stimulation of neutrophil phagocytosis
- Responsible for autoimmunity and early graft rejection

## Type III (immune complex mediated)

- Antigen–antibody complexes combine with complement to produce insoluble immune complexes
- Immune complexes are deposited in the tissues
- Damage results from platelet aggregation, activation of complement and coagulation factors
- Responsible for immune complex diseases (Box 2.1)

## Type IV (cell mediated, delayed hypersensitivity)

- Mediated by $T_{DH}$ cells
- Contact with antigen stimulates release of cytokines
- Can lead to granuloma formation
- Responsible for tuberculin skin reaction, delayed graft rejection and graft-versus-host disease

# Autoimmunity

This is the process in which antibodies are produced against the body's own antigens.

## Aetiology of autoimmunity

- Microbial antigens cross-react with host tissues to stimulate an autoimmune response
- Alteration of self antigens
- Attachment of foreign hapten to self molecule, forming hapten carrier complexes
- Deficiency of $T_S$ cells
- Spontaneous emergence of clones of cells capable of mounting an autoimmune response

## Causes of positive rheumatoid factor

### Autoimmune disease (Table 2.7)
- Rheumatoid arthritis
- Sjögren's syndrome
- SLE
- Systemic sclerosis
- Dermatomyositis
- Polyarteritis nodosa
- Juvenile chronic arthritis
- Chronic active hepatitis
- Cryptogenic fibrosing alveolitis
- Mixed connective tissue disease
- Behçet's disease

---

**Box 2.1: Immune complex diseases**

Serum sickness
Drug-induced haemolytic anaemia
Extrinsic allergic alveolitis
Post-streptococcal glomerulonephritis
Infective endocarditis nephritis
Syphilis nephritis
Hepatitis B nephritis
Quartan malaria
Schistosomiasis
Wegener's granulomatosis
Polyarteritis nodosa
Mixed essential cryoglobulinaemia
Cutaneous vasculitis
SLE nephritis
Rapidly progressive nephritis

### Table 2.7: Autoimmune diseases

| Disease | Autoantibody |
| --- | --- |
| Hashimoto's thyroiditis | Thyroglobulin |
| Graves' disease | Long-acting thyroid stimulator (LATS) |
|  | Thyroid microsomal |
| Pernicious anaemia | Parietal cell |
|  | Intrinsic factor |
| Coeliac disease | Endomysial |
|  | Gliaden |
|  | Reticulin |
| Autoimmune Addison's disease | Adrenal cell |
| Chronic active hepatitis | Smooth muscle |
| Primary biliary cirrhosis | Mitochondrial |
| Myasthenia gravis | Acetylcholine |
| Goodpasture's syndrome | Glomerular basement membrane (GBM) |
| Rheumatoid arthritis | Rheumatoid factor |
| Mixed connective disease | Ribonucleoprotein |
| CREST syndrome | Centromere |
| Sjögren's syndrome | Ro, la |
| Dematomyositis | Jo, mi, PM |
| SLE | Single- and double-stranded DNA |
|  | Histone, RNA |
|  | Phospholipid (cardiolipin, lupus anticoagulant) |
|  | Ro, la, SM |
|  | ANCA |
|  | Ribonucleoprotein |
| Drug-induced lupus | Histone |
| Vasculitis | ANCA |
| Scleroderma | Scl-70 |

## Infection
- TB
- Syphilis
- Leprosy
- HIV
- Viral hepatitis
- Rubella
- EBV
- Infective endocarditis
- Kala azar

## Miscellaneous
- Asbestosis
- Sarcoid
- Malignancy

- Waldenström's macroglobulinaemia
- Glomerulonephritis
- Renal transplant
- Advanced age
- Blood transfusion
- Coalworker's pneumoconiosis
- Myocardial infarction
- Essential mixed cryoglobulinaemia

## Causes of positive ANCA

- Wegener's granulomatosis
- Polyarteritis nodosa
- Churg–Strauss syndrome

- SLE
- Atrial myxoma
- HIV infection
- Rheumatoid arthritis

## Causes of positive ANA

- <u>Collagen vascular disease</u>
- Chronic liver disease
- Hashimoto's thyroiditis
- Thymoma
- Myasthenia gravis
- Pernicious anaemia
- TB
- Leprosy
- Pulmonary fibrosis
- Lymphoma
- Malignancy
- Ulcerative colitis
- Advanced age

# Transplantation

- *Autograft*: tissue transplant within the same individual, e.g. skin graft
- *Isograft*: tissue transplant between monozygotic identical twins
- *Allograft*: tissue transplant between different non-identical individuals
- *Xenograft*: transplantation of animal tissue into human, e.g. porcine heart valves
- *Heterotopic*: a graft inserted into a different type of tissue
- *Isotopic*: a graft inserted into the same type of tissue, e.g. corneal grafts
- *Orthotopic*: a graft inserted into the same type of tissue but in a different anatomical position, e.g., skin graft from thigh to arm
- ABO compatibility essential
- Main obstacle to successful transplantation is HLA compatibility
- HLA-D antigen matching is the most important

# Graft rejection

*Hyperacute:* occurs within hours or days of transplantation
Mediated by preformed B-cell antibodies
*Early acute*: occurs 10–30 days post transplantation
Mediated by T lymphocytes (cell mediated response)
*Chronic*: occurs over a period of months or even years
Mediated by immunoglobulins or cell-mediated response

# Graft-versus-host disease (GVHD)

- Occurs because of the presence of competent T lymphocytes in the graft tissue
- These T cells react against the HLA antigens of the recipient
- Common after transplants involving skin, liver, gastrointestinal tract and bone marrow
- Does not occur following heart or kidney transplants
- May be acute or chronic

*Acute GVHD*: develops shortly after transplantation
Maculopapular rash, hepatitis, diarrhoea, erythroderma may develop
Treated with high-dose steroids
*Chronic GVHD*: develops several months after transplantation
Not always preceded by acute GVHD
Sclerodermatous skin changes, obstructive liver disease may develop
Treated with immunosuppressive agents (azathioprine)

---

**Box 2.2: Cytotoxic agents**

**Alkylating agents**
Nitrogen mustard
Melphalan
Cyclophosphamide
Busulphan
Chlorambucil
Nitrosoureas
Cisplatin
Carboplatin

**Antimetabolites**
Methotrexate
5-Fluorouracil
Mercaptopurine
Thioguanine
Cytosine arabinoside

**Plant alkaloids**
Vinca alkaloids
Epidodophyllotoxins
Taxoids

**Antibiotics**
Anthracyclines
Doxorubicin
Daunorubicin
Bleomycin

# Immunosuppression

## Steroids

- Effects mediated by inhibition of monocytes, macrophages and phagocytic function

## Cytotoxic agents (Box 2.2)

- Major action is killing of cells capable of self-replication. Effects achieved by interference with protein and DNA synthesis. May also act as steroid-sparing agents
- Increased risk of sepsis, myelosuppression, malignancy

*Alkylating agents*: form irreversible crosslinks with DNA
*Antimetabolites*: closely related analogues of normal components of DNA synthesis inhibit DNA synthesis
*Plant Alkaloids*: inhibit cell division or DNA synthesis
*Antibiotics*: intercalate between nucleotide bases in DNA

## Non-cytotoxic agents

- Do not exert effect by killing of self-replicating cells. No effect on DNA or protein synthesis
- More used in transplantation than tumour therapy, and as steroid-sparing agents

*Cyclosporin*: fungal metabolite. Inhibits T-cell activation. Major side effect renal impairment
*Tacrolimus*: macrolide. Similar action to cyclosporin but more potent. Similar side effects

# Tumour immunology

Tumour cells are cells transformed by virus or by physical or chemical means.

*Oncogenes*: genes that cause transformation of cells and rapid uncontrolled cell proliferation
*In normal cells they are switched off*
*In tumour cells they are switched on*

- Some tumours arise as a result of

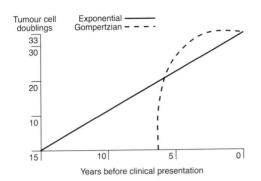

Years before clinical presentation

**Fig. 2.4: Growth characteristics of tumours showing typical exponential increase in tumour cell numbers as well as more rapid Gompertzian growth**

clonal expansion of a single transformed cell
- Tumour cells exhibit marked heterogenicity with regard to growth rate, surface antigen expression, expression of biochemical markers and resistance to chemotherapeutic agents
- In normal tissues, self-renewing stem cells are constantly developing into mature cells. This process is regulated so that the number of new cells produced equals the number lost. There is a constant turnover of cells, but the number of mature cells remains constant (except during periods of growth)
- In tumours, the normal regulatory mechanisms of cell turnover are impaired. This leads to unrestrained growth of a cell population (tumour)
- Tumour growth is usually exponential
- Tumours become clinically apparent after 32 doublings of cell numbers
- Some tumours may grow more rapidly when they are small (Gompertzian growth) (Fig. 2.4)
- Tumour cells express tumour-associated antigens (TAA) on their cell surfaces (Table 2.8)
- TAA stimulate humoral and cell-mediated immune responses

# HIV immunology

HIV is comprised of a cylindrical core surrounded by a bilayered lipid envelope.

*Core*: made of capsid protein (p24), which encases two strands of viral RNA and viral enzymes
Viral enzymes include reverse transcriptase, integrase and protease
*Envelope*: bilayered lipid membrane
Glycoproteins inserted into envelope
Glycoproteins carry receptor sites for CD4 antigens (Class II HLA)

**Table 2.8: Common tumour markers**

| Marker | Tumour |
|---|---|
| Carcinoembryonic antigen (CEA) | Gastrointestinal tract |
| Ca125 | Ovary |
| α-Fetoprotein | Hepatocellular |
| Human chorionic gonadotrophin (HCG) | Choriocarcinoma, teratoma |
| Prostate-specific antigen (PSA) | Prostate |
| Acid phosphatase | Prostate |

**Box 2.3: Immunological
abnormalities in HIV infection**

Reduced CD4 lymphocyte levels
Impaired skin allergy responses
Reduced CD8 lymphocyte levels
Reduced NK cell levels
Raised immunoglobulin levels
Raised circulating immune complexes
Reduced monocyte/macrophage function
Raised cytokine levels

# Mode of infection (Fig. 2.5)

- On entry to host cell, reverse transcriptase makes a DNA copy of the RNA genome
- The DNA formed integrates with the host cell DNA
- There are two types of reproduction of the virus:
  *Latent (non-productive)*: a quiescent stage, during which virus prepares to replicate
  *Productive*: new virus particles are made and released from the host cell by budding
- In the weeks following infection, there is a rapid increase in viral load and dissemination
- This period may be associated with a transient seroconversion illness
- The host then mounts a cell-mediated immune response leading to a fall in viral load

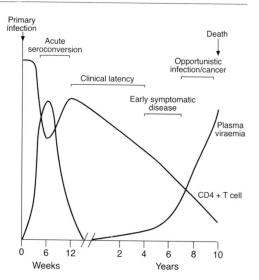

**Fig. 2.5: Timescale of CD4 counts,
viral load and clinical features
in HIV infection**

- A period of latency then ensues during which virus particles continue to replicate
- During this time CD4 levels fall progressively as they are attacked and destroyed by the virus
- Destruction of CD4 cells is the primary immune abnormality in HIV infection
- As CD4 levels fall viral load again increases, leading to clinical manifestation of AIDS

# 3 Genetics

## Contents

## Chromosome structure

In somatic cells there are 23 pairs of chromosomes (46):

*Chromosome*: a continuous molecule of DNA coding for many thousands of genes

Each chromosome has a short arm (p) and a long arm (q)

*Gene*: a segment of DNA that codes for the synthesis of a single polypeptide

*DNA*: a double helical structure comprised of two chains of nucleotide sequences

*Nucleotide*: compound consisting of three components: a nitrogenous base, a pentose sugar, 1–3 phosphate groups

There are five types of nucleotide:

*Purine bases*: adenine (A)
guanine (G)

*Pyrimidine bases*: cytosine (C)
thymidine (T)
uracil (U)

In DNA, the nucleotides are specifically paired, such that adenine always binds with thymidine and guanine always binds with cytosine (see Fig. 3.1).

| A | T | C | G | A | T | C | G | A | T | C | G |
| T | A | G | C | T | A | G | C | T | A | G | C |

**Fig. 3.1: Base sequence and pairings in human DNA**

The bonds between the bases are hydrogen bonds:

*Exon*: a sequence of bases that codes for a gene

*Intron*: a sequence of bases that does not code for a gene

*DNA replication*: occurs during the S phase of the cell cycle

This is preceded by the G1 phase (cells prepare to duplicate chromosomes)

After the S phase is the G2 phase (cells prepare to divide)

Cell division occurs during the M (mitotic) phase

DNA replication is catalysed by the enzyme DNA polymerase

The two nucleotide sequences unwind and peel apart

New daughter strands form, as shown in Fig. 3.2

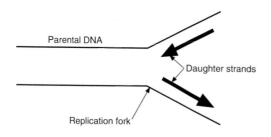

Parental DNA

Daughter strands

Replication fork

**Fig. 3.2: DNA replication showing mechanism of daughter strand production**

# Protein synthesis

The following sequence of events is required for protein synthesis:

DNA ⟶ RNA ⟶ Polypeptide ⟶ Protein
    ↑           ↑   chain
Transcription Translation

## Transcription

- The process whereby RNA is synthesised from DNA
- Takes place in the nucleus
- RNA consists of a single strand of nucleotide sequences

---

**Box 3.1: Inhibitors of protein synthesis**

**Antibiotics:** Rifampicin, streptomycin, tetracycline, chloramphenicol, erythromycin

**Pyrimidine analogues:** 5-fluorouracil, cytosine arabinoside

**Purine analogues:** mercaptopurine, adenine arabinoside, thioguanine

**Alkylating agents:** cyclophosphamide, chlorambucil, melphalan

**Others:** vincristine, bleomycin, methotrexate, doxorubicin, etoposide, hydroxyurea, cisplatin, carboplatin

---

- The nitrogenous bases in RNA are the same as in DNA except that uracil replaces thymidine
- Transcription is catalysed by RNA polymerase
- Transcription produces three types of RNA:
  mRNA – the template for polypeptide synthesis
  tRNA – required for translation
  rRNA – ribosomal RNA required for translation

## Translation

- The process of synthesis of protein on the mRNA template
- Takes place in the cytoplasm on the ribosomes (rRNA)
- Each tRNA carries a three-base coding region (anticodon) which pairs specifically with a corresponding sequence of three bases on the mRNA (codon)
- The tRNA therefore binds to the mRNA
- The tRNA takes the mRNA to the ribosomal RNA and polypeptide chain formation begins
- Polypeptide chain formation begins with the amino acid methionine
- The polypeptide chain gradually elongates
- Chain formation is terminated by the presence of three specific codons (stop codons)

# Methods of gene analysis

## DNA probe hybridisation

*Probe*: a piece of single-stranded DNA used to detect homologous sequences

in DNA samples
- Radiolabelling of probe allows its detection
- There are three methods of producing probes:
  from mRNA using reverse transcriptase enzyme
  from cloned DNA
  from DNA fragments

**Box 3.2: Uses of cloned DNA**

Isolation of individual genes
Probe preparation
Pharmaceutical production of proteins:
  Insulin, Growth hormone, Hepatitis B vaccine, Interferon, Erythropoietin
Prenatal diagnosis
Gene therapy

# Gene mapping

- A method of identifying DNA sequences

*Restriction enzymes*: bacterial enzymes that recognise specific DNA sequences and cleave DNA at these sites to produce DNA fragments
*Restriction fragment length polymorphisms (RFLP)*: produced by variations in non-coding DNA sequences. If these variations occur at restriction enzyme cleavage sites, it produces DNA fragments of different sizes (RFLP)
*Southern blotting*: used for analysis of DNA sequences
  Three steps involved: restriction enzymes cleave DNA
  DNA fragments separated by electrophoresis
  DNA fragments identified using probes

# Gene cloning (Box 3.2)

- Insertion of foreign DNA into carriers (bacteriophages, plasmids or cosmids)
  *Bacteriophages*: viruses that multiply in bacteria
  *Plasmids*: extrachromosomal DNA molecules which replicate autonomously in bacteria
  *Cosmids*: artificial vectors that are hybrids between bacteriophages and plasmids

*Cloning process:* DNA cleavage by restriction enzymes
  DNA fragments inserted into carrier
  carrier introduced into host cell
  Cells allowed to replicate
  Carrier DNA extracted and amplified

# Polymerase chain reaction (PCR)

- Method of amplifying DNA that allows identification of small amounts of DNA
- DNA is denatured by heating to produce two single strands (primers)
- DNA polymerase is added to the primers
- The process is repeated many times
- After each cycle the amount of DNA is doubled
- Can be performed on any tissue (alive or dead)
- Useful for prenatal diagnosis and diagnosis of viral infections

# Chromosomal abnormalities

## Abnormalities of chromosome number

- *Down's syndrome*: trisomy 21
- *Edward's syndrome*: trisomy 18

**Box 3.3: Examples of deletions**

Cri du chat (5p–)
Wolf syndrome (4p–)
Wilms' tumour (11p–)
Retinoblastoma (13q–)
Prader–Willi syndrome (15q–)

**Box 3.4: Autosomal dominant conditions**

Achondroplasia
Adult polycystic kidney disease
Charcot–Marie–Tooth disease
Ehlers–Danlos syndrome
Fascioscapulohumeral dystrophy
Gardner's syndrome
Hereditary haemorrhagic telangiectasia
Hereditary spherocytosis
Huntington's chorea
Intestinal polyposis
Marfan's syndrome
Myotonic dystrophy
Neurofibromatosis
Osteogenesis imperfecta
Tuberous sclerosis
Retinoblastoma
Hepatic porphyrias
Erythropoietic porphyrias
Von Willebrand's disease

- *Patau's syndrome*: trisomy 13
- *Turner's syndrome*: monosomy X (45XO)
- *Noonan's syndrome*: 45XY
- *Klinefelter's syndrome*: 47 XXY, XXXYY, XXYY
- *Testicular feminisation*: 46XY
- *Psychopathic personality*: 47XYY

# Abnormalities of chromosome structure

*Deletion*: loss of part of the chromosome (Box 3.3)
    p– (loss of short arm)
    q– (loss of long arm)
*Translocation*: transfer of material from one chromosome to another
    14/21 translocation can lead to Down's syndrome
*Robertsonian translocation*: translocation between the long arms of two chromosomes that are joined at the centromere
*Philadelphia chromosome*: 22q– translocated to chromosome 9

*Insertion*: the addition of material to a chromosome
    Usually associated with translocation

# Single gene abnormalities

## Autosomal dominant inheritance

- Both sexes are equally affected
- No carrier state
- Both homozgotes and heterozygotes are phenotypically affected
- 50% of offspring are affected (Fig. 3.3)
- Risk identical in successive pregnancies
- Variable penetrance leads to variable phenotypic severity

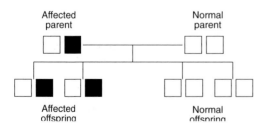

**Fig 3.3: Autosomal dominant inheritance**

## Box 3.5: Autosomal recessive conditions

$\alpha_1$-Antitrypsin deficiency
Agammaglobulinaemia
Albinism
Alkaptonuria
Congenital adrenal hyperplasia
Congenital erythropoietic porphyria
Cystic fibrosis
Gaucher's disease
Galactosaemia
Glycogen storage diseases
Hartnup's disease
Homocystinuria
Hurler's syndrome
Infantile polycystic disease
Niemann–Pick disease
Phenylketonuria
Refsum's disease
Sickle cell disease
Tay –Sachs disease
Thalassaemia
Wilson's disease
Xeroderma pigmentosa
Werdnig–Hoffman disease

- Usually associated with structural abnormalities (Box 3.4)

## Autosomal recessive inheritance

- Both sexes equally affected
- Phenotypic presentation only in homozygotes
- Heterozygotes are carriers (phenotypically unaffected)
- If both parents carry the gene (Fig. 3.4):
  25% of offspring affected
  25% of offspring normal
  50% of offspring carriers
- If one parent carries the gene:
  50% of offspring normal;

## Box 3.6: X-linked dominant conditions

Vitamin D-resistant rickets
Incontinentia pigmenti
Goltz syndrome
Aicardi syndrome

  50% of offspring carriers
- Increased risk of transmission in consanguinous marriages
- Usually associated with metabolic abnormalities (Box 3.5)
- Conditions usually more severe than autosomal dominant conditions

## X-linked dominant inheritance

- Affects both females and males, but F > M
- Males affected more severely than females
- No carrier state
- In homozygous females:
  all offspring affected
- In heterozygous females:
  50% of sons normal, 50% of sons affected;
  50% of daughters normal, 50% of daughters affected
- In affected males:
  all daughters affected;
  all sons normal (no male–male transmission)

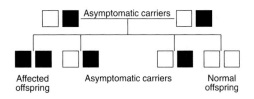

**Fig. 3.4: Autosomal recessive inheritance**

## Box 3.7: X-linked recessive conditions

Agammaglobulinaemia
Becker's muscular dystrophy
Colour blindness
Combined immunodeficiency
Duchenne muscular dystrophy
Fragile X syndrome
G6PD deficiency
Haemophilia A and B
Hypophosphataemic rickets
Hunter's syndrome
Ichthyosis
Lesch–Nyhan syndrome
Nephrogenic diabetes insipidus

# X-linked recessive inheritance

- Affected cases are males and homozygous females
- Only females are carriers
- In homozygous females:
  all sons affected;
  50% of daughters carriers, 50% of daughters normal
- In heterozygous females:
  50% of daughters carriers, 50% of daughters normal;

## Box 3.8: Polygenic conditions

Breast cancer
Club foot
Congenital heart disease
Congenital dislocation of the hip
Cleft lip
Diabetes mellitus
Hirschsprung's disease
Neural tube defects
Pyloric stenosis
Rheumatoid arthritis
Schizophrenia

50% of sons affected, 50% of sons normal
- In affected males:
  50% of daughters carriers, 50% of daughters normal;
  all sons normal (no male–male transmission)

# Polygenic inheritance

- Observed phenotype is due to the additive effects of many different gene loci
- Environmental factors may be involved
- Everyone has a liability to develop a particular malformation
- If the liability exceeds a certain threshold, the malformation manifests
- Risk of manifestation increases if:
  Previous offspring affected
  First-degree relative affected
  Relatives severely affected

# Prenatal diagnosis (Table 3.1)

## Diseases that can be diagnosed prenatally

- Adult polycystic disease
- Becker's muscular dystrophy
- Cystic fibrosis
- Duchenne muscular dystrophy
- Down's syndrome
- Gangliosidoses
- G6PD deficiency
- Haemophilia A and B
- Hunter's syndrome
- Huntington's chorea
- Hypophosphatasia
- Lesch–Nyhan syndrome

## Table 3.1: Techniques of prenatal diagnosis

| Procedure | Timing | Disorder detected |
|---|---|---|
| Ultrasound | From 16 weeks | Anatomical defects |
| Maternal α-fetoprotein | 16 weeks | Neural tube defects (raised) |
| | | Down's syndrome (low) |
| Amniocentesis | 16–20 weeks | Enzyme defects |
| | | Chromosomal abnormalities |
| | | Neural tube defects |
| | | Single gene defects |
| Chorionic villus sampling | 8–10 weeks | Enzyme defects |
| | | Chromosomal abnormalities |
| | | Single gene defects |
| Fetoscopy | 16–20 weeks | Anatomical defects |
| | | Fetal haematological disorders |
| | | Fetal skin disorders |
| | | Organ biopsies |

**Box 3.9: Diseases where gene therapy has been attempted**

Adenosine deaminase deficiency
(immunodeficiency)
Thalassaemia
Sickle cell disease
Phenylketonuria
Haemophilia A
Cystic fibrosis
Duchenne muscular dystrophy

**Box 3.10: Indications for prenatal diagnosis**

Women aged > 35 years
Raised maternal serum α-fetoprotein
Family history of neural tube defects
Family history of chromosomal disorder
Carriers of X-linked recessive diseases who
    want termination
For genetic prediction of above conditions

- Menkes' syndrome
- Metachromatic leukodystrophy
- Myotonic dystrophy
- Neurofibromatosis
- Neural tube defects
- Niemann–Pick disease
- Osteogenesis imperfecta
- Phenylketonuria
- Sickle cell disease
- Tay–Sachs disease
- Tuberous sclerosis
- Thalassaemia

# Clinical case scenarios

## Marfan's syndrome

- The patient is tall
- The limbs are disproportionately long
- The fingers and toes are elongated (arachnodactyly)
- There is a high arched palate
- There is upwards deviation of the lens
- Chest wall muscles are underdeveloped, causing deformities (pigeon chest, pectus excavatum)

**Table 3.2: Differences between Marfan's syndrome and homocystinuria**

| Feature | Marfan's syndrome | Homocystinuria |
| --- | --- | --- |
| Lens dislocation | Upwards | Downwards |
| Mental retardation | No | Yes |
| Osteoporosis | No | Yes |
| Aortic regurgitation | Yes | No |
| Positive urine cyanide nitroprusside test | No | Yes |

- There may be kyphoscoliosis

- Other features to look for:
  Signs of aortic regurgitation
  Mitral valve prolapse
  Thoracotomy scar (valve surgery, aneurysm repair)
  Heterochromia of the iris
  Blue sclerae
  Hyperextensible joints
  Pneumothorax (spontaneous)
  Signs of infective endocarditis
  Inguinal/femoral herniae
  Spectacles (myopia)

# Ehlers–Danlos syndrome

- The skin is hyperextensible, elastic and thin
- The joints are hyperextensible

- Other features to look for:
  multiple scars, particularly over knees (thin skin, easily torn, poor healing)
  pseudotumours, particularly over knees (calcified haematomas)
  purpura

epicanthal folds
flat feet
kyphoscoliosis
blue sclerae
pneumothorax (spontaneous)
mitral valve prolapse
signs of infective endocarditis

# Down's syndrome

- The patient has short stature
- The nasal bridge is flattened
- There are epicanthic folds
- The mouth often hangs open to reveal macroglossia
- There may be a single palmar crease
- The fingers and toes are short

- Other features to look for:
  mental retardation
  dementia (Alzheimer's type)
  atrial septal defect
  Fallot's tetralogy
  thoracotomy scar (cardiac surgery)
  alopecia
  hyperextensible joints
  generalised hypotonia

# Turner's syndrome

- The patient is female
- The patient has short stature
- The neck is short and webbed
- There is a cubitus valgus deformity
- The nipples are widely spaced
- The secondary sexual characteristics are underdeveloped
- The fourth metacarpals are short

- Other features to look for:
  lymphoedema
  low hairline
  high arched palate
  coarctation
  atrial septal defect

ventricular septal defect
aortic stenosis
strabismus
ptosis
thoracotomy scar
diabetes mellitus
premature ageing

# Klinefelter's syndrome

- The male secondary sexual characteristics are underdeveloped
- The testes are small
- There is gynaecomastia
- There is female-like fat distribution
- There may be mild mental retardation (usually normal)

# 4 Microbiology

## Contents

# Bacteria

## Structure of bacteria

Bacteria are unicellular organisms with the following features:

### Cell wall
- Surrounds bacterial cell contents
- Determines shape of bacterial cell
- Prevents bacterial cell from bursting
- Composed of mucopeptide (peptidoglycan)
- Gram staining reactions are determined by the amount of mucopeptide in the walls (Gram-positive organisms' walls have 50–90%, Gram-negative 5–10%)
- Gram-positive organisms also have techoic acid in their walls
- Gram-negative organisms also have a layer of phospholipid–polysaccharide–protein complex surrounding the cell wall
- Some bacterial cell walls have fimbriae or pili to aid adhesion and reproduction

### Protoplast
- Found inside the cell wall
- Consists of cytoplasm, cytoplasmic membrane, ribosomes (RNA) and the nuclear body or chromosome (DNA)

### Flagellae
- Possessed by some bacteria (Box 4.1)
- Long, thin, threadlike appendages
- Arise from the protoplast and project through the cell wall
- Composed of protein
- Not stainable unless thickened
- Allows motility of bacterial cell

---

**Box 4.1: Flagellate bacteria**

---

*Clostridium botulinum*
*Clostridium tetani*
*Salmonella* spp.
*Enterobacter* spp.
*Yersinia pseudotuberculosis*
*Yersinia enterocolitica*
*Pseudomonas* spp.

### Spores

- Round oval structures
- Heat-resistant coats
- Produced as a reaction to unfavourable growth conditions
- Have low water content and minimal metabolic activity
- Not capable of reproduction
- Formed by *Bacillus* and *Clostridium* species

### Shape

See classification table (Table 4.1)
- *Cocci*: spherical
- *Bacilli*: rod-shaped
- *Vibrios*: curved rods
- *Spirochaetes*: corkscrew-like spirals

### Alternative forms

- *Protoplasts*: bacteria converted by the action of lysozymes
  No cell wall, leading to loss of rigidity, shape and osmotic resistance
  Survive only in suitable hypertonic media
  Unable to reproduce
- *Spheroplasts*: bacteria with residual but damaged cell walls
- *L forms*: mutant bacteria with no cell wall
  Fragile and delicate
  Able to reproduce
  *Mycoplasma* is an example

## Staining reactions

See classification table (Table 4.1)
- *Gram stain*: most commonly used
  Uses methyl or gentian violet followed by iodine
- *Gram-positive*: resist decolorisation by ethyl alcohol or acetone
- *Gram-negative*: give up dye and counterstained with red carbol fuchsin or safranin
- *Ziehl–Neelsen stain*: organisms stained red by hot carbol fuchsin
  Resist decolorisation by ethyl alcohol or 20% sulphuric acid (acid fast)
  Counterstain with methylene blue or malachite green
  Responsible for staining of mycobacteria
- *Alberts (Neissers) stain*: allows identification of metachromatic (volutin) granules
  Characteristically found in *Corynebacterium diphtheriae*

## Bacterial physiology

### Metabolic needs (Table 4.2)

Most bacteria grow best in alkaline environment (*Lactobacillus* prefers an acidic environment).
- *Constitutive enzymes*: produced in all circumstances
- *Inducible enzymes*: produced in response to special circumstances
- *Phototrophs*: derive energy from sunlight
- *Chemotrophs*: derive energy from oxidation of chemical compounds
- *Chemo-organotrophs*: parasites that use organic compounds
- *Aerobes*: require oxygen for growth
- *Obligate aerobes*: unable to grow in the absence of oxygen
- *Facultative aerobes*: able to grow with or without oxygen, but grow best in aerobic conditions
- *Anaerobes*: require oxygen-free environment to grow
- *Microaerophiles*: grow best in the presence of a little oxygen
- *Carboxyphiles*: require a higher concentration than normal of $CO_2$ to grow
- *Psychrophiles*: grow best at low temperature
- *Thermophiles*: grow best at high temperature

## Table 4.1: Classification of bacteria

| Gram-positive | Gram-negative | Non-Gram-staining |
|---|---|---|
| **Cocci** | **Cocci** | *Mycobacteria* |
| *Streptococcus* | *Neisseria* | |
| *Staphylococcus* | | Spirochaetes: *Treponema* |
| | | *Borrelia* |
| **Bacilli** | **Bacilli** | *Leptospira* |
| *Corynebacterium* | Enterobacteria: *Escherichia coli* | |
| *Bacillus* | *Klebsiella* | *Mycoplasma* |
| *Lactobacillus* | *Salmonella* | |
| *Clostridium* | *Shigella* | |
| *Listeria* | *Proteus* | |
| | *Yersinia* | |
| **Branching bacteria** | *Citrobacter* | |
| *Streptomyces* | *Serratia* | |
| *Actinomyces* | *Enterobacter* | |
| *Nocardia* | | |
| | Parvobacteria: *Haemophilus* | |
| | *Bordetella* | |
| | *Brucella* | |
| | *Legionella* | |
| | *Francisella* | |
| | *Bartonella* | |
| | Anaerobes: *Bacteroides* | |
| | *Fusobacterium* | |
| | *Pseudomonas* | |
| | Cat scratch bacillus | |
| | **Vibrios** | |
| | *Vibrio cholera* | |
| | *Campylobacter* | |

## Table 4.2: Oxygen requirements of bacteria

| Aerobes | Facultative aerobes | Microaerophiles | Anaerobes | Carboxyphiles |
|---|---|---|---|---|
| *Corynebacterium* | *S. pyogenes* | *Lactobacillus* | Enterococci | *S. pneumoniae* |
| *Bacillus* | *S. viridans* | *Campylobacter* | Bacillus | *Neisseria* |
| *Neisseria* | *Staphylococcus* | | *Clostridia* | Parvobacteria |
| Enterobacteria | | | Enterobacteria | |
| Parvobacteria | | | *Bacteroides* | |
| *Pseudomonas* | | | *Vibrio cholerae* | |
| *Nocardia* | | | Spirochaetes | |
| *Vibrio cholerae* | | | Actinomyces | |
| *Listeria* | | | *Streptomyces* | |
| *Mycobacterium TB* | | | *Lactobacillus* | |

---

**Box 4.2: Exotoxin-producing bacteria**

*Streptococcus pyogenes*
*Staphylococcus aureus*
*Corynebacterium diphtheriae*
*Bacillus cereus*
*Clostridium botulinum*
*Clostridium tetani*
*Clostridium perfringens*
*Clostridium difficile*
*Escherichia coli* (EHEC, ETEC)
*Vibrio cholerae*

---

**Box 4.3: Enzyme-producing bacteria**

*Streptococcus pyogenes* (streptolysin, streptokinase, hyaluronidase, DNAase)
*Staphylococcus aureus* (coagulase, catalase, β-lactamase, hyaluronidase, DNAase)
*Neisseria gonorrhoeae* (β-lactamase)
*Escherichia coli* (β-lactamase)
*Clostridium perfringens* (phospholipase)

---

- All chemotrophs contain pigments
- Pigments are composed of flavoproteins and cytochromes

## Growth characteristics

Different bacteria require different energy substrates and conditions in order to flourish. These different requirements can be met in vitro by altering the environment and the content of the agar on which they are grown.

- *Simple nutrient agar*: limited use
- *Blood agar*: nutrient agar plus 5–10% horse blood
  Allows identification of streptococci subtypes according to haemolytic changes
  *β-Haemolysis*: characterised by the presence of clear colourless zone around colonies. Represents complete haemolysis
  Characteristic of *Streptococcus pyogenes*, *S. agalactiae*, enterococci
  *α-Haemolysis*: characterised by the presence of opaque zone around colonies
  Represents partial haemolysis
  Characteristic of *Streptococcus pneumoniae*, *S. viridans*, enterococci
- *Chocolate agar*: heated blood agar
  Particularly good for identification of *Neisseria meningitidis*
- *MacConkey's agar*: contains bile salts and lactose
  Used for differentiation between enterobacteria (Table 4.3)

- *Mesophiles*: grow best at temperature between 20 and 40°C

## Metabolic products

### Exotoxins
These are heat-labile proteins with enzymic activity, released into the environment.
- Produced mainly by Gram-positive organisms (Box 4.2)
- Exotoxins released into the intestinal lumen are called enterotoxins

### Endotoxins
- Produced exclusively by Gram-negative organisms
- Derived from phospholipid–polysaccharide–protein complex surrounding cell wall
- More heat stable than exotoxins
- Only liberated upon death of the organism
- Mediate damage by stimulating coagulation cascade and causing cardiovascular collapse

### Aggressins
- Enzymes produced by bacteria that invoke an antibody response (Box 4.3)

### Pigments
- Phototrophs trap the energy of sunlight using pigments

**Table 4.3: Lactose-fermenting characteristics of bacteria**

| Lactose fermenters | Non-lactose fermenters |
|---|---|
| *Escherichia coli* | *Salmonella* |
| *Klebsiella* | *Shigella dysenteriae* |
| *Shigella sonnei* | *Shigella flexneri* |
| | *Shigella boydii* |
| | *Proteus* |
| | *Yersinia* |

- *Blood agar and tellurite*: useful for identification of *Corynebacterium diphtheriae*
- *Bordet–Gengou medium*: used for identification of *Bordetella pertussis*
- *Lowenstein Jensen medium*: used for growth of *Mycobacterium tuberculosis*
- *Loeffler's serum*: useful for identification of *Corynebacterium diphtheriae*
- *Deoxycholate citrate agar (DCA)*: suppresses most bacteria except *Salmonella* and *Shigella*
- *Selenite F broth*: useful for identification of *Salmonella*
- *Thiosulphate–citrate–bile salts–sucrose (TCBS) agar*: useful for identification of *Vibrio cholerae*

When bacteria are provided with a suitable environment and nutrients, a typical growth pattern is seen (Fig. 4.1).

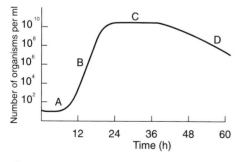

**Fig. 4.1: Growth curve of bacteria in a liquid medium**

*Lag phase (A):* bacterial cells adapt to new environment; cells increase in size but not in number

*Logarithmic phase (B):* bacterial cells divide and increase in number; can be maintained if culture medium renewed (continuous culture)

*Stationary phase (C):* rate of new cell production equals rate of cell loss; cell loss occurs as a result of exhaustion of nutrients and accumulation of toxic metabolites

*Phase of decline (D):* bacterial cell numbers decline owing to accumulation of toxic metabolites

## Reproduction

Bacteria reproduce by binary fission to produce two identical organisms. Genotypic variation may occur due to:

- *Mutation* of bacterial cell DNA
- *Transduction*: if bacterial cell culture is infected with a bacteriophage, the DNA of the bacteriophage's previous host may become incorporated into the bacterial cell DNA and hence passed on. In lysogenic conversion, the bacteriophage's own DNA becomes incorporated into the bacterial cell DNA
- *Conjugation*: transfer of DNA from one bacterial cell to another. This occurs due to the presence of special plasmids (extranuclear DNA) called transfer factors, which are capable of forming sex fimbriae.

Sex fimbriae allow a bacterial cell to attach itself to another cell.

This is one method by which bacteria develop antibiotic resistance.

**Table 4.4: Streptococcal infections**

| Lancefield group | Streptococcus subtype | Infections |
|---|---|---|
| A | *pyogenes* | Pharyngitis |
| | | Scarlet fever |
| | | Otitis media |
| | | Sinusitis |
| | | Rheumatic fever |
| | | Erysipelas |
| | | Impetigo |
| | | Lymphangitis |
| B | *agalactiae* | Neonatal infection |
| D | Enterococci | UTI, septicaemia, endocarditis |
| | *pneumoniae* | Pneumonia, meningitis, otitis media |
| | *viridans* | Endocarditis, cerebral abscess, empyema |

# Specific bacterial infections

## *Streptococcus (Table 4.4)*

## *Staphylococcus (Table 4.5)*

## *Tetanus* Clostridium tetani

- Faecal–oral transmission
- Incubation period up to 3 weeks
- Pathogenicity determined by production of neurotoxin
- Neurotoxin inhibits release of acetylcholine, leading to interference of synaptic reflexes in spinal cord, leading to disinhibition and muscular spasm

*Clinical features*: begins with muscle spasm around wound
Trismus heralds the onset of generalised tetanus
Autonomic involvement may ensue

- Risk of developing tetanus greater if soil present in wound
- Prognosis worse if incubation period short and rapid onset of first spasm

*Treatment*:
Local wound debridement
Human immunoglobulin containing antitoxin
Metronidazole
Benzodiazepenes for muscular spasm

*Prevention in patients with wounds*:
Immunised – tetanus toxoid booster
Non-immunised – tetanus toxoid plus antitoxin plus penicillin

## *Gonorrhoea* Neisseria gonorrhoeae

- Sexually transmitted disease
- Incubation period 2–7 days

**Table 4.5: Staphylococcal infections**

| Invasive | Toxin mediated |
|---|---|
| Impetigo | Toxic shock syndrome |
| Carbuncles | Scalded skin syndrome |
| Surgical wound infections | Food poisoning |
| Septicaemia | |
| Pneumonia (cavitating) | |
| Endocarditis | |

- Symptoms in men: urethritis
- Symptoms in women:
  Usually asymptomatic
  May cause vaginal discharge, dysuria, abdominal pain
  Dissemination more common
- Anal intercourse: proctitis
- Oral sex: pharyngitis usually asymptomatic

  *Complications*: generalised papular–pustular rash
  pelvic inflammatory disease
  peritonitis
  septicaemia
  infertility
  urethral stricture
  septic arthritis
  meningitis
  endocarditis
  myocarditis
  pericarditis
  peri-hepatitis (FitzHugh–Curtis syndrome)

  *Treatment*: penicillin plus probenecid
  ciproxin and septrin are alternatives

## Typhoid *salmonella typhi + paratyphi*

- Faecal–oral transmission
- Incubation period usually 10–14 days
- Organism multiplies mainly in Peyer's patches of the intestine

*Symptoms*:
  *during 1st week* – headache, dry cough, constipation, relative bradycardia
  *during 2nd week* – splenomegaly, rose spots (in only 50%)
  *during 3rd week* – diarrhoea

*Complications*:
  intestinal perforation
  intestinal haemorrhage
  myocarditis
  bone marrow suppression
  osteomyelitis

  meningitis
  chronic carriage in gallbladder

*Diagnosis*:
  *during 1st week* – blood culture, bone marrow
  *during 2nd week* – urine, faeces, bone marrow

*Treatment*: ciproxin first choice
  Chloramphenicol, amoxil, septrin, trimethoprim are alternatives

## Whooping cough
- Airborne droplet transmission
- Incubation period 7–10 days
- Most common in children < 5 years
- More severe in those < 1 year
- After 2–3 days, characteristic coughing spasms develop
- Illness lasts up to 2 months

*Complications*:
  Secondary pneumonia
  Cerebral hypoxia during spasms leading to seizures
  Subconjunctival haemorrhages, periorbital bruising, frenal ulcer

*Treatment*: if given during catarrhal phase, erythromycin may reduce infectivity or shorten illness
  No treatment is of benefit when coughing spasms begin

## Lyme disease
- Transmitted by the tick *Ixodes dammini*

  *Clinical features*: initially presents with rash of erythema chronicum migrans, fever, lymphadenopathy and migratory arthralgia
  1–24 weeks after rash, recurrent asymmetrical large joint arthritis
  Subsequent features include focal neurological signs, myelopathy, meningoencephalitis, carditis

*Treatment*: penicillin or tetracycline
   given early may shorten illness and
   limit progression

## Brucellosis
- Transmitted by close contact with cattle
  or ingestion of unpasteurised milk
- Most common in vets, farmers,
  abattoir workers
- Incubation period 3 weeks

   *Clinical features:* swinging fever
      back pain (spondylitis)
      hepatosplenomegaly
      acute monoarthritis
      meningoencephalitis
      endocarditis
      epididymo-orchitis
      depression

   *Treatment*: doxycycline plus rifampicin
      or streptomycin
      6 weeks' treatment for un-
      complicated cases
      12 weeks' treatment if
      complications

## Legionnaire's disease
- Transmission by airborne droplets
- Incubation period 2–10 days
- Organism thrives in air-conditioning
  and humidifying systems that form
  aerosols
- Usually produces outbreaks rather
  than isolated cases
- Most cases occur in the summer
- Mostly in the middle-aged and older
  people

   *Clinical features*: severe pneumonia
      with haemoptysis
      haematuria, renal failure
      bloody diarrhoea and vomiting
      abdominal pain
      hyponatraemia
      hypoalbuminaemia
      transaminasaemia

raised alkaline phosphatase
hypocalcaemia
neutrophilia
lymphopenia

*Pontiac fever*: mild upper respiratory
   tract infection
*Treatment*: erythromycin (plus
   rifampicin if severe)
   ciproxin is an alternative

## Leptospirosis
- Transmitted by contact with infected
  rat urine
- Incubation period 1–2 weeks

   *Clinical features*: prodromal illness of
      myalgia (especially calves),
      jaundice, fever, followed by
      hepatitis-like illness with associated
      neutrophilia
      May develop meningitis,
      haematuria, headache, epistaxis,
      renal failure

   *Treatment*: penicillin

## Mycoplasma pneumonia (Box 4.4)
- Airborne droplet transmission
- Incubation period 1–3 weeks
- Usually affects people aged 15–30
  years
- Most common during autumn
- Cough often dry
- Typically white cell count normal
- Cold agglutinins present in 50%

## Syphilis *Treponema pallidum*
- Sexually transmitted disease
- May be divided into five stages:

   *Primary*: primary lesion is chancre
      (painless ulcer)
      Usually appears 10–90 days after
      infection
      May occur on genitalia or in anus
      or pharynx

## Box 4.4: Features of mycoplasma infection

**Haematological**
Autoimmune haemolytic anaemia
Cold agglutinins
Thrombocytopenia
Disseminated intravascular coagulation
Splenomegaly

**Gastroenterological**
Gastroenteritis
Hepatitis
Pancreatitis

**Neurological**
Meningitis
Encephalitis
Transverse myelitis
Peripheral neuropathy
Cerebellar ataxia

**Rheumatological**
Arthralgia
Myalgia
Polyarthritis

**Cardiovascular**
Pericarditis
Myocarditis
Pericardial effusion

**Dermatological**
Erythema nodosum
Erythema multiforme

**Renal**
Interstitial nephritis
Glomerulonephritis

*Secondary*: may take up to 3 months to develop
Characterised by bacteremia leading to general systemic upset
Most commonly presents with generalised papular rash resembling psoriasis
Also characterised by presence of highly infectious perianal warts (condylomata lata)
Alopecia may occur
Arthralgia, hepatosplenomegaly, acute meningitis, cranial nerve palsies may occur

*Latent period*: if untreated, about 2 years after infection the disease goes into remission
During this period there are no clinical symptoms or signs

*Tertiary*: characterised by the presence of gummata (destructive granuloma)
May be found in any organ

*Quaternary*: characterised by the development of neurosyphilis or cardiovascular disease
Neurosyphilis may present as:

*Chronic meningovascular syphilis*:
10–12 years after primary infection
Chronic basal meningitis

*General paralysis of the insane (GPI)*:
15– 20 years after primary infection
Dementia, extensor plantars, Argyll Robertson pupils *Small, non reactive constriction, ocular convergence unequal side, irregular outline*
*Tabes dorsalis*: 10–25 years after primary infection
Posterior column degeneration leading to sensory ataxia
Lightning pains in the legs, cutaneous paraesthesia or hyperaesthesia
Loss of deep pain sensation
Neuropathic (Charcot) joints

Neurogenic bladder, flexor
plantars, Argyll Robertson pupils
Tabetic crises (abdominal pain
and vomiting)

*Syphilitic amyotrophy*: anterior horn
cell degeneration of spinal cord

Cardiovascular disease presents as end-
arteritis obliterans, leading to aneurysm of
ascending aorta

## Diagnosis of syphilis
### Non-treponemal tests (VDRL, RPR)
Detect cardiolipin antibody in patient's
serum
Become positive 2–3 weeks after
infection
Become negative during therapy or
latent phase of untreated disease
Indicative of acute infection
Beware of false positive results (Box 4.5)

### Treponemal tests (FTA, TPHA)
• Detect specific antibody against
treponemal antigen
• Positive early in infection
• Remain positive after therapy and
during latent phase
• Indicative of chronic infection

*Primary syphilis*: FTA positive, TPHA
may be positive or negative
Non-treponemal tests negative

*Secondary syphilis*: all tests positive

*Latent syphilis*: treponemal tests positive
Non-treponemal tests negative
*Tertiary and Quaternary syphilis*:
treponemal tests positive for years
Non-treponemal tests negative

## Treatment of syphilis
• *Primary, secondary, early latent disease*:
procaine penicillin for 14 days
• *Tertiary, quaternary, late latent disease*:

---

**Box 4.5: Causes of false positive VDRL**

Malaria
Leprosy
Tuberculosis
Leptospirosis
Hepatitis
Rheumatoid arthritis
SLE
Pregnancy
Post immunisations
Autoimmune conditions

---

procaine penicillin plus probenecid
• *Penicillin allergy*: erythromycin or
doxycycline

*Jarisch–Herxheimer reaction*: caused by
endotoxin release from dying
spirochaetes
Transient fever following first
penicillin dose
More common in secondary
disease, more serious in tertiary
disease
Attenuated by prednisolone before
penicillin injection

## Tuberculosis
• Transmission by airborne droplets
• Primary infection leads to lymph node
involvement and subpleural
consolidation (Ghon focus)
• Affects mid and lower zones
• Any of the following may occur:
*Ghon focus* heals, leaving residual
pulmonary fibrosis and calcification
of lymph nodes
In some patients infection is
reactivated (post primary TB) which
usually produces apical lung
disease, consisting of either
cavitation, bronchiectasis,
consolidation, fibrosis or pleural
thickening (caseating granulomas)
Reactivation related to poor

immunity (advanced age, alcohol abuse, malnutrition, sepsis, steroids, pregnancy)

Reactivated TB highly infectious when patient is producing large quantities of purulent sputum

Primary lesion invades bloodstream, leading to miliary TB consisting of multiorgan involvement

TB meningitis common in such patients

CXR shows miliary mottling

Primary lung lesion may cavitate, leading to pleural effusion

Primary lymph node involvement may progress to cause bronchial obstruction

## Diagnosis of TB

- *Microscopy*: tissue samples or sputum using Ziehl–Neelsen stain
- *Culture*: using Lowenstein–Jensen medium. Takes 6 weeks
- *Skin testing*: dependent on integrity of cell-mediated immunity

Can be carried out in 3 ways:

1. *Mantoux test*: standard amount of old tuberculin or purified protein derivative injected intradermally
   Test read after 72 hours
   Positive test indicated by area of induration > 6mm
2. *Heaf test*: quicker multiple puncture technique
   Test read after 4–7 days
   Reactions graded 0–4
   Grades 0,1 – negative
   Grades 2-4 – positive
3. *Tine test*: variant of Heaf test but less reliable

*Positive skin test indicates*: previous primary infection (natural immunity/BCG)
Active infection (may be negative in early or miliary infection)

---

### Box 4.6: Diagnosis of extrapulmonary TB

Three early-morning urine specimens
Liver biopsy
Lymph node biopsy
Bone marrow aspirate and trephine
Lumbar puncture
Laparoscopy and biopsy
Joint aspiration
Bone biopsy
Stool specimens in immunosuppressed patients

---

## Treatment of TB

- Major drugs used: rifampicin, isoniazid, pyrazinamide, ethambutol

  *Pulmonary TB*: triple or quadruple therapy for 2 months followed by isoniazid and rifampicin for 4 months

  *Miliary TB/TB meningitis*: treatment for 1 year

- Corticosteroids used in:
  cachectic patients
  TB meningitis
  intracerebral tuberculoma
  pleural/pericardial effusions
  hypersensitivity to drugs

## Leprosy

- Transmission by airborne droplets from patients with lepromatous leprosy
- No evidence of transmission by direct contact
- Outcome of infection dependent on host immunity
- If macrophages are able to kill bacteria, there is little or no clinical disease
- Five clinical patterns of disease are described (Table 4.6):

**Table 4.6: Features of different leprosy patterns**

| Feature | Tuberculoid | Lepromatous |
|---|---|---|
| Skin lesions | Few (1–3) | Large numbers |
| Nerve involvement | Local | Diffuse |
| Number of bacilli | Few | Vast numbers |
| Lepromin test | +++ | – |
| Erythema nodosum leprosum | – | +++ |

*Paucibacillary*:
   Tuberculoid
   Borderline tuberculoid

*Multibacillary*:
   Borderline
   Borderline lepromatous
   Lepromatous

### Diagnosis of leprosy
- Cannot be cultured in vitro
- In vivo culture can be performed using mouse foot pads, armadillos or hedgehogs
- Tissue can be obtained from skin smears or nerve biopsies
- Microscopy using Ziehl–Neelsen stain

### Treatment of leprosy
- *Paucibacillary*: rifampicin + dapsone
- *Multibacillary*: rifampicin + dapsone + clofazimine
- All treatments should be continued for at least 2 years until skin smears show no bacilli

# Viruses

See classification table (Table 4.7).

# Virus structure and physiology

*Virion*: virus particle
*Active virus*: able to invade and replicate in host cell
*Inactivated virus*: unable to replicate in host cell

- Basic structure consists of nucleic acid core (genome) surrounded by a protein coat (capsid)
- Some viruses possess a loose membranous envelope composed of lipids, protein and carbohydrate
- Viruses are replicated by host cells
- Process begins with attachment and adsorption of virus to host cell surface (via envelope)
- Once adsorbed, the virus enters host cell by a process similar to phagocytosis (penetration)
- The capsid is then removed (uncoating) and the nucleic acid released into the host cell
- More viruses are then produced by the host cell
- Some viruses are made within the cytoplasm, some within the host cell nucleus
- New viruses are then released from the host cell either by budding (which preserves the host cell) or following lysis of the host cell (cytopathic effect)

*Inclusion bodies*: accumulation of virus material in host cell
   Visible on light microscopy
   May be cytoplasmic or nucleic
   Usually contain active virus but may only be due to post-replication debris

*Latency:* after acute infection virus

## Table 4.7: Classification of viruses

| DNA viruses | RNA viruses |
|---|---|
| ***Envelope, double-stranded*** | ***Envelope, double-stranded*** |
| Herpes viruses: | Orthomyxoviruses: Influenza |
|   Herpes simplex | Paramyxoviruses: |
|   Varicella zoster |   Parainfluenza |
|   Cytomegalovirus |   Respiratory syncytial virus |
|   Epstein–Barr virus |   Mumps |
|   Human herpes virus 6 |   Measles |
| Pox viruses: | Toga viruses: |
|   Vaccinia |   Rubella |
|   Variola (smallpox) |   α viruses |
|   Orf | Flaviviruses: |
| ***Envelope, single-stranded*** |   Dengue fever |
| Parvo viruses |   Yellow fever |
| Hepatitis viruses: B, D |   Hepatitis C |
| ***Non-enveloped, double-stranded*** | Bunyaviruses: |
| Adeno viruses |   Sandfly fever virus |
| Papova viruses: Papilloma virus |   Hantavirus |
| | Arenaviruses: |
| |   Lymphocytic choriomeningitis virus |
| |   Lassa fever |
| | Filoviruses: |
| |   Marburg virus |
| |   Ebola virus |
| | Retroviruses: Lenti virus (HIV 1,2) |
| | Oncoviruses: HTLV |
| | Rhabdovirus: Rabies |
| | Coronavirus |
| | ***Non-enveloped, double-stranded*** |
| | Reo viruses: |
| |   Rota virus |
| |   Reo virus |
| | ***Non-enveloped, single-stranded*** |
| | Picornaviruses: |
| |   Rhino virus |
| |   Coxsackie viruses |
| |   Polio virus |
| |   Echovirus |
| |   Hepatitis A |
| | Calci viruses: |
| |   Norwalk agent |
| |   Hepatitis E |
| | Astrovirus |

**Table 4.8: Features of common viral infections**

| Virus | Incubation period (days) | Infectivity | Rash | Complications | Immunity |
|---|---|---|---|---|---|
| Chickenpox | 13–17 | Few days before rash until cessation of appearance of new lesions | Begins centripetally Appears in crops Macule–papule–vesicle–pustule–scab | Secondary bacterial infection Pneumonia Encephalitis DIC | Lifelong to chickenpox Reactivation leads to shingles |
| Measles | 8–11 | 2 days before symptoms until 4 days after rash disappears | Begins peripherally Maculopapular Koplik's spots in mouth | Otitis media Pneumonia Encephalitis Subacute sclerosing panencephalitis | Lifelong |
| Mumps | 18 | 7 days before symptoms until 1 week later | – | Orchitis Infertility Encephalitis Pancreatitis Polyarthritis | Lifelong in most |
| Glandular fever | 7–14 | Prolonged excretion may occur in saliva | Maculopapular rash induced by ampicillin | Hepatitis Splenic rupture Thrombocytopenia Autoimmune haemolytic anaemia Meningoencephalitis Chronic fatigue | Lifelong |

EBV

**Table 4.8 continued**

| Virus | Incubation period (days) | Infectivity | Rash | Complications | Immunity |
|-------|-------------------------|-------------|------|---------------|----------|
| Influenza | 1–3 | 1 day before until 3–7 days after | – | Secondary bacterial pneumonia<br>Myositis<br>Myocarditis<br>Pericarditis<br>Guillain–Barré syndrome<br>Encephalitis | Strain specific |
| Herpes simplex | 1–2 | Direct contact with skin lesions | Vesicular<br>HSV 1: gingivostomatitis<br>HSV 2: genital | Secondary bacterial infection<br>Encephalitis<br>Eczema herpeticum<br>Pneumonia<br>Hepatitis | Reactivation occurs |
| Shingles | Variable | Direct contact with lesions | Vesicular<br>Localised to dermatomes (most commonly truncal) | Secondary bacterial infection<br>Dissemination<br>Postherpetic neuralgia (more common following ophthalmic or disseminated infection) | Second infection rare |

remains dormant in the host cells without causing damage
Virus may be reactivated later to cause reinfection (herpes viruses)

*Persistent infection*: some viruses persist and replicate in host cells
Manage to escape host's immune responses
Often leads to immune complex formation

*Slow viruses*: atypical viruses
Long incubation period (often years)
Lead to a chronic degenerative process
Usually affect the CNS

*Transformation*: some viruses stimulate host cell to become 'malignant' and replicate rapidly

*Bacteriophages*: viruses that are parasitic upon bacteria (live in bacteria)
Usually DNA viruses
Phage may replicate in host cell and, on release, cause lysis of bacterial cell
Some phages become incorporated into the host cell chromosome and are reproduced synchronously with the bacterial cell (lysogeny)

*Pathogenicity of viruses*: immune complex formation (type III hypersensitivity reactions)
Cytopathic effects, alteration of host cellular function,
Stimulation of transformation
Chronic degenerative process

# Specific viral infections

## Rabies
- Transmitted in saliva of infected animals (dog, cat, fox, bat)
- All mammals die except bats
- Virus initially replicates in salivary glands and travels from point of entry to brain
- Virus replicates again in the brain leading to an encephalitis
- Incubation period proportional to length of journey from bite to brain and hence site of bite
- Incubation period 20–60 days (may be up to 1 year)

*Clinical features:* Initially non-specific prodromal symptoms (headache, fever, anorexia)
After 2–3 days patient becomes agitated and confused
This is followed by a rapid progression to hydrophobia and hypersalivation
Pharyngeal and respiratory muscle spasms lead to bizarre breathing patterns
Late features include ascending paralysis, respiratory failure, arrhythmias

*Diagnosis*: corneal smears, skin biopsy
Inclusion bodies (Negri bodies) may be seen

*Treatment*: long incubation period allows immunisation and treatment with rabies-specific immunoglobulin, which may stave off disease
If biting animal healthy after 10 days, treatment can be discontinued
No treatment once disease progresses

## Dengue fever
- Transmitted by *Aedes aegypti* mosquito
- Incubation period 7 days

*Clinical features*: begins with fever, headache, eye pain, backache, limb pain, followed by a generalised erythematous macular rash

Leucopenia commonly occurs
In haemorrhagic variant the patient
is more ill with thrombocytopenia,
mucosal haemorrhage and
hypovolaemic shock

*Treatment*: supportive

### Yellow fever
- Transmitted by *Haemagogus* and *Aedes aegypti* mosquitoes
- Monkeys may also harbour the virus and be involved in a transmission cycle
- Incubation period 6 days
- Liver is main site of infection, leading to hepatitis

*Clinical features*: begins with headache, fever, limb pains
Other features include proteinuria, coagulation abnormalities, mucosal haemorrhage, thrombocytopenia, leucopenia, cardiac failure, renal failure

*Treatment*: supportive

### Viral haemorrhagic fevers

*Clinical features*: incubation period 5–17 days
Characterised by bleeding tendency, leading to purpura, mucosal haemorrhage and organ haemorrhage in severe cases
May progress to multiorgan failure in severe cases
Not all patients develop clinical disease: if they do, it is often mild and self-limiting

*Treatment*: supportive
Ribavarin may help if used early in Lassa fever

**Table 4.9: Oncogenic viruses**

| Virus | Associated malignancy |
| --- | --- |
| HTLV | Lymphoma |
| HIV | Kaposi's sarcoma |
|  | B-cell lymphoma |
| Hepatitis B | Hepatoma |
| Hepatitis C | Hepatoma |
| EBV | Burkitt's lymphoma |
| Papillomavirus | Cancer of cervix |

# Rickettsia and Chlamydia

- Small bacteria similar in size to viruses
- They contain RNA and DNA
- They are susceptible to antibiotics (tetracycline, chloramphenicol)
- They are unable to replicate outside the host cell (obligate intracellular organisms)
- They stain Gram negative

**Box 4.7: Causes of viral haemorrhagic fevers**

**Bunyaviruses**
Hanta
Crimean–Congo haemorrhagic fever
Rift Valley haemorrhagic fever
California encephalitis

**Filoviruses**
Marburg virus
Ebola virus

**Arenaviruses**
Lymphocytic choriomeningitis virus
Lassa virus
Junin (Argentinian haemorrhagic fever)
Machupo (Bolivian haemorrhagic fever)
Guananto (Venezuelan haemorrhagic fever)
Sabia (Brazilian haemorrhagic fever)

**Table 4.10: Classification of *Rickettsia***

| Disease | Organism | Reservoir | Vector | Eschar |
|---------|----------|-----------|--------|--------|
| ***Typhus group*** | | | | |
| Epidemic typhus | *R. prowazeki* | Humans | Lice | No |
| Endemic typhus | *R. typhi* | Rats | Fleas, lice | No |
| Scrub typhus | *R. tsutsugamushi* | Rodents | Mites | Yes |
| | | | | |
| ***Spotted fever group*** | | | | |
| Rocky mountain spotted fever | *R. rickettsi* | Rodents, dogs | Ticks | No |
| Boutonneuse fever | *R. conori* | Rodents, dogs | Ticks | Yes |
| Rickettsial pox | *R. akari* | Mice | Mites | Yes |

- *Rickettsia* and *Coxiella* are pleomorphic and have a variety of shapes
- *Chlamydia* are spherical

## Rickettsia (Table 4.10)

- Primarily intestinal parasites of bloodsucking arthropods
- Human infection follows direct inoculation into bites or inhalation of arthropod faeces
- They produce endotoxins
- Composed of three groups: typhus group, spotted fever group, Q fever (*Coxiella burnetii*)

## Q fever

- Transmitted by close contact with domestic animals
- Incubation period 20 days
- Influenza-like illness but may progress to cause pneumonia, meningo-encephalitis, hepatitis
- Chronic untreated infection may cause osteomyelitis, endocarditis, pericarditis, myocarditis, peripheral neuropathy
- Treatment with tetracycline

## Chlamydia

*Chlamydia psittaci*: many serotypes. Zoonosis leading to psittacosis, ornithosis, pneumonia

*Chlamydia trachomatis*: L1, 2, 3 – sexually transmitted, leading to lymphogranuloma venereum
A, B, C – contact transmission, leading to trachoma
D–K – sexually transmitted, leading to Reiter's syndrome, pelvic inflammatory disease (PID)

# Protozoa

## Structure and physiology of protozoa

- Unicellular organisms
- Larger than bacteria
- Reproduce by binary fission, sexual or asexual lifecycles

### Lifecycles
- All protozoa pass through stages of development until maturity is reached
- Cycles of development are unidirectional
- In some cases different stages of development require a different host

*Direct development*: single host required
*Indirect development*: two or more hosts
required

*Definitive host:* parasites reproduce
sexually
*Intermediate host*: all other hosts
*Reservoir host*: any host that can
maintain parasitic lifecycle in the
absence of humans

- Asexual reproduction may occur in
any host

## Pathogenicity

- Dependent on site of infection,
numbers of organisms and
physiological state of host

*Trauma/invasion*: direct mucosal
damage, e.g. amoebic dysentery

*Toxins*: neurotoxin produced in
Chagas' disease

*Immunological*: may stimulate cellular
and humoral responses or cause
autoimmunity
This occurs in Chagas' disease and
schistosomiasis

# Specific protozoal infections

See classification table (Table 4.11).

## Amoebiasis

- *Entamoeba histolytica* has two forms: a
motile trophozoite and an encysted
trophozoite (infective form)
- Faecal–oral spread
- Several clinical presentations:
  1. *Non-invasive*: confined to lumen of
  colon
  Asymptomatic
  2. *Invasive*: causes colonic ulceration
  and amoebic dysentery
  Amoeboma may develop as a late
  complication
  Amoeboma consists of a mass of
  granulation tissue
  Usually found at caecum
  3. *Disseminated*: metastatic
  haematogenous spread leads to

## Table 4.11: Classification of protozoa

| **Gut protozoa** | **Genital tract protozoa** |
|---|---|
| *Giardia lamblia* | *Trichomonas vaginalis* |
| *Cryptosporidium* | |
| *Entamoeba histolytica* | **Free-living protozoa** |
| *Blastocystis hominis* | *Naegleria fowleri* |
| *Balantidium coli* | *Acanthamoeba* |
| *Isospora belli* | |
| *Sarcocystis* | **Non-pathogenic gut protozoa** |
| | *Entamoeba coli* |
| **Tissue/blood protozoa** | *Entamoeba hartmanni* |
| *Toxoplasma gondii* | *Endolimax nana* |
| *Pneumocystis carinii* | *Iodamoeba bütschilii* |
| *Plasmodium* | *Chilomastix mesneli* |
| *Trypanosoma* | |
| *Leishmania* | |
| *Babesia* | |

hepatic abscess formation
Usually a solitary abscess in right
lobe of liver, but may occur
elsewhere

## Diagnosis

- *Amoebic dysentery*: identification of motile
  trophozoites in stools or rectal biopsy
  Serology positive in 60%
- *Amoeboma*: identification of cysts in
  stools
  Serology positive in 90%
- *Disseminated*: identification of
  intrahepatic lesion
  Serology positive in > 95%

## Trypanosomiasis

### African (sleeping sickness)

- *Trypanosoma gambiense* and *trypanosoma
  rhodesiense*
- Transmitted by the tsetse fly
- Inflammation around bite and
  regional lymphadenopathy
- Other features: hepatosplenomegaly,
  jaundice, purpura, pneumonia,
  myocarditis, pericarditis,
  parkinsonism, epilepsy, personality
  changes

### American (Chagas' disease)

- *Trypanosoma cruzi*
- Transmitted by the tsetse fly
- Acute infection produces regional
  lymphadenopathy and a lump at the
  bite site (chagoma)

- Periorbital oedema indicates
  conjunctival route of entry
- Other features of acute infection:
  hepatosplenomegaly, myocarditis,
  cardiomyopathy, meningoencephalitis
- Chronic infection leads to:
  cardiomyopathy, megaoesophagus
  (mimics achalasia), megacolon

## Leishmaniasis (Table 4.12)

- Obligate intracellular parasites
- Transmitted by bites from sandflies

  *Cutaneous*: granulomatous skin
  infections producing chronic
  painless ulceration

  *Visceral*: produces hepatosplenomegaly,
  weight loss, lymphadenopathy,
  hypersplenism, hypoalbuminaemia,
  raised globulin, polyclonal IgG

## Malaria

- Transmitted by anopheline mosquito
- Four types: *Plasmodium falciparum, P.
  malariae, P. vivax, P. ovale*

### Lifecycle (Fig. 4.2)

- Each liver schizont produces 40 000
  merozoites
- Hypnozoites remain dormant in the
  liver and may initiate cycles in the
  future, leading to relapse
- No hypnozoites are produced by *P.
  falciparum* or *P. malariae*

**Table 4.12: Classification of leishmaniasis**

| Location | Cutaneous | Visceral (kala azar) |
|---|---|---|
| Old World | *L. tropica* | *L. donovani* |
| | *L. major* | *L. infantum* |
| | *L. aethiopica* | |
| | *L. infantum* | |
| New World | *L. mexicana* | *L. donovani* |
| | *L. brazilienis* | |
| | *L. peruviana* | |

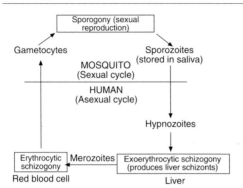

**Fig. 4.2: Lifecycle of the malaria parasite**

- Asexual reproduction produces fever
  *falciparum*: asexual cycles every 36–48 hours (subtertian malaria*)*
    *vivax and ovale*: asexual cycles every 48 hours (tertian malaria)
    *malariae*: asexual cycles every 72 hours (quartan malaria)

- *vivax, ovale and malariae*: invade 1–2% of red blood cells
- *falciparum*: severity of illness proportional to number of red blood cells invaded

- *Sickle cell trait:* protects against falciparum malaria

## Treatment of malaria
- *No hypnozoite stage*: treatment of erythrocytic phase sufficient
- *If hypnozoites*: need treatment for both asexual phases
- *vivax and ovale*: chloroquine + primaquine (for hepatic phase)
- *malariae*: chloroquine
- *falciparum*: quinine with or without sulphadoxine and pyrimethamine (single dose)
  High incidence of chloroquine resistance

## Prophylaxis of infection
- *Low-risk areas*: chloroquine or proguanil hydrochloride

**Box 4.8: Complications of falciparum malaria**

**CNS**
Impaired consciousness
Convulsions
Coma

**Renal**
Acute renal failure

**Liver**
Hepatomegaly
Hepatitis

**Haematological**
Intravascular haemolysis (Blackwater fever)

**Metabolic**
Hypoglycaemia

**Respiratory**
Pulmonary oedema

- *Medium-risk areas*: chloroquine + proguanil hydrochloride
- *High-risk areas*: mefloquine first choice; chloroquine and proguanil hydrochloride as alternatives
- Prophylaxis should be taken for at least 1 week (preferably 2–3 weeks) prior to travelling and should be continued for 4 weeks after returning

# Fungi

See classification table (Table 4.13).

## Structure

- Commonly multicellular
- Thick walls due to chitin

  *Moulds*: filamentous fungi which grow as tubular branching filaments (hyphae)

### Table 4.13: Classification of fungi

| Superficial | Deep |
|---|---|
| Pityriasis versicolor (Malassezia furfur) | Blastomycosis |
| *Candida* | Histoplasmosis |
| Dermatophytes (Trichophyton | Coccidiomycosis |
| Epidermophyton | Paracoccidiomycosis |
| Microsporum) | *Aspergillus* |
| | *Candida* |
| | Cryptococcus |
| | Mucormycosis |
| | Sporotrichosis |
| | Maduromycosis |

Hyphae be    e interwoven to form networks    elia)

*Yeasts*: spherical or oval cells that reproduce by budding

*Dimorphic fungi*: able to assume either yeast or mycelia depending on environment

## Growth

- Fungi are predominantly aerobic but some ferment carbohydrate to produce alcohol in anaerobic conditions
- Fungi grow readily on Sabouraud's agar
- Many moulds produce potent toxins (aflatoxin)

### Box 4.9: Precipitants of candida infection

Damaged skin
T-cell deficiency
Broad-spectrum antibiotics
Corticosteroids
Oral contraceptive use
Severe illness
Debilitation
Neutropenia
Pregnancy

## Reproduction

- Virtually all fungi are capable of producing asexual spores
- *Conidia*: produced in large numbers for dissemination
- *Arthrospores*: produced in small numbers for survival in extreme conditions

  *Superficial mycoses*: only invade the outer layer of skin and sometimes the dermis (mycetoma)

  *Deep mycoses*: can cause disseminated invasive infection
  Usually do so only in immuno-compromised patients

## Specific fungal infections

### Aspergillus fumigatus
#### Otomycosis
- Chronic otitis media

### Allergic bronchopulmonary aspergillosis
- Allergic response to inhaled *Aspergillus*
- Initially elicits a type I hypersensitivity reaction
- Later stimulates a type III (immune complex) reaction
- Produces acute dyspnoea, asthma and pulmonary eosinophilia

## Table 4.14: Classification of helminths

| Trematodes (flukes) | Cestodes (tapeworms) | Nematodes (roundworms) |
|---|---|---|
| **Intestinal** | **Intestinal** | **Intestinal** |
| *Fasciolopis* | *Taenia saginata* | *Ascaris lumbricoides* |
| *Metagonimus* | *Diphyllobothrium latum* | *Ancylostoma* |
| *Heterophyes* | (fish tapeworm) | *Trichuris* |
| | *Hymenolepis nana* | *Necator* |
| **Hepatic** | | *Strongyloides* |
| *Fasciola* | **Larval tissue infection** | *Enterobius vermicularis* (threadworm) |
| *Opisthorchis* | *Taenia solium* (cystercicosis) | *Trichenella* |
| | *Echinococcus granulosus* | |
| **Pulmonary** | (hydatid disease) | **Adult larval infection** |
| *Paragonimus* | | *Wucheria bancrofti* (filiariasis) |
| | | *Brugia* |
| **Haematological** | | *Loa loa* |
| Schistosomes | | *Onchocerca* |
| | | *Dracunculus* |
| | | **Larval tissue infection** |
| | | *Toxocara canis* |

- Diagnosis: skin testing
- Treatment: corticosteroids

### *Aspergilloma*
- Produces a mass of *Aspergillus* that forms in lung cavities
- No lung invasion
- Typical lesions have crescent of air around the lesion
- Diagnosis: serology to detect antibody response
- Treatment: excision

### *Invasive aspergillus*
- Occurs in immunocompromised patients
- Disseminated invasive disease
- Diagnosis: tissue sampling
- Treatment: amphotericin B

# Helminths

See classification table (Table 4.14).

# Flukes

- Bilaterally symmetrical
- Flattened dorsoventrally
- Three body layers
- No true body cavities
- Possess a simple digestive system
- All transmitted by freshwater snails
- Hermaphrodites (usually)

# Roundworms

- Bilaterally symmetrical
- More tubular structure
- Possess a primitive digestive system
- Separate sexes
- Intestinal parasites produce eggs which are excreted in the host faeces to undergo maturation outside the host

## Tapeworms

- Bilaterally symmetrical

- Flattened dorsoventrally
- Three body layers
- No true body cavities
- Hermaphrodites
- No digestive system
- Gain nutrients by absorption through the skin
- Adult has a head (scolex) with 2–3 suckers and hooks
- The body (strobilia) is long and thin and consists of many proglottis units
- The tail end proglottides are sexually mature and are eventually dropped off and excreted in the host faeces

# Reproduction of helminths

- Asexual reproduction by internal budding
- Sexual reproduction by self-fertilisation in hermaphrodites (usually occurs in human host)

# Pathogenicity of helminths

- *Mechanical*: mechanical blockage of intestinal tract (*ascaris*) or lymphatics (*filiarias*)
- *Traumatic/Invasive*: skin penetration may occur in *Strongyloides* or hookworm infections
- *Physiological*: gut helminths may utilise host nutrients (B12 deficiency, fish tapeworm; anaemia, hookworm)
- *Immunological*: allergic reaction may be stimulated by hydatid cyst fluid Schistosomiasis stimulates delayed hypersensitivity reactions

# Specific helminth infections

## *Schistosomiasis*
- Most important of the fluke parasites
- Three species: *Schistosoma mansoni, S. japonicum, S. haematobium*
- Adult parasites live in abdominal veins
- Separate sexes
- Eggs laid in capillaries draining intestine (*mansoni, japonicum*) or bladder (*haematobium*)
- Most eggs excreted in faeces or urine
- Some eggs enter blood and pass to liver (*mansoni, japonicum*) or lungs (*haematobium*)
- This leads to granuloma formation around eggs and clinical symptoms
- Some eggs stay in the intestine to produce symptoms
- Severity of clinical presentation proportional to number of eggs
- Excreted eggs hatch in fresh water and the resultant larvae infect freshwater snails
- In snails there is an asexual phase of reproduction producing cercariae
- Cercariae are capable of penetrating unbroken human skin

## *Clinical features*
- Migration and maturation of organisms usually asymptomatic except in the non-immune, who may develop Katayama fever

  *S. mansoni*: mainly causes colonic disease (haemorrhage, polyps, intestinal obstruction, protein-losing enteropathy, granulomatous infiltration)
  May also cause liver disease (hepatosplenomegaly, fibrosis, portal hypertension)
  CNS (posterior fossa lesions) and spinal cord (transverse myelitis, spinal artery occlusion,

compression, cauda equina lesions)

*S. japonicum*: mainly causes small and large bowel disease
Often produces intestinal strictures
Implicated in the pathogenesis of colonic carcinoma
Clinically similar to *S. mansoni*
CNS involvement more common

*S. haematobium*: mainly causes bladder and lung disease
Implicated in the pathogenesis of squamous cell bladder carcinoma
May also cause pulmonary hypertension, cor pulmonale
May also cause perianal and scrotal skin infection
Chronic infection may cause tramline calcification of bladder and ureters
*Diagnosis*: cysts in stools or urine
Serology
Eosinophilia (blood, CSF)

### Hydatid disease
- Tapeworm of dogs
- Ingested eggs release onchospheres, which penetrate the gut mucosa to disseminate via the blood or lymphatics to other organs
- In the organs they produce cystic lesions
- Commonest sites of infection are liver and lungs
- Cysts may occur in any organ
- Commonly cyst wall calcifies

### Hookworm
- Gastrointestinal infection with either *Ancylostoma* or *Necator*
- Eggs in the soil mature to produce larvae
- Larvae enter through the host's skin and pass to the lungs, where they grow
- After maturation organisms enter the upper small intestine. Here they hook onto the gut lining and cause slow blood loss, leading to iron deficiency
- Further eggs are produced and excreted in the faeces
- *Ancylostoma* can also be ingested directly with food

### Ascaris lumbricoides
- *Ascaris* organisms live in the upper small intestine
- Eggs are excreted in the faeces
- Transmission is faecal–oral
- Eggs are able to resist high temperature (up to 60%)
- Larvae develop inside the eggs
- Larvae penetrate gut lining, enter blood and travel to the lungs
- They grow in the lungs and eventually migrate up the respiratory tree, to be swallowed and re-enter the intestine
- May be associated with few symptoms
- Main symptom is bowel obstruction, but may also cause biliary or pancreatic obstruction

### Filiariasis
- Transmitted by *Culex*, *Aedes* or *Anopheles* mosquitos
- Larvae pass through the host skin and enter lymphatics
- Here they mature into adults
- Clinical features produced by lymphatic obstruction leading to lymphoedema
- Adult worms are long-lived, leading to chronic disease that may last many years
- Severity of symptoms proportional to number of organisms present

# Infection control

- Three main principles:
  1. Eliminate source of responsible organism (eradication of infected animal)

**Table 4.15: Properties of common disinfectants**

| Class of compound | Examples | Activity against bacteria | Activity against viruses and rickettsiae | Activity against fungi | Human toxicity |
|---|---|---|---|---|---|
| **Environmental disinfectants** | | | | | |
| Clear phenolics | Hycolin, Stericol | All | Some | Good | Moderate |
| Chloroxylenols | Dettol | Some | Nil | Nil | Moderate |
| Hypochlorites | Domestos, Milton | All | Good | Good | Moderate |
| Dichloroisocynurates | Kirbychlor, Presept | All | Good | Good | Moderate |
| Quaternary ammonium compounds | Cetrimide | Most | Some | Good | Slight |
| **Skin disinfectants** | | | | | |
| Diguanides | Chlorhexidine, Savlon | Most | Slight | Good | Slight |
| Alcohol | Isopropyl alcohol, ethanol | All | Good | Good | Moderate |
| Iodine and iodophors | Betadine | All | Good | Good | Slight/Moderate |
| Hexachlorophane | Sterzac | Most | Nil | Nil | Slight |
| Triclosan | Manusept, Phisomed | Most | Nil | Nil | Nil |
| **Instrument disinfectants** | | | | | |
| Aldehydes | Glutaraldehyde, formaldehyde | All | Good | Good | Moderate/ Marked |

2. Prevent transmission of organism (control of migration or quarantine, attention to hygiene)
3. Raise host resistance to organism (attention to general health, prophylactic treatment, immunisation)

## Sterilisation/disinfection

*Sterilisation*: killing or removal of all microorganisms including spores
*Disinfection*: use of chemicals to eliminate microorganisms but not spores (Table 4.15)

### Methods of sterilisation
- *Dry heat*: burning, oven
- *Moist heat*: autoclave, steamer
- *Radiation*: ultraviolet light, X-rays, γ-rays
- *Filtration*: air filters

### Methods of disinfection
- *Bactericidal*: kill bacteria
- *Bacteriostatic*: prevent multiplication

## Immunisation

See Table 4.16.

## Active

- Administration of antigen which stimulates recipient's own immunological mechanisms
- Initially initiates a slow primary antibody response (IgM)
- Re-exposure at a later date leads to a rapid secondary antibody response (IgG)
- For long-lasting immunity, periodic boosters may be required
- Aims to provide an immunisation regimen that mimics natural infection

---

**Box 4.10: Contraindications to live vaccine use**

Immunodeficiency
Immunosuppression
High-dose corticosteroids
Pregnancy
Malignancy

---

- Vaccines may be given by different routes to stimulate natural infection
- If infectious agent has many strains a single-strain vaccine may not prevent the illness
- Adjuvants (alum) may be added to vaccine to delay absorption and prolong duration of effectiveness
- Active vaccines provide prophylaxis and are of no therapeutic use if no previous exposure to antigen, in view of the slow primary antibody response

## Passive

- Administration of preformed antibody
- If formed in animals they are potential allergens and may stimulate type I or type III hypersensitivity reactions
- Vaccines are immediately effective
- Duration of effectiveness is short
- Only of use for short-term prophylaxis or treatment of existing infection

## Types of vaccine

### Active
- Live attenuated *(live organisms, limited virulence)*
  Tuberculosis
  Polio virus (Sabin)
  Measles
  Mumps
  Rubella
  Influenza

Yellow fever
- Dead *(suspension of dead organisms)*
  Whooping cough
  Typhoid
  Paratyphoid
  Polio virus (Salk)
  Hepatitis A
  Hepatitis B
  Meningococcus
  Pneumococcus
  Haemophilus b (Hib)
  Anthrax
  Cholera
  Influenza
  Rabies
- Toxoid *(purified microbial toxins)*
  Diphtheria
  Tetanus
  Botulism

## Passive
Rabies
Hepatitis A
Hepatitis B
Diphtheria
Tetanus
Measles
Rubella
CMV
Chickenpox

**Box 4.11: Notifiable diseases**

Anthrax
Cholera
Diphtheria
Dysentery (amoebic or bacillary)
Acute encephalitis
Food poisoning
Viral haemorrhagic fever
Viral hepatitis
Leprosy
Leptospirosis
Malaria
Measles
Meningitis
Meningococcal septicaemia (without meningitis)
Mumps
Ophthalmia neonatorum
Paratyphoid fever
Plague
Acute poliomyelitis
Rabies
Relapsing fever
Rubella
Scarlet fever
Smallpox
Tetanus
Tuberculosis
Typhoid
Typhus
Whooping cough
Yellow fever

**Table 4.16: Differences between active and passive immunisation**

| Feature | Active | Passive |
|---|---|---|
| *Immunising agent* | Live or dead organisms, toxoids | Sera from immunised animals/humans |
| *Rapidity of protection* | 3-week delay if no previous exposure | Immediate |
| *Duration of protection* | Several years | Few months |
| *Uses* | Long-term prophylaxis Treatment only if previous exposure | Short-term prophylaxis Treatment |

## Table 4.17: UK vaccination schedule

| Age | Vaccines |
| --- | --- |
| 2 months | Diphtheria |
| | Tetanus |
| | Whooping cough |
| | Polio |
| | Haemophilus b |
| 3 months | Diphtheria |
| | Tetanus |
| | Whooping cough |
| | Polio |
| | Haemophilus b |
| 4 months | Diphtheria |
| | Tetanus |
| | Whooping cough |
| | Polio |
| | Haemophilus b |
| 1 year | Measles |
| | Mumps |
| | Rubella |
| Preschool | Diphtheria |
| | Tetanus |
| | Polio |
| | Measles |
| | Mumps |
| | Rubella |
| 10–14 years | Tuberculosis (if tuberculin negative) |
| School leaving | Diphtheria |
| | Tetanus |
| | Polio |
| Adults | Diphtheria: 10 years after primary course |
| | Tetanus: 10 years after primary course and 10 years later |
| | Polio: every 10 years for at risk groups (health care workers, travelers to endemic regions, lab staff working with virus) |

### Box 4.12: Modes of action of antibiotics

**Inhibition of bacterial cell wall synthesis**
Penicillins
Cephalosporins

**Inhibition of bacterial cell protein synthesis**
Aminoglycosides
Chloramphenicol
Tetracyclines
Erythromycin

**Inhibition of bacterial cell DNA synthesis and replication**
Rifampicin
Quinolones
Metronidazole

**Inhibition of microbial enzymes**
Sulphonamides
Trimethoprim
Rifampicin

# Antimicrobial treatments

## Antibiotics

- *Minimal inhibitory concentration*: smallest drug concentration that inhibits organism growth
- *Minimal bactericidal concentration*: smallest drug concentration that kills the organism
- *Antibiotic resistance*: arises as a result of several mechanisms:

  1. Relative impermeability of cell wall (Gram-negative organisms resistant to Penicillin as they are unable to penetrate envelope
  2. Low affinity between antibiotic and bacterial receptors

3. Ability of bacteria to use alternative metabolic pathways unaffected by antibiotics
4. Ability of bacteria to produce enzymes that inactivate or destroy antibiotic (β-lactamases)
5. Chromosomally determined resistance via conjugation of DNA via plasmids

# Antiviral agents

- *Acyclovir:* activated by contact with virally infected cells
Harmless to uninfected host cells
Active against DNA viruses only
Inhibits DNA polymerase
Only effective against replicating virus and does not eliminate dormant virus
Useful against herpes simplex and varicella zoster viruses
- *Ganciclovir:* similar mode of action to aciclovir
Potentially harmful to uninfected host cells
Toxicity greater than aciclovir, leading to bone marrow suppression
Used for treatment of CMV infections in immunocompromised patients

- *Antiretroviral drugs:* zidovudine (AZT)
Nucleoside analogues which inhibit reverse transcriptase of HIV
- *Ribavarin:* nucleoside analogue
Active against a wide spectrum of DNA and RNA viruses
Used for severe RSV infection and some viral haemorrhagic fevers
- *Amantadine:* activity only against influenza A virus
May shorten duration of symptoms
- *Idoxuridine:* thymidine analogue
Interferes with DNA synthesis
Used topically for herpes infections
Too toxic for parenteral use
- *α-Interferon:* produced by T lymphocytes
Inhibits replication of hepatitis B and C viruses
Inhibits viral assembly
Many side effects, including flu-like symptoms, bone marrow suppression

# Antifungal agents

- *Amphotericin B:* polyene antifungal produced by streptomyces
Fungistatic by interfering with cell wall
Not absorbed from the GI tract

**Table 4.18: Antibiotic classification**

| Bactericidal (kill organism) | Bacteriostatic (prevent multiplication, allow host defences to kill organism) |
|---|---|
| Nitrofurantoin | Sulphonamides |
| Penicillin | Trimethoprim |
| Cephalosporins | Metronidazole |
| Aminoglycosides | Quinolones |
| Chloramphenicol | Tetracyclines |
| Erythromycin | Ethambutol |
| Rifampicin | |
| Fusidic acid | |
| Isoniazid | |
| Pyrazinamide | |

Acts in synergy with flucytosine
Active against all fungi except *Candida*

- *Nystatin:* polyene antifungal
  Acts in a similar way to amphotericin B
  Not absorbed from the GI tract
  Main use for superficial *Candida* infections
- *Flucytosine:* synthetic pyrimidine analogue
  Active form is 5-fluorouracil
  Incorporates into RNA and inhibits protein synthesis
  Active against yeasts
  Resistance may develop if treatment protracted
- *Griseofulvin:* produced by *Penicillium* species
  Inhibits microtubule formation
  Absorbed from the GI tract and deposited in keratin of skin
  Active against superficial dermatophytes
- *Imidazoles:* synthetic compounds
  Inhibit ergosterol synthesis and disrupt fungal cell walls
  Effective for superficial infections only
  Ketoconazole, miconazole, clotrimazole
- *Triazoles:* active against systemic infections
  Also pass blood–brain barrier and effective against cryptococcal meningitis
  Fluconazole

## Antiprotozoal agents

- *Metronidazole:* effective against amoeba, *Giardia*
- *Tinidazole:* alternative to metronidazole
- *Dilanoxide furoate:* used in conjunction with tinidazole or metronidazole
- *Amphotericin B:* effective against *Naegleria fowleri*, acanthamoeba, kala azar
- *Pyrimethamine:* used in conjunction with sulphadiazine and folinic acid for *Toxoplasma*

- *Pentamidine:* activity against *Pneumocystis, Trypanosoma gambiense,* kala azar
- *Suramin:* used with melarsoprol for treatment of *Trypanosoma gambiense*
- *Nifurtimox/Benzonidazole:* used for the treatment of *Trypanosoma cruzi*
- *Sodium stibogluconate/pentavalent antimony:* used in cutaneous and visceral Leishmaniasis
- *Septrin:* first-line treatment for *Pneumocystis* infection

## Antihelminth agents

- *Intestinal nematodes:* mebendazole, albendazole, thiabendazole
- *Tissue nematodes:* ivermectin, diethylcarbamazine, suramin
- *Larval nematodes:* diethylcarbamazine
- *Trematodes:* praziquantel, oxamniquine, metrifonate
- *Intestinal cestodes:* praziquantel, niclosamide
- *Larval cestodes:* praziquantel, albendazole, mebendazole

# Congenital infections

## Toxoplasmosis

- Early maternal infection may lead to stillbirth, microcephaly, choroidoretinitis, hydrocephalus, intracerebral calcification, hepato-splenomegaly, thrombocytopenia
- Infection in the third trimester causes no harm

## Rubella

- Particularly serious if contracted in the first trimester: stillbirth, low

percentage of measurements occur
- *Quartiles*: the 25th and 75th centiles
- *Interquartile range:* the difference between the 25th and 75th centiles
- *Standard deviation (SD)*: a measure of the scatter of values around the mean
SD = √V
- *Variance (V)*: the average squared deviation of a set of values from the mean V = SD$^2$
- *Standard error of the mean (SEM):* gives an estimate of the standard deviation that would be  obtained from the means of a large number of samples drawn from the population. Provides some measure of how well the results from the study subjects reflect the true situation in the entire population
Equal to the standard deviation divided by the square root of the number of observations
- *Confidence interval*: range of values which we can be confident includes the true value

# Normal (Gaussian) distribution

This is a frequency distribution which is unimodal and symmetrical (Fig. 5.1).

- In a normal distribution the mean, median and mode are equal.

    One  standard deviation from the mean includes 68% of the observations.
    Two  standard deviations from the mean include 95% of the observations.
    Three standard deviations from the mean include 99.7% of the observations.

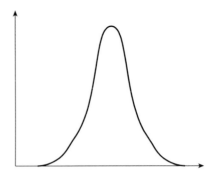

**Fig. 5.1:  The normal distribution curve**

- In a positively skewed distribution the mean > median > mode
- In a negatively skewed distribution the mean < median < mode
- The normality of data can be assessed by using a scatter plot or the Shapiro–Wilk test

## *Scatter plot*
- In a scatter plot the individual results are represented graphically (Fig. 5.2)

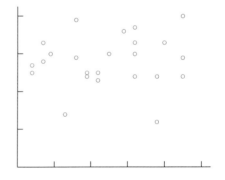

**Fig. 5.2:  A scatter plot**

# Design of research studies

- *Prospective*: data are collected forwards in time from the start of the study

Patient consent and participation required
- *Retrospective*: data are collected backwards in time from the start of the study
Data collected from existing records without patient participation
- *Longitudinal*: observations are made and repeated over time
- *Cross-sectional*: single observations are made at one point in time
- *Observational*: measurements are collected without influencing course of events (no intervention). Case control and cohort studies are examples
- *Case control study*: takes a group with a certain characteristic and looks backwards for causal factors
- *Cohort study*: takes a group with a certain characteristic and follows them forward in time and observes outcomes
- *Experimental*: measurements are collected following intervention
- *Randomised trial*: subjects are randomly divided into groups receiving different interventions
- *Controlled trial*: a trial that uses a comparison group that does not receive the intervention
- *Bias*: factors that influence and distort the results
- *Confounding variable*: a variable that leads to bias
- *Blinding*: patient and/or observer are unaware of the type of intervention

# Hypothesis testing

- *Null hypothesis*: there is no difference between two observed populations and any difference that is observed is due to chance
- *Chi-squared ($\chi^2$) test*: tests the null hypothesis and measures the difference between the observed and expected frequencies
- *p value*: the probability that the null hypothesis is true
- *Significance:* the degree by which the results disagree with the null hypothesis. In other words, a measure of how confident we can be that a result obtained is a true one and not obtained by chance. Given by the p value. A significant result is one with a p value < 0.05.
- *Type 1 error*: an error which causes rejection of the null hypothesis when it is true
Suggests a treatment is effective when it is not (false positive result)
- *Type 2 error*: an error which causes acceptance of the null hypothesis when it is false
Suggests a treatment is not effective when it is (false negative result)

# Types of statistical test (Box 5.1)

- *Parametric tests*: tests used to analyse data that are normally distributed

---

**Box 5.1: Parametric and Non-parametric tests**

**Parametric tests**
*t*-test
Analysis of variance (ANOVA)
Two-way analysis of variance

**Non-parametric tests**
Mann–Whitney U test
Wilcoxon rank sum test
Kruskal–Wallis test
Friedman's two-way analysis of variance
Chi-squared test
Fisher's exact test

- *Non-parametric tests*: tests used to analyse data that are not normally distributed

# Correlation and regression

Correlation and regression are methods for assessing the relationship between two continuous variables.

- *Correlation*: indicates the type and degree of relationship
- *Correlation coefficient*: a numerical measure of the relationship
  Values range from −1 to +1, depending on the relationship (Fig. 5.3)
- *Regression*: provides a more detailed description of the relationship
  Allows prediction of the amount of change of one variable as a result of change in another variable
- *Regression equation*: y = a + bx (for a straight line) (Fig. 5.4)

  y = dependent variable (one that is affected)
  x = independent variable (one that causes change in dependent variable)
  a = the y axis intercept value
  b = the slope of the line

# Screening (Fig. 5.5)

- *Sensitivity:* the proportion of positives that are correctly identified by the test ($a/[a+c]$)
- *Specificity*: the proportion of negatives that are correctly identified by the test ($d/[b+d]$)
- *Positive predictive value*: the proportion

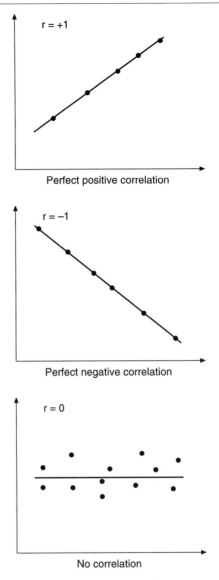

**Fig. 5.3: Correlation coefficient**
Scatter plots showing the relationship between two continuous variables and the correlation between the two variables, indicated by the gradient of a best-fit straight line through the plot where the gradient is equal to the correlation coefficient ($r$).

of patients with positive tests that are correctly diagnosed ($a/[a+b]$)

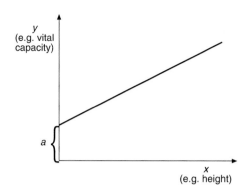

Fig. 5.4: Graphical representation of a regression equation

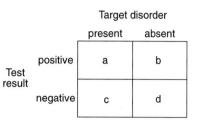
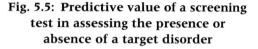

Fig. 5.5: Predictive value of a screening test in assessing the presence or absence of a target disorder

- *Negative predictive value*: the proportion of patients with negative tests that are correctly diagnosed $(d/[c+d])$
- As sensitivity increases (low false negative rate) specificity decreases (high false positive rate). In other words, a test with high sensitivity and low specificity will not miss any true positives but will incorrectly identify some as positive, e.g. polymerase chain reaction
- As sensitivity decreases (high false negative rate) specificity increases (low false positive rate). In other words, a test with low sensitivity and high specificity will miss some true positives but will not incorrectly identify some as positive, e.g. venograms

---

**Box 5.2: Features of an ideal screening test**

Simple
Cheap
Quick
Non-invasive
Reproducible
Applicable to all
High sensitivity
High specificity
High positive predictive value
High negative predictive value

---

# Population statistics

- *Population*: a group of subjects being studied
- *Sample*: a selected portion of that population
- *Incidence*: number of new cases occurring in a certain time period
- *Prevalence*: number of cases existing at a certain point in time
- *Rates*: the proportion of new cases occurring in a certain period
- *Absolute risk*: rate of occurrence, i.e. incidence
- *Relative risk*: the proportion of incidences in those exposed compared to those not exposed
- *Attributable risk*: the difference in incidences between those exposed and those not exposed
- *Relative risk reduction (RRR)*: the proportional reduction in rates between experimental (experimental event rate [EER]) and control (control event rate [CER]) groups. Calculated as (EER−CER/CER)
- *Absolute risk reduction (ARR)*: the absolute difference between experimental and control groups (EER−CER)
- *Number needed to treat (NNT)*: the number of patients who need to be treated to achieve one favourable outcome. Calculated as 1/ARR

# 6 Metabolic medicine

## Contents

## Metabolic bone disease

### Calcium homoeostasis

#### Functions of calcium
- Structural
- Control of neuromuscular excitability
- Release of synaptic neurotransmitters
- Control of muscular contraction
- Coenzyme for coagulation factors
- Intracellular second messenger

#### Causes of hypocalcaemia
- Osteomalacia
- Chronic renal failure
- Hypoparathyroidism
- Dietary deficiency (low calcium intake, high phytic acid intake: chapatis, wholemeal bread)
- Pseudohypoparathyroidism
- Hypomagnesaemia
- Acute pancreatitis
- Transient neonatal hypocalcaemia
- Massive transfusion with citrated blood
- Chronic liver disease
- Hypoproteinaemia
- Respiratory alkalosis

**Table 6.1: Normal distribution of calcium**

| Site | Amount (mmol) |
|------|---------------|
| Bone | 25 000 |
| Extracellular fluid | 25 |
| Serum | 2.25–2.60 |
| Intracellular fluid | 25 |

#### Causes of hypercalcaemia
- Primary hyperparathyroidism
- Malignancy (with or without bone metastases)
- Volume depletion
- Sarcoidosis
- Milk–alkali syndrome
- Hypervitaminosis D
- Multiple myeloma
- Thyrotoxicosis
- Adrenocortical insufficiency
- Phaeochromocytoma
- Thiazide diuretics, lithium
- Immobility
- Pagets disease
- Tertiary hyperparathyroidism: renal transplant
- Acromegaly

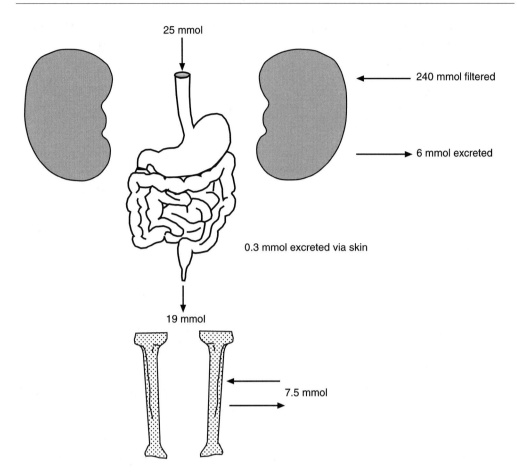

**Fig. 6.1: Normal daily calcium exchange**

**Table 6.2: Distribution of serum calcium**

| Site | % |
|------|---|
| *Ultrafiltrable* | 53 |
| Ionised | 47 |
| Complexed (phosphate, bicarbonate, citrate) | 6 |
| *Protein bound* | 47 |
| Albumin | 37 |
| Globulin | 10 |

# Phosphate homoeostasis

- Phosphate is a major intracellular anion
- It is present in virtually all foods
- Its main function is structural (88% of total body phosphate found in bone)
- In bone it combines with calcium to form hydroxyapatite
- It also acts as a major acidic buffer
- The metabolism of phosphate generally follows the inverse of calcium metabolism

## Causes of hyperphosphataemia
- Acute renal failure
- Chronic renal failure
- Excessive intake (undiluted cow's milk, parenteral nutrition)
- Hypoparathyroidism
- Pseudohypoparathyroidism
- Acromegaly
- Vitamin D intoxication
- Catabolic states
- Haemolytic anaemia
- Metabolic acidosis

## Causes of hypophosphataemia
- Hyperparathyroidism
- Vitamin D deficiency
- Inadequate intake (parenteral nutrition)
- During recovery from diabetic ketoacidosis
- Alcohol withdrawal
- Vitamin D-resistant (hypo-phosphataemic) rickets
- Magnesium salts
- Aluminium salts
- Malnutrition
- Malabsorption
- Renal tubular acidosis
- Malignancy

# Magnesium homoeostasis

Magnesium acts as a cofactor for many enzyme reactions and is involved in the control of muscular contractions.
- Average daily intake = 10 mmol
- Average daily requirements = 8 mmol

## Causes of hypermagnesaemia
- Acute renal failure
- Chronic renal failure
- Excessive intake (iatrogenic, parenteral nutrition)

## Causes of hypomagnesaemia
- Malnutrition

**Table 6.3: Normal distribution of magnesium**

| Site | Amount (mmol) |
| --- | --- |
| Bone | 500 |
| Intracellular fluid | 490 |
| Extracellular fluid | 10 |

- Malabsorption
- Severe diarrhoea
- Inadequate intake (parenteral nutrition)
- Alcohol abuse
- Renal tubular acidosis
- Chronic diuretic therapy
- Diabetic ketoacidosis
- Cisplatin
- Hepatic cirrhosis
- Renal dialysis
- Acute pancreatitis
- Parathyroidectomy

# Hormonal control of bone minerals

## Parathyroid hormone (PTH)
- 84 amino acid polypeptide hormone
- Produced and stored in parathyroid glands

## Vitamin D (calcitriol or 1,25-dihydroxycholecalciferol)
- Potent steroid hormone
- Produced almost solely by the kidney (Fig. 6.2)

## Calcitonin
- 32 amino acid polypeptide hormone
- Produced by C (parafollicular) cells of thyroid gland
- Actions of little clinical significance
- No syndromes associated with excess or deficiency

**Table 6.4:  Actions of major hormones controlling bone metabolism**

| Effect | Parathyroid hormone | Vitamin D | Calcitonin |
|---|---|---|---|
| Calcium resorption from bone | Increased | Increased | Decreased |
| Calcium absorption from gut | Increased | Increased | – |
| Phosphate absorption from gut | Increased | Increased | – |
| Urinary calcium | Increased * | Decreased | – |
| Urinary phosphate | Increased | – | Increased |
| Other effects | Increased $1_\alpha$ hydroxylation<br>Bicarbonaturia<br>Metabolic acidosis | – | – |

*Although calcium reabsorption by the kidney is increased, bone resorption is the more prominent effect. The increased calcium load leads to a net increase in urine calcium.

**Table 6.5:  Biochemical findings in metabolic bone disease**

| Disease | Serum calcium | Serum phosphate | Alkaline phosphatase | Urinary hydroxyproline |
|---|---|---|---|---|
| Osteomalacia | Reduced | Reduced | Increased | Normal |
| Osteoporosis | Normal | Normal | Normal | Normal |
| Paget's disease | Normal | Normal | Increased | Increased |
| Primary hyperparathyroidism | Increased | Reduced | Normal | Normal |
| Secondary hyperparathyroidism | Reduced | Increased | Normal | Normal |
| Tertiary hyperparathyroidism | Increased | Reduced | Normal | Normal |

# Hyperparathyroidism and hypoparathyroidism

## Causes of hyperparathyroidism
### Primary
- Parathyroid adenoma
- Parathyroid hyperplasia
- Parathyroid carcinoma

### Secondary (appropriate physiological increase in PTH)
- Hypocalcaemia

### Tertiary (inappropriate autonomous increase in PTH)
- Chronic hypocalcaemia
- Post renal transplant

## Causes of hypoparathyroidism
### Congenital
- Di George's syndrome

### Acquired
- Surgical removal
- Idiopathic
- Autoimmune
- Haemochromatosis
- Parathyroid infiltration

# Osteomalacia

## Causes of osteomalacia
### Vitamin D deficiency
- Inadequate dietary intake
- Inadequate exposure to UV light
- Malabsorption
- Chronic liver disease
- Liver enzyme-inducing drugs
- Chronic renal failure
- Hereditary vitamin D-dependent rickets

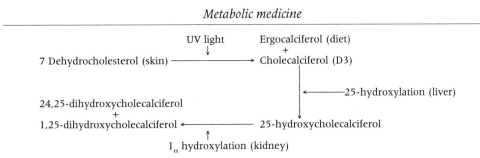

**Fig. 6.2: Production of vitamin D**

*Hypophosphataemia*

*Chronic metabolic acidosis*

*Osteoblast defects,*
- Hypophosphatasia
- Biphosphonate therapy
- Aluminium intoxication

*Malignancy*
- Sarcoma
- Neurofibromatosis
- Haemangioendothelioma

## Osteoporosis

### Causes of osteoporosis
<u>Advanced age</u>

*Endocrine*
- Premature ovarian failure
- Cushing's syndrome
- Diabetes mellitus
- Hypogonadism
- Hypopituitarism
- Hyperthyroidism
- Primary hyperparathyroidism
- Adult growth hormone deficiency

*Drugs*
- Alcohol abuse
- Prolonged heparin therapy
- Corticosteroids (>7.5 mg for > 3 months)

*Miscellaneous*
- Malabsorption

- Immobility
- Chronic inflammatory arthropathy
- Weightlessness
- Chronic liver disease

# Disorders of lipid metabolism
## Cholesterol and triglycerides

- Exogenously derived from diet (especially meat, eggs, dairy products)
- Endogenously derived from hepatic synthesis
- Cholesterol synthesised from acetyl CoA, for which the rate-limiting enzyme is hydroxymethylglutaryl coenzyme A reductase (HMG CoA reductase)

**Box 6.1: Other hormones involved in bone metabolism**

Glucocorticoids
Growth hormone
Somatomedins
Thyroid hormones
Androgens
Oestrogens
Insulin
Prostaglandin $E_2$
Cytokines

- Not water soluble, therefore transported in plasma by lipoproteins

# Free fatty acids (FFA)

*Saturated*: palmitic acid, stearic acid
*Unsaturated*: oleic acid, linoleic acid, arachidonic acid
*Esterified*: glycerides (glycerol)
*Essential*: polyunsaturated, cannot be synthesised (linoleic acid, linolenic acid)

# Phospho/sphingolipids

- Triglycerides with one fatty acid residue replaced by a nitrogenous base
- Synthesised in the gastrointestinal tract and liver
   *Phospholipids*: phosphatidylcholine, phosphatidylethanolamine, phosphatidylinositol
   *Sphingolipids*: ceramides, cerebrosides, gangliosides, sphingomyelin

# Normal lipid metabolism

## Exogenous pathway

- Follows ingestion of dietary fat
- In the duodenum dietary fat stimulates the production of pancreozymin–cholecystokinin
- This stimulates the production of bile salts
- Pancreatic lipases hydrolyse triglycerides into free fatty acids
- Bile salts emulsify the free fatty acids into micelles
- Small free fatty acids are absorbed directly into the portal circulation, bound to albumin
- Larger free fatty acids are absorbed into mucosal cells and re-esterified into triglyceride

### Table 6.8: Functions of lipids

| Cholesterol | Triglycerides | Phospholipids | Sphingolipids |
|---|---|---|---|
| Cell membrane stability | Nutritional value | Cell membrane stability | Component of white matter of CNS |
| Steroid hormone synthesis | | | |
| Lipoprotein production | | | |
| Bile acid production | | | |

- Chylomicrons are synthesised in mucosal cells and take up triglyceride
- Chylomicrons enter the lymphatic system and transport triglyceride to the tissues
- In the tissues, triglyceride is metabolised into free fatty acids
- Chylomicron remnants are then taken up by the liver

## Endogenous pathway

- Follows hepatic production of triglyceride
- VLDL is synthesised in the liver and transports triglyceride to the tissues
- In the tissues, triglyceride is metabolised
- As triglyceride is lost from VLDL, IDL is formed
- IDL is either taken up by the liver or further depleted of triglyceride to form LDL

- LDL transports cholesterol to the tissues and is then taken up by the liver
- HDL is produced in the liver and opposes the actions of LDL
- (VLDL: very low density lipoprotein; IDL: intermediate density lipoprotein; HDL: high density lipoprotein)

## Lipoproteins

- Spherical particles
- Hydrophobic core of triglyceride and cholesterol
- Hydrophilic coat of phospholipid and apoproteins
- Apoproteins are synthesised in the liver
- Six classes of apoprotein (A–F)
- Lipoproteins are classified according to density (Table 6.7)

### Table 6.7: Lipoprotein classification

| Lipoprotein | Major apoprotein | Function |
| --- | --- | --- |
| Chylomicron | A1, B48, C, E | Transport of exogenous triglyceride to tissues |
| VLDL | B100, C, E | Transport of endogenous triglyceride to tissues |
| IDL | B100, C, E | Intermediary between VLDL and LDL |
| LDL | B100 | Transport of cholesterol from liver to tissues |
| HDL | A, C, E | Transport of cholesterol from tissues to liver |
| Lipoprotein a | B100, a | Prevents thrombolysis and promotes thrombosis |

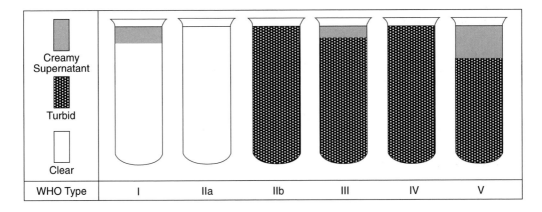

**Fig. 6.3: Appearance of fasting serum samples after standing overnight at 4°C in various hyperlipoproteinaemic states**

## Causes of raised HDL levels
- Increasing age
- Exercise
- Fish diet
- Moderate alcohol consumption

## Causes of reduced HDL levels
- Progesterone
- Androgens

- Smoking
- Obesity
- High dietary carbohydrate

## Causes of hypolipoproteinaemia
- Abetalipoproteinaemia
- Tangier disease

**Table 6.8: Classification of primary hyperlipidaemias**

| Abnormality | I | IIa | IIb | III | IV | V |
|---|---|---|---|---|---|---|
| Chylomicrons | ++ | – | – | + | – | ++ |
| VLDL | Normal | Normal | ++ | + | ++ | ++ |
| LDL | Normal | ++ | ++ | Reduced | Normal | Normal |
| Cholesterol | + | ++ | ++ | ++ | + | + |
| Triglyceride | +++ | Normal | ++ | ++ | ++ | ++ |
| Atherogenic risk | No | Yes | Yes | Yes | No | No |
| Inheritance | Autosomal recessive | Autosomal dominant | Autosomal dominant | – | Autosomal dominant | Autosomal recessive |
| Primary defect | Lipoprotein lipase deficiency apoCII deficiency | LDL receptor defect | LDL receptor defect | apoE abnormality | Over-production of VLDL | Lipoprotein deficiency apoCII deficiency |

**Table 6.9: Causes of secondary hyperlipidaemia**

| Disease/Condition | Raised cholesterol | Raised triglyceride |
|---|---|---|
| Hypothyroidism | ✓ | |
| Alcohol abuse | | ✓ |
| Diabetes mellitus | ✓ | ✓ |
| Nephrotic syndrome | ✓ | ✓ |
| Liver disease | ✓ | |
| Pregnancy | | ✓ |
| Acute pancreatitis | | ✓ |
| Oral contraceptives | | ✓ |
| Glycogen storage diseases (I, III, VI) | | ✓ |
| Chronic renal failure | | ✓ |
| Thiazide diuretics | ✓ | |
| Myeloma | ✓ | ✓ |
| Obesity | | ✓ |
| Acute porphyria | ✓ | |
| SLE | | ✓ |
| β-blockers | | ✓ |

**Table 6.10: Lipid-lowering drugs**

| Class | Examples | LDL | Triglyceride | HDL | Indications |
|---|---|---|---|---|---|
| Resins | Cholestyramine Colestipol | Reduced | Increased | – | Hypercholesterol-aemia |
| Statins (HMG CoA reductase inhibitors) | Simvastatin Pravastatin Cerivastatin | Reduced | Reduced | Increased | Hypercholesterol-aemia |
| Fibrates | Gemfibrozil Bezafibrate | Reduced | Reduced | Increased | Mixed hyperlipid-aemia |
| Nicotinic acid derivatives | Acipimox | Reduced | Reduced | Increased | Mixed hyperlipidaemia |
| Fish oils | Ω-3 marine oils | Increased | Reduced | – | Hypertriglycerid-aemia |

**Table 6.11: Disorders of phospholipid metabolism**

| Disease | Defective enzyme | Blocked pathway | Effect |
|---|---|---|---|
| Tay–Sachs | Hexosaminidase A | Ganglioside GM2 to GM3 | Increased gangliosides GM3 |
| Gaucher's | β-glucosidase | Glucocerebroside to galactose | Increased glucocerebrosides |
| Niemann–Picks | Sphingomyelinase | Sphingomyelin to ceramide | Increased sphingomyelin |
| Fabry's | α-galactosidase | Trihexoside to ganslioside GM3 | Increased trihexoside |
| Farber's | Ceramidase | Ceramide to sphingosine | Increased ceramide |
| Sandhoff's | Hexosaminidase A, B | Ganglioside GM2 to GM3 | Increased gangliosides |
| Metachromic leukodystrophy | Arylsulphatase A | Catabolism of sulphides to ceramide | Metachromic deposits |
| Globoid cell leukodystrophy | β-galactosidase | Catabolism of sulphides to ceramide | Increased galactocerebrosides |

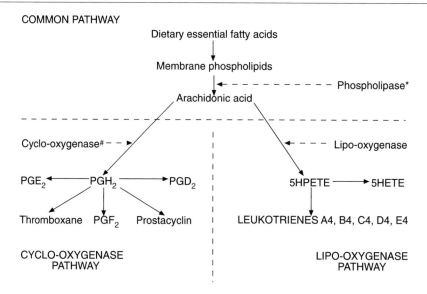

**Fig. 6.4: Metabolic pathway of production of prostanoids**
*\* inhibited by steroids     # inhibited by aspirin*

# Prostanoid metabolism

## Prostaglandins

- 20-carbon unsaturated fatty acids containing a 5-carbon cyclopentane ring
- Different prostaglandins identified by different cyclopentane rings

**Box 6.4: Functions of prostanoids**

Increased vascular permeability
Chemotaxis for neutrophils and eosinophils
Smooth muscle contraction
Uterine muscle contraction (PGE2)
Stimulate platelet aggregation
Involved in type 1 hypersensitivity reactions
Vasodilatation (prostacyclin)
Inhibit platelet aggregation (prostacyclin)
Modulation of hormone actions

- Each subset determined by degree of unsaturation of hydrocarbon ring

## Leukotrienes

- Synthesised by leukocytes

# Disorders of carbohydrate metabolism

## Normal carbohydrate metabolism

- Dietary carbohydrate consists mainly of starch, amylose, amylopectin (polysaccharides), cellulose, sucrose, lactose, maltose (disaccharides) and glucose, fructose (monosaccharides)

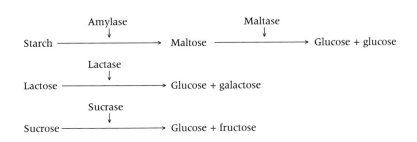

**Fig. 6.5: Normal carbohydrate metabolism**

- Dietary carbohydrate is partially hydrolysed by salivary amylase
- In the gut, further hydrolysis by disaccharidases leads to the production of the monosaccharides (glucose, fructose, galactose)
- Monosaccharides are absorbed either by an active process (glucose, galactose) or by passive diffusion (fructose)
- Glucose is either oxidised via the Embden–Meherhof pathway to produce energy (ATP); converted to glycogen and stored; or converted to triglyceride, amino acids or proteins

# Complex carbohydrates

## Glycoproteins
- Proteins with oligosaccharides covalently attached to the protein chain
- Act as membrane proteins

**Table 6.12: Glycogen storage diseases**

| Type | Name | Defective enzyme | Blocked pathway | Main storage site |
|---|---|---|---|---|
| I | Von Gierke's | Glucose-6-phosphatase | Glucose-6-phosphate to glucose and phosphate | Liver |
| II | Pompe's | Lysosomal a-glucosidase | Glycogen to glucose | Liver |
| III | Forbes' | Amylo 1,6-glucosidase debranching enzyme | Dextran to glucose | Liver |
| IV | Andersen's | 1,4a glucan branching enzyme | Dextran to glucose | Liver |
| V | McCardle's | Muscle phosphorylase | Glycogen to glucose-1-phosphate | Muscle |
| VI | Hers | Phosphorylase | Glycogen to glucose-1-phosphate | Liver |
| VII | Tauri | Phosphofructokinase | Fructose-6-phosphate to fructose-1,6-diphosphate | Muscle |
| IX | – | Phosphorylase kinase | Glycogen to glucose-1-phosphate | Liver |
| X | – | Phosphorylase kinase | Glycogen to glucose-1-phosphate | Liver, muscle |
| XI | – | None | – | Liver |
| 0 | – | Glycogen synthetase | Glucose to glycogen | Deficient liver glycogen |

**Table 6.13: Other disorders of carbohydrate metabolism**

| Disorder | Defective enzyme | Blocked pathway | Accumulation of |
|---|---|---|---|
| Galactosaemia | Galactose-1-phosphate-uridyl transferase | Galactose-1-phosphate to glucose-1-phosphate | Galactose-1-phosphate |
| Fructose intolerance | Fructose-1-phosphate aldolase | Fructose-1-phosphate and fructose-1,6-diphosphate to glyceraldehyde | Fructose |
| Essential fructosuria | Fructokinase | Fructose to fructose-1-phosphate | Fructose |
| Fructose-1,6-diphosphatase deficiency | Fructose 1,6 diphosphatase | Fructose-6-phosphate to fructose-1,6-diphosphatase and vice versa | Fructose-6-phosphate, fructose-1,6 diphosphate |
| Galactokinase deficiency | Galactokinase | Galactose to galactose-1-phosphate | Galactose |

**Table 6.14: Mucopolysaccharidoses**

| Disease | Defective enzyme | Accumulating proteoglycan | Main sites affected |
|---|---|---|---|
| Hurler's | Iduronidase | Dermatan sulphate<br>Heparan sulphate | CNS<br>Skeleton<br>Viscera |
| Hunter's | Iduronate sulphatase | Dermatan sulphate<br>Heparan sulphate | CNS<br>Skeleton<br>Viscera |
| Sanfilippo | Glucosaminidase | Heparan sulphate | CNS |
| Morquio | Galactosidase | Keratan sulphate | Skeleton |

# Glycolipids

- Lipids with oligosaccharides covalently attached
- Act as cell surface antigens

# Proteoglycans

- Consist of a core of protein
- Glycosaminoglycans are covalently attached to the core
- Important components of connective tissue

- Examples include: chondroitin sulphate, dermatan sulphate, hyaluronate

# Glycosaminoglycans

- Linear polysaccharides consisting of alternating hexosamine and uronic acid or galactose
- Examples include: galactosamine, glucuronic acid

# Disorders of protein metabolism

## Classification of amino acids

### Essential (cannot be synthesised)
- Isoleucine
- Leucine
- Valine
- Phenylalanine
- Tyrosine
- Tryptophan
- Methionine
- Cysteine
- Arginine
- Histidine
- Lysine

### Non-essential (synthesised in vivo)
- Alanine
- Aspartic acid
- Hydroxyproline
- Glutamic acid
- Glycine
- Proline
- Serine
- Tyrosine
- Cysteine
- Hydroxylysine

## Protein
- Linear unbranched polymers of different amino acids
- Amino acids joined by peptide bonds
- Biological action of proteins determined by the following:

    *Primary structure*: order of amino acids in polypeptide chain
    *Secondary structure*: spatial relationship of neighbouring amino acids, produced by twisting
    *Tertiary structure*: spatial relationship between distant amino acids produced by arrangement of layers, crystals, fibres
    *Quaternary structure*: spatial relationship between individual polypeptide chains

## Normal protein metabolism
- Dietary protein is hydrolysed in the stomach by pepsin to produce short peptide chains
- The short peptide chains are further broken down by trypsin and chymotrypsin (brush border peptidases) to produce dipeptides and free amino acids
- Free amino acids are actively absorbed in the small intestine and transported to the liver

## Fate of free amino acids
- Protein production
- Transamination (conversion into different amino acid)
- Oxidation via tricarboxylic acid cycle to produce $CO_2$ and water
- Metabolism to urea via urea cycle

## Causes of aminoaciduria

### Generalised
- Amino acid infusion
- Liver failure
- Inborn errors of metabolism
- Fanconi syndrome

### Specific
- Cystinuria
- Hartnup's disease

**Table 6.15: Inborn errors of protein metabolism**

| Disorder | Defective enzyme | Blocked pathway |
|---|---|---|
| Alkaptonuria | Homogentisic acid oxidase | Homogentisic acid to maleyacetoacetic acid |
| Homocystinuria | Cystathionine synthetase | Homocysteine to serine and cystathionine |
| Maple syrup urine disease | Branched chain ketoacid decarboxylase | Leucine, isoleucine and valine to CoA and acetoacetate |
| Phenylketonuria | Phenylalanine hydroxylase | Phenylalanine to tyrosine |
| Tyrosinaemia | Fumarylacetoacetase | Fumarylacetoacetic acid to fumaric acid and acetoacetic acid |

# Causes of Fanconi syndrome

## *Inherited*

- Cystinosis
- Galactosaemia
- Hereditary fructose intolerance
- Glycogen storage disease type 1
- Tyrosinaemia type 1
- Fructose-1,6-diphosphatase deficiency
- Wilson's disease
- Osteogenesis imperfecta
- Congenital renal tubular acidosis
- Congenital haemolytic anaemias: sickle cell disease, thalassaemia, spherocytosis
- Busby syndrome
- Luder–Sheldon syndrome
- Paine's syndrome

## *Acquired*

- Poisons: *mercury*, *lead*, cadmium, uranium, zinc, toluene, arsenic,

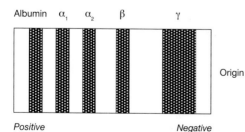

Albumin   α₁   α₂   β        γ

Origin

Positive                    Negative

**Fig. 6.6: Normal protein electrophoresis**

**Box 6.5: Abnormalities of CRP**

**Increased CRP**
*Acute inflammation*
Trauma, Burns
Bacterial infection
Myocardial infarction
Stroke
Connective tissue diseases

*Chronic inflammation*
Bacterial infection
Cryoglobulinaemia
Waldenstrom's macroglobulinaemia
Myeloma
Connective tissue disease
Crohn's disease
Malignancy

**Decreased CRP**
Lymphoma
Nephrotic syndrome
Ulcerative colitis
Scleroderma

bismuth, Paraquat
- Drugs: outdated tetracycline, salicylates, cisplatin
- Renal disease: acute tubular necrosis, nephrotic syndrome, renal transplant rejection, potassium depletion nephropathy
- Nutritional deficiencies: vitamins B₁₂, C, D, kwashiorkor

**Table 6.16: Classification of plasma proteins**

| Protein | Examples | % in plasma | Functions |
|---|---|---|---|
| Albumin | – | 50–70 | Maintenance of plasma volume<br>Maintenance of distribution of ECF<br>Carrier for bilirubin, calcium, thyroxine, free fatty acids, drugs<br>Minor role as a buffer |
| $\alpha_1$-globulins | *$\alpha_1$-Antitrypsin*<br>Thyroid-binding globulin<br>HDL<br>Transcortin<br>Oromucoid | 2–6 | Inhibition of proteolytic enzymes<br>Thyroid hormone transport<br>Lipid transport<br>Cortisol transport |
| $\alpha_2$-globulins | *$\alpha_2$-Macroglobulin*<br>Caeruloplasmin<br>VLDL<br>Haptoglobins | 5–11 | Inhibition of proteolytic enzymes<br>Copper transport<br>Lipid transport<br>Binding of free haemoglobin released from haemolysed red blood cells (low levels in haemolytic anaemia) |
| $\beta$-globulins | Transferrin<br>LDL<br>Fibrinogen<br>Plasminogen<br>C3, C4<br>$\beta_2$ Microglobulin | 7–16 | Iron transport<br>Lipid transport<br>Fibrinolysis<br><br>Inflammation, immune protection<br>Measure of GFR |
| $\gamma$-globulins | *Immunoglobulins*<br>Factor VIII<br>$\alpha$-Fetoprotein<br>CRP | 11–21 | Immune competence<br>Blood coagulation<br>Neural tube formation<br>Marker of acute inflammation |

- Primary hyperparathyroidism
- Sjögren's syndrome

# Acute-phase proteins

## *Proteins increased in acute inflammation*
- CRP
- Fibrinogen
- Plasminogen
- Protein S
- $\alpha_1$-acid glycoprotein
- Haptoglobins
- Ferritin
- $\alpha_1$-antitrypsin
- Complement
- Prealbumin
- Oromucoid
- Caeruloplasmin

### Proteins decreased in acute inflammation
- Transferrin
- α-Fetoprotein
- Insulin-like growth factor
- Albumin

## Causes of hypoalbuminaemia

### Decreased synthesis
- Malnutrition
- Chronic liver disease

### Increased volume of distribution
- Fluid overload
- Increased capillary permeability (septicaemia, hypoxia)

### Increased loss
- Nephrotic syndrome
- Protein-losing enteropathy
- Haemorrhage
- Catabolic states (burns, sepsis, fever, trauma, malignancy)

## Porphyrias

- Defects in porphyrin metabolism
- Characterised by increased δ-aminol-aevulinic acid (ALA) synthase activity
- Classified according to site of enzyme defect (Table 6.17)
  *Acute*: normal or reduced porphobilinogen (PBG) deaminase activity
  Primarily present with neurological manifestations
  *Chronic*: increased PBG deaminase activity
  Primarily present with photo-sensitivity

---

**Box 6.6:  Other causes of raised urinary porphyrins**

Alcohol
Lead poisoning
Cholestatic liver disease
Iron deficiency anaemia
Sideroblastic anaemia
Hereditary tyrosinaemia
Dubin–Johnson syndrome
Gilbert's syndrome
Schizophrenia

## Features of an acute porphyria attack

### Gastrointestinal
- Abdominal pain
- Vomitimg
- Constipation

### Cardiovascular
- Tachycardia
- Hypertension
- Cardiac failure

---

**Box 6.7:  Precipitants of an acute porphyria attack**

| Antibiotics | Anticonvulsants |
|---|---|
| Rifampicin | Phenytoin |
| Sulphonamides | Barbiturates |
| Chloramphenicol | Primidone |
| Tetracyclines | |
| Dapsone | **Other drugs** |
| Griseofulvin | Alcohol |
| Pyrazinamide | Chloroquine |
| | Sulphonylureas |
| **Miscellaneous** | Methyldopa |
| Pregnancy | Ergots |
| Stress | Danazol |
| Premenstruation | Imipramine |
| Sepsis | Progesterone |
| Starvation | Oral contraceptives |
| | Pentazocine |
| | Thiopentone |

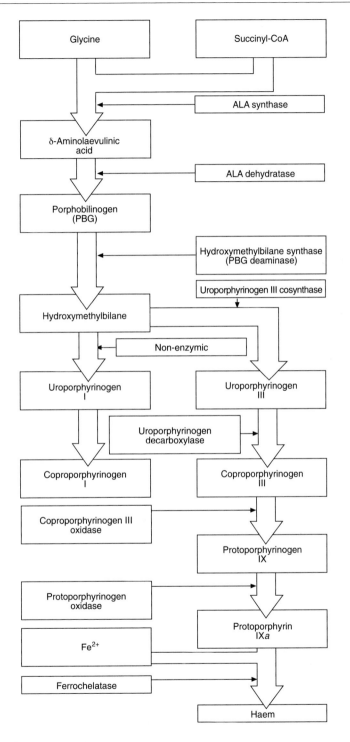

**Fig. 6.7: Porphyrin metabolism**

**Table 6.17: Classification of porphyrias**

| Type | Condition | Inherited | Defective enzyme | Skin | CNS | Urinary porphyrins |
|------|-----------|-----------|------------------|------|-----|--------------------|
| Acute | Acute intermittent porphyria | Autosomal dominant | PBG deaminase | – | + | PBG, ALA |
| Acute | Hereditary coproporphyria | Autosomal dominant | Coproporphrinogen III oxidase | + | + | PBG, ALA, coproporphyrinogen |
| Acute | Variegate porphyria | Autosomal dominant | Protoporphrinogen oxidase | + | + | PBG, ALA, protoporphyrin |
| Chronic | Porphyria cutanea tarda | No | Uroporphrinogen decarboxylase | + | – | Uroporphyrinogen |
| Chronic | Congenital erythropoietic porphyria | Autosomal recessive | Uroporphyrinogen III cosynthase | + | – | Uroporphyrinogen, coproporphyrinogen |
| Chronic | Erythropoietic porphyria | Autosomal dominant | Ferrochelatase | + | – | Protoporphyrin |

## Neuropsychiatric
- *Peripheral neuropathy*
- Seizures
- Depression
- Psychosis
- Proximal myopathy

## Metabolic
- Hyponatraemia
- SIADH

# Treatment of acute porphyria attack

- Strict fluid balance
- Avoid precipitant causes
- High carbohydrate intake
- i.v. haematin (reduces ALA synthase activity)

*Analgesia*: opiates, paracetamol, brufen, indomethacin
*Hypertension and tachycardia*: β-blockers
*Psychiatric manifestations*: phenothiazines
*Seizures*: benzodiazepines
*Sepsis*: ampicillin, gentamicin
*Vomiting*: stemetil, domperidone, cyclizine

# Disorders of purine metabolism

## Uric acid metabolism

- Uric acid produced by breakdown of purine bases
- Only 10% of uric acid obtained from diet

**Table 6.18: Causes of hyperuricaemia**

| Increased production | Reduced excretion | Miscellaneous |
|---|---|---|
| **Increased synthesis** | Idiopathic | Ischaemic heart disease |
| Idiopathic | Chronic renal failure | Hyperlipidaemia |
| Hypoxanthine guanine | Lead nephropathy | Obesity |
| phosphoribosyl transferase | Hyperparathyroidism | Impaired glucose |
| (HGPRT) deficiency | Volume depletion | tolerance |
| (Lesch–Nyhan syndrome) | Nephrogenic diabetes insipidus | |
| Phosphoribosyl pyrophosphate | Hypertension | |
| (PRPP) synthetase overactivity | Sickle cell disease | |
| Ribose-5-phosphatase | Hypothyroidism | |
| overproduction | Bartter's syndrome | |
| Glucose-6-phosphatase | Down's syndrome | |
| deficiency | Chronic beryllium poisoning | |
| | | |
| **Increased turnover** | Sarcoidosis | |
| Myeloproliferative disorders | Drugs: Diuretics, ethambutol, | |
| Lymphoproliferative disorders | low-dose salicylates, | |
| Chronic haemolytic anaemia | pyrazinamide, | |
| Severe exfoliative psoriasis | Angiotensin | |
| Secondary polycythaemia | Exercise | |
| Gaucher's disease | Alcohol | |
| Infectious mononucleosis | Starvation | |
| Carcinomatosis | Ketoacidosis | |
| Cytotoxic drugs | | |

- Uric acid filtered at glomeruli
- 90% reabsorbed in proximal and distal convuluted tubules
- 75% uric acid excreted via kidney
- Uric acid circulates in plasma as monosodium urate

# Nutrition

## Complications of artificial enteral nutrition

*Major*
- Aspiration pneumonia
- Upper gastrointestinal haemorrhage
- Septicaemia
- Peritonitis
- Mortality

*Minor*
- Wound infection
- Diarrhoea
- Vomiting
- Abdominal pain
- Oesophagitis
- Increased gastro-oesophageal reflux
- Nasal septal necrosis (nasogastric tubes)
- Tube blockage
- Tube dislodgement
- Accidental tube removal

## Complications of parenteral nutrition

*Line problems*
- Blockage
- Sepsis
- Dislodgement

**Table 6.19: Vitamins and trace elements**

| Vitamin | Solubility | Major source | Function | Causes of deficiency | Features of deficiency | Features of excess |
|---|---|---|---|---|---|---|
| A | Fat | Carrots, dark green leafy vegetables, pumpkin, mango, fish oil, margarine, liver, eggs | Maintenance of mucosal surfaces Production of mucus Immune competence Retinal function | Poor diet Inflammatory bowel disease | Night blindness Xerophthalmia Immune incompetence | Headache Seizures Myalgia Hepatomegaly Teratogenesis |
| Thiamine (B₁) | Water | Fortified flour, cereals, milk, eggs, yeast extract, fruit | Carbohydrate metabolism Maintenance of cardiac muscle and peripheral nerves | Poor diet Alcohol abuse | Peripheral neuropathy ptic atrophy 'rnicke–Korsakoff's syndrome High-output cardiac failure Beri-beri | None |
| Riboflavin (B₂) | Water | Milk, cheese, eggs, cereals, liver, kidney | Control of intracellular oxidation Maintenance of skin | Protein–energy Malnutrition Alcohol abuse Pregnancy | Mucosal dryness Anaemia | None |
| Nicotinic acid (niacin) | Water | Liver, kidney, milk, cheese, eggs, beef, pork, chicken, coffee, peas, beans, yeast extract | Energy utilisation Maintenance of skin | Malabsorption Hartnup's disease Carcinoid syndrome Protein-losing states | Pellagra | Vasodilatation |

**Table 6.19 continued**

| Vitamin | Solubility | Major source | Function | Causes of deficiency | Features of deficiency | Features of excess |
|---|---|---|---|---|---|---|
| Pyridoxine (B$_6$) | Water | Liver, meat, fish, cereals, milk, peanuts | Amino acid metabolism | Malabsorption Alcohol abuse Isoniazid | Glossitis, dry skin Cognitive impairment Peripheral neuropathy Premenstrual tension Sideroblastic anaemia | Peripheral neuropathy |
| Ascorbic acid (C) | Water | Citrus fruit, potatoes, green vegetables | Antioxidant Maintenance of connective tissue Increased iron absorption | Poor diet Alcohol abuse Smoking | Scurvy | Hyperoxaluria |
| E | Fat | Vegetable oils, cereals, eggs | Antioxidant Maintenance of RBC membrane | Malabsorption Inadequate TPN Abetalipoproteinaemia | Haemolytic anaemia Peripheral neuropathy | Nausea |
| K | Fat | Vegetables, peas, beans, liver | Blood coagulation | Cholestatic liver disease Malabsorption Warfarin | Hypothrombinaemia | Hyperbilirubinaemia |
| Copper | – | – | Cofactor for cytochrome oxidase Antioxidant | Premature infants fed only with cows' milk | Anaemia, Neutropenia Osteomalacia Menkes' syndrome | Wilson's disease (increased tissue copper deposition) |

**Table 6.19 continued**

| Vitamin | Solubility | Major source | Function | Causes of deficiency | Features of deficiency | Features of excess |
|---|---|---|---|---|---|---|
| Zinc | – | Herrings, beef, liver, eggs, nuts | Cofactor for carbonic anhydrase and other enzymes<br>Antioxidant | Malabsorption<br>Inadequate TPN | Acrodermatitis enteropathica<br>Impaired wound healing | None |
| Selenium | – | – | Cofactor for glutathione peroxidase<br>Antioxidant | Stress<br>Acute-phase response<br>Inadequate TPN | Cardiomyopathy (keshan disease) | None |
| Chromium | – | – | – | Inadequate TPN | Glucose intolerance | None |
| Cobalt | – | – | Component of vitamin $B_{12}$ | Inadequate TPN | None | Cardiomyopathy |
| Fluorine | – | Water, toothpaste | Component of bones and teeth | Inadequate dental hygiene/water supplementation | Dental caries | Fluorosis |
| Nickel | – | – | Maintenance of membranes | Inadequate TPN | None | None |

- Tissue necrosis
- Thrombosis

### Metabolic
- Electrolyte abnormalities
- Hyperglycaemia
- Acidosis
- Fatty liver
- Hepatic cirrhosis
- Hypophosphataemia
- Trace element deficiency
- Osteomalacia
- Renal failure

# Enzymology

## Causes of raised serum alkaline phosphatase

### Physiological
- Childhood
- Pregnancy (last trimester)

### Pathological
- Paget's disease
- Osteomalacia
- Healing fractures
- Biliary tract obstruction
- Congestive cardiac failure
- Hepatic cirrhosis
- Hepatic tumours
- Hepatic infiltration
- Hepatic abscess
- Acute hepatitis
- Chronic hepatitis
- Bone tumours
- Primary hyperparathyroidism
- Chronic renal failure
- Osteomyelitis
- Inflammatory bowel disease
- Choriocarcinoma

## Causes of raised serum transaminases

- Acute hepatitis
- Acute myocardial infarction
- Trauma
- Chronic hepatitis
- Biliary tract obstruction
- Acute pancreatitis
- Chronic renal failure
- Haemolytic anaemia
- Congestive cardiac failure
- Crush injury
- Tissue hypoxia
- Skeletal muscle disease
- Physiological (neonates)
- Septicaemia

## Causes of raised serum angiotensin-converting enzyme

- Active sarcoid
- Liver disease
- Leprosy
- Berylliosis
- Asbestosis
- Silicosis

## Causes of raised serum γ-glutamyl transpeptidase

- Biliary tract obstruction
- Alcohol abuse
- Acute hepatitis
- Chronic hepatitis
- Hepatic cirrhosis
- Acute pancreatitis
- Liver enzyme-inducing drugs
- Congestive cardiac failure

# 7 Haematology

## Contents

## Haemopoiesis

Haemopoiesis is the process of blood cell formation.

### Main sites

- 0–6 weeks' gestation: yolk sac
- 6–24 weeks' gestation: fetal liver and spleen
- 24 weeks' gestation onwards: bone marrow
- Hepatic haemopoiesis declines during the third trimester and ceases 2 weeks after birth
- At birth all bone marrow is haemopoietic
- During childhood most of the marrow is replaced by fatty tissue
- In normal adults haemopoiesis is confined to the proximal femur and humerus, vertebrae, skull, sternum, ribs, sacrum and pelvis
- In disease the fatty marrow can resume haemopoiesis, as can the liver and spleen (extramedullary haemopoiesis)

### Stem cell differentiation

- All blood cells are derived from pluripotent stem cells
- The stem cells are capable of self-renewal and their numbers remain constant in normal adults
- The stem cells pass through several stages of maturation (Fig. 7.1)
- At each stage of development the cells progressively lose multipotential and become committed to one cell line
- There are four main cell lineages: erythroid, granulocytic, lymphoid, megakaryocytic

Stem cells $\longrightarrow$ Multipotent progenitor cells $\longrightarrow$ Committed progenitor cells $\longrightarrow$ Precursor cells $\longrightarrow$ End cells

**Fig. 7.1: Maturation of stem cells**

Pronormoblast → Early → Intermediate → Late → Reticulocyte → Mature
                        Normoblast   normoblast    normoblast                   RBC

**Fig. 7.2: Erythropoiesis**

# Erythropoiesis (Fig. 7.2)

The earliest recognisable erythroid cell in the bone marrow is the pronormoblast.

- One pronormoblast leads to the development of 16 mature red blood cells (RBC)
- At each stage there is progressive loss of nuclear material and an increase in haemoglobin
- Reticulocytes are the first erythroid cells to circulate in the peripheral blood in normal adults
- Reticulocytes still contain rRNA, but no nuclear DNA
- Reticulocytes spend 1–2 days circulating before maturing into non-nucleated RBC in the spleen
- The presence of normoblasts in the peripheral blood indicates extramedullary haemopoiesis

## Mature RBC

- Biconcave non-nucleated disc, diameter 8 μm
- Membrane consists of a bipolar lipid layer (mainly phospholipid)
- Biconcave shape maintained by structural proteins (especially spectrin)
- Energy as adenosine triphosphate (ATP) produced via anaerobic glycolytic (Embden–Meyerhof) pathway
- Reducing power produced from Embden–Meyerhof pathway (reduced-form nicotinamide adenine dinusleotide: NADH) and hexose monophosphate shunt (NADPH)
- Lifespan of RBC is 120 days
- RBC destroyed extravascularly by macrophages of the reticuloendothelial system (liver, spleen, bone marrow)
- RBC breakdown leads to:

*iron*
- recirculated and reused

*amino acids*
- reused for protein synthesis

*protoporphyrin*
- small amount CO produced and excreted via lungs
- mainly degraded to bilirubin
- bilirubin conjugated in liver
- excreted in bile as glucuronides
- in gut converted to stercobilin and stercobilinogen
- some reabsorbed and excreted in urine as urobilin and urobilinogen

## Haemoglobin synthesis

- One RBC contains 640 million haemoglobin molecules
- Each haemoglobin molecule consists of four polypeptide (globin) chains and four haem molecules
- Each haem molecule consists of protoporphyrin and ferrous iron ($Fe^{2+}$)
- Haem synthesis controlled by aminolaevulinic acid (ALA) synthetase
- Haem synthesis takes place in mitochondria
- 65% of haemoglobin synthesised in erythroblasts, 35% in reticulocytes
- Major switch to adult haemoglobin occurs 3–6 months after birth (Table 7.1)

## Regulation of erythropoiesis

Erythropoiesis is controlled by erythropoi-etin.

## Actions of erythropoietin

- Increases the number of stem cells committed to erythropoiesis

**Table 7.1: Normal human haemoglobins**

| Haemoglobin | Embryo/fetus | At birth | Adult | Globin structure |
|---|---|---|---|---|
| A | No | 10–50% | 97% | $\alpha_2\beta_2$ |
| A2 | No | Trace | 2.5% | $\alpha_2\delta_2$ |
| F | Yes | 50–90% | 0.5% | $\alpha_2\gamma_2$ |
| Gower 1 | Yes | No | No | $\zeta_2\epsilon_2$ |
| Gower 2 | Yes | No | No | $\alpha_2\epsilon_2$ |
| Portland | Yes | No | No | $\zeta_2\gamma_2$ |

- Increases haemoglobin synthesis
- Decreases maturation time of RBC precursors
- Releases reticulocytes into peripheral blood earlier

## Substances needed for erythropoiesis

- Metals: iron, manganese, cobalt, zinc
- Vitamins: $B_{12}$, $B_6$ (pyridoxine), thiamine, riboflavin, pantothenic acid, C, E, folate
- Hormones: erythropoietin, androgens, thyroxine
- Amino acids

## Causes of impaired erythropoiesis

- Marrow disease: aplasia, infiltration
- Haematinic deficiency
- Erythropoietin deficiency: chronic renal disease
- Reduced tissue oxygen consumption: hypothyroidism, protein deficiency
- Chronic inflammatory or malignant disease

# Granulopoiesis

- Granulopoiesis is limited before birth
- Only mature cells are normally found in the peripheral blood
- Process regulated by leukopoietins

## Granulocytes

- Multilobed nuclear cells, 12–15 μm in diameter
- Cytoplasm contains two types of granule:
  *Primary:* contain myeloperoxidase, acid phosphatase, acid hydrolases
  *Secondary:* contain alkaline phosphatase, lysozyme
- Mature granulocytes circulate for 10 hours before migrating into tissues

## Monocytes

- Large mononuclear cells, 16–20 μm in

---

**Box 7.1: Tests of erythropoiesis**

| Test | Finding in impaired erythropoiesis |
|---|---|
| Marrow cellularity | Reduced |
| Myeloid:erythroid ratio (normally 2.5–12:1) | Increased |
| Plasma iron turnover (using $^{59}$Fe-radiolabelled iron) | Increased |
| Iron incorporation into circulating RBC (using $^{59}$Fe) | Poor |
| Carbon monoxide excretion | Increased |
| Reticulocyte count | Reduced |
| Serum LDH | Raised |
| Red cell lifespan (using $^{51}$Cr-labelled RBC) | Reduced |

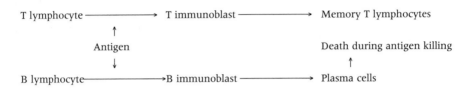

(a) Myeloblast⟶ Promyelocyte ⟶ Myelocyte ⟶ Metamyelocyte ⟶ Mature cell

(b) Myeloblast⟶ Promonocyte ⟶ Monocyte ⟶ Immature macrophage ⟶ Mature macrophage

**Fig. 7.3: Steps in the production (a) of neutrophils, eosinophils and basophils; (b) of monocytes**

T lymphocyte ⟶ T immunoblast ⟶ Memory T lymphocytes

↑ Antigen

Death during antigen killing

↓ ↑

B lymphocyte ⟶ B immunoblast ⟶ Plasma cells

**Fig. 7.4: Production of lymphocytes**

diameter
- Cytoplasm contains granules similar to granulocytes
- Mature cells circulate for 20–40 hours before entering the tissues to mature as macrophages
- Macrophage lifespan may be as long as several months or years

## Eosinophils
- Similar to granulocytes
- Cytoplasmic granules are coarser and rarely more than three nuclear lobes
- Blood transit time longer than that of granulocytes

## Basophils
- Only occasionally seen in the peripheral blood
- Cytoplasmic granules contain histamine and heparin
- In the tissues they become mast cells

# Lymphopoiesis

- The production of lymphocytes begins in the first trimester
- By the second trimester the fetal blood contains mature cells

- In the fetus the main sites are the yolk sac, liver, spleen, bone marrow and thymus
- Postnatally the main sites are the bone marrow and thymus
- Lymphocytes that leave the bone marrow are not fully functional
- Final maturation takes place when they meet antigens and become immunoblasts
- A further group of follicle centre cells (FCC) develop in lymphoid tissue (follicular germinal centres) in response to antigen stimulation

*T cells* make up 70% of all lymphocytes
Two types: T4 (helper) and T8 (cytotoxic) cells
*B cells* make up 10% of all lymphocytes
*Non-T non-B cells* make up 20% of all lymphocytes

# Megakaryopoiesis

Platelet production follows the following process:

Megakaryoblast ⟶ Megakaryocyte ⟶ Platelet

- Each megakaryocyte produces 4000

mature platelets
- Megakaryopoiesis is regulated by thrombopoietin

## Mature platelet
- Platelet size is 1–2 μm
- Platelet lifespan is 7–10 days
- Surrounded by mucopolysaccharide surface coat

| Box 7.2: Functions of haemopoietic cells | |
| --- | --- |
| Red blood cells | Carriage of $O_2$ (1g of haemoglobin carries 1.39ml $O_2$ Carriage of $CO_2$ (30% carbaminohaemoglobin, 60% bicarbonate) |
| Granulocytes | Chemotaxis Phagocytosis Killing of bacteria |
| Monocytes/ macrophages | As for granulocytes Also act as antigen-presenting cells May adopt specific functions in different tissues |
| Eosinophils | Parasitic phagocytosis Involved in hypersensitivity reactions |
| Basophils | Involved in type I hypersensitivity reactions |
| T lymphocytes | Responsible for cell-mediated immunity T4 cells involved in antigen presentation (recognise class II HLA antigens) T8 cells involved in cytotoxicity (recognise class I HLA antigens) |
| B lymphocytes | Responsible for humoral immunity Production of antibodies |
| Platelets | Formation of haemostatic plugs |

- This overlies a trilaminar plasma membrane
- Discoid shape maintained by internal microtubule skeleton
- Cytoplasm contains two types of granule:
    *Electron-dense granules*: contain nucleotides, calcium, serotonin
    *α Granules*: contain platelet factor IV, platelet growth factor, β-thromboglobulin, fibrinogen, acid hydrolases, fibronectin, factor V, von Willebrand factor

# Anaemia

## Classification of anaemia

### Microcytic (low MCV)
- Iron deficiency
- Thalassaemia
- Chronic disease
- Sideroblastic anaemia

### Normocytic (normal MCV)
- Chronic disease
- Acute haemorrhage
- Haemolytic anaemia
- Aplastic anaemia
- Combined microcytic and macrocytic anaemia

### Macrocytic (raised MCV)
- Megaloblastic anaemia
- Alcohol
- Liver disease
- Hypothyroidism
- Reticulocytosis
- Cytotoxic drugs
- Aplastic anaemia
- Pregnancy
- Myelodysplasia
- Myeloma
- Respiratory failure

**Box 7.3: Shifts of dissociation curve**

| Left | Right |
|------|-------|
| Low $PCO_2$ | Raised $PCO_2$ |
| Alkalosis | Acidosis |
| Low 2,3-DPG | Raised 2,3-DPG |
| (diphosphoglycerate) | Raised temperature |
| Hypothermia | Anaemia |
| Polycythaemia | |

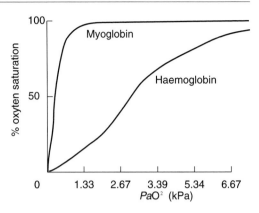

**Fig. 7.5: Oxygen dissociation curve**

# Important clinical points about anaemia

- The development of anaemia depends on the balance between circulating plasma volume and circulating haemoglobin mass
- Reductions in plasma volume may mask anaemia (e.g., in dehydration)
- Increases in plasma volume may cause anaemia even if haemoglobin mass normal (e.g., splenomegaly)
- The presence of clinical features depends on the following:

*Speed of onset of anaemia*: slowly progressive anaemia may be asymptomatic

*Severity of anaemia*: mild anaemia often asymptomatic

*Age of patient*: older people generally tolerate anaemia less well

# Iron deficiency anaemia

## Iron metabolism
- Average Western diet contains 10–15mg/day of iron
- Only 5–10% of dietary iron is absorbed in normal adults (0.5–1.5mg/day)
- In iron deficiency or pregnancy, up to 20–30% of dietary iron may be absorbed
- Iron is absorbed in the ferrous form ($Fe^{3+}$) in the duodenum and jejunum

by an active process
- When iron enters the intestinal luminal cells some ferritin is formed (apoferritin + $Fe^{3+}$)
- The rest is transported in the plasma bound to transferrin in the ferric form
- Most of the plasma iron comes from the reticuloendothelial system (macrophages)
- Iron is released by macrophages in a diurnal variation
- Plasma iron levels therefore have a diurnal variation (higher in the morning)
- Iron is converted from the ferrous form to the ferric form by caeruloplasmin
- Iron is stored in the bone marrow, liver and spleen as ferritin and haemosiderin (Table 7.2)
- Average iron losses (mainly via the intestine) are 1 mg/day
- During menstruation losses may

**Box 7.4: Failure to respond to oral iron**

Continued haemorrhage
Poor compliance
Incorrect diagnosis
Coexistent additional type of anaemia
Severe malabsorption
Use of slow-release preparations

increase to 2 mg/day
- During pregnancy losses may be as high as 3 mg/day

### Causes of iron deficiency
- Blood loss
    Uterine
    Gastro-intestinal
    Trauma
- Increased demands
    Prematurity
    Growth
    Pregnancy
- Malabsorption
- Dietary insufficiency

# Anaemia of chronic disease

- Usually multifactorial:
    Decreased release of iron from
        macrophages
    Bone marrow erythroid hypoplasia
    Decreased RBC survival
    Decreased erythropoietin production
- No response to iron therapy

### Causes of anaemia of chronic disease
- Chronic inflammatory diseases
    Chronic sepsis
    Connective tissue disorders
    Inflammatory bowel disease
    Sarcoid
- Malignancy
- Chronic renal failure

**Table 7.2: Distribution of body iron**

| Site | Amount (g) |
| --- | --- |
| Haemoglobin | 2.4–3.5 |
| Ferritin/haemosiderin | 1–1.25 |
| Myoglobin | 0.12–0.25 |
| Haem enzyme | 0.01 |
| Plasma (transferrin bound) | 0.0005 |
| **Total** | **4–5** |

**Box 7.5: Factors affecting iron absorption**

**Factors increasing absorption**
Ferrous form ($Fe^{3+}$)
Inorganic iron
Acidic environment
Solubilising agents (sugars, amino acids)
Iron deficiency
Increased erythropoiesis
Pregnancy
Primary haemochromatosis

**Factors reducing absorption**
Ferric form ($Fe^{2+}$)
Organic iron
Alkalis (antacids)
Precipitating agents (phosphates)
Iron excess
Decreased erythropoiesis
Infection
Tea
Desferroxamine

# Sideroblastic anaemia

This is a refractory anaemia characterised by the presence of ring sideroblasts (abnormal erythroblasts).

- Results from a defect in haem synthesis
- Hereditary forms due to a congenital enzyme defect
- Acquired forms due to mutation of erythroid progenitor cells
- May transform into acute myeloid leukaemia
- Some patients respond to pyridoxine

### Causes of sideroblastic anaemia
*Hereditary*
*Acquired*
- Primary idiopathic
- Malignant infiltration of bone marrow
- Drugs: isoniazid, cycloserine, pyrazinamide, chloramphenicol
- Toxins: alcohol, lead

- Vitamin B$_6$ deficiency
- Connective tissue disorders
- Malabsorption

# Haemolytic anaemias

These are anaemias resulting from an increase in the rate of destruction of RBC.

## Causes of haemolytic anaemias
### Hereditary
- Membrane defects: <u>hereditary spherocytosis</u>, hereditary eliptocytosis
- Enzyme defects: <u>G6PD deficiency</u> (Box 7.6), pyruvate kinase deficiency
- Haemoglobin defects: <u>sickle cell anaemia</u>, <u>thalassaemias</u>, Hb C, Hb D, Hb E

### Acquired
- *Warm autoimmune (IgG)*
  <u>Idiopathic</u>
  Viral infection
  Autoimmune disorders
  Lymphoproliferative disorders: CLL, lymphomas
  Drugs: methyldopa, L-dopa, mefanamic acid
- *Cold autoimmune (IgM)*
  <u>Idiopathic</u>
  <u>Mycoplasma pneumoniae</u>

---

**Box 7.6: Agents precipitating haemolysis in G6PD deficiency**

<u>Drugs</u>: antimalarials, analgesics (NSAIDS, paracetamol)
Antibiotics (sulphonamides, penicillin, antituberculous agents, nitrofurantoin, chloramphenicol),
Miscellaneous (dapsone, vitamin K, probenecid, quinidine)
Infections
Acute illness
Fava beans

---

  EBV
  Lymphoma
  Paroxysmal cold haemoglobinuria: syphilis, viral infection
- *Isoimmune*
  <u>Haemolytic transfusion reaction</u>
  Haemolytic disease of the newborn
- *Drug-induced immune*
  Methyldopa, L-dopa, penicillin, cephalosporins, sulphonamides, phenacetin, mefanamic acid, quinidine, chlorpropramide, rifampicin, isoniazid
- *Non-immune*
  <u>Microangiopathic haemolytic anaemia: disseminated intravascular coagulation</u>
  RBC trauma: cardiac prostheses, burns, march haemoglobinuria
  Hypersplenism
  Paroxysmal nocturnal haemoglobinuria
  Vitamin E deficiency
  Infection: malaria, bartonella, clostridia
  Metabolic: uraemia, liver disease, hypophosphataemia
  Toxins: lead, chlorate, copper, nitrobenzenes, naphthalene
  Venoms: snake bites, spider bites

# Sickle cell anaemia

- In the β-globulin chains, valine replaces glutamine
- The resultant HbS is insoluble and crystallises if O$_2$ tension is low
- Course punctuated by acute crises (Box 7.7)
- Painful crises precipitated by infection, dehydration, cold exposure, trauma
- Haemolytic crises accompany painful crises
- Aplastic crises precipitated by infection (especially parvovirus)
- Sequestration crises are the most

**Box 7.7: Types of sickle crises**

Painful (thrombotic):
   generalised pain
   localised bone pain
   abdominal
   pulmonary
   neurological
Aplastic
Haemolytic
Sequestration: spleen, liver

serious

## Management of sickle crises
- Attempt to identify underlying cause
- Bed rest, rehydration
- Oxygen therapy
- Analgesia (usually strong opiate analgesics required)
- Broad-spectrum antibiotics
- Blood transfusion:
   Only if severe symptomatic anaemia
   May need exchange transfusion

# Thalassaemia syndromes

## Types of thalassaemia
### α-Thalassaemias
- Hydrops fetalis (4 gene deletion)
- Haemoglobin H (3 gene deletion)
- α-Thalassaemia trait
- Hb constant spring

### β-Thalassaemias
- β-Thalassaemia major (homozygous)
- β-Thalassaemia trait (heterozygous)

### Thalassaemia intermedia
- β-Thalassaemia with more HbF production
- Severe β-thalassaemia trait
- HbE
- Hb Lepore

- Coexistent α-thalassaemia trait and β-thalassaemia major

# Aplastic anaemia

- Characterised by reduced numbers of haemopoietic pluripotent stem cells
- Usually results in pancytopenia, but selective cytopenias may occur

## Causes of aplastic anaemia
### Congenital
- Fanconi's anaemia
- Diamond–Blackfan syndrome (isolated RBC aplasia)

### Acquired
- Idiopathic
- Infection: viral hepatitis, EBV, parvovirus
- Ionising radiation
- Chemicals: benzene, organic solvents, TNT, insecticides, DDT, hair dyes
- Drugs: antibiotics (sulphonamides, chloramphenicol)
   cytotoxics
   anti-inflammatories: phenylbutazone, penicillamine, gold, indomethacin
   antithyroid agents: carbimazole, thiouracils
   anticonvulsants: phenytoin
   psychotropics: phenothiazines, dothiepin
   diuretics: thiazides
   miscellaneous: arsenic, chlorpropramide, chloroquine, antihistamines
- Autoimmune disease
- Pregnancy
- Paroxysmal nocturnal haemoglobinuria

## Causes of pancytopenia
- Aplastic anaemia
- Bone marrow infiltration: carcinomatosis

**Table 7.3: Investigation of anaemia (continues on facing page)**

| | Iron deficiency | Anaemia of chronic disease | Sideroblastic anaemia | Extra-vascular haemolysis |
|---|---|---|---|---|
| MCV | Low | Normal/low | Low (congenital) High (acquired) | Normal |
| MCH | Low | Normal/low | Low (acquired) High (congenital) | Normal |
| Serum iron | Low | Low | High | Normal |
| TIBC | High | Low | Normal | Normal |
| Serum ferritin | Low | Normal/high | High | Normal |
| Bone marrow | Absent iron | Low iron in erythroblasts | Erythroid hyperplasia Ring sideroblasts | Erythroid hyperplasia |
| Haemoglobin electrophoresis | Normal | Normal | Normal | Normal |
| Serum folate | Normal | Normal | Normal/low | Normal/low |
| Serum $B_{12}$ | Normal | Normal | Normal | Normal |
| Reticulocytes | Low | Normal | Normal | High |
| Direct Coombs' test | Negative | Negative | Negative | Positive |
| Blood film | Hypochromia Poikilocytosis Anisocytosis Microcytosis Target cells | Normal or iron deficiency | Iron deficiency or megaloblastic changes | Micro spherocytes Fragmented cells |
| Serum bilirubin | Normal | Normal | Normal/high | High |
| Serum LDH | Normal | Normal | Normal/high | High |
| WBC | Normal | Normal | Normal/low | Normal |
| Platelets | Normal | Normal | Normal/high /low | Normal |
| Urine bile pigments | Normal | Normal | Normal/high | High |
| Faecal bile pigments | Normal | Normal | Normal/high | High |
| Osmotic fragility | No | No | No | Yes |
| RBC survival | Normal | Normal | Normal | Reduced |
| Haemoglobinaemia | No | No | No | No |
| Haemoglobinuria | No | No | No | No |
| Haemosiderinuria | No | No | No | No |
| Methaemalbuminaemia | No | No | No | No |

## Table 7.3 (continued)

| Intravascular haemolysis | Sickle cell anaemia | Thalassaemias | Aplastic anaemia | $B_{12}$ deficiency | Folate deficiency |
|---|---|---|---|---|---|
| Normal | Low | Low | Normal/high | High | High |
| Normal | Low | Low | Normal/high | High | High |
| Normal | Normal | Normal/high | Normal | Normal | Normal |
| Normal | Normal | Normal | Normal | Normal | Normal |
| Normal | Normal | Normal/high | Normal | Normal | Normal |
| Erythroid hyperplasia | Erythroid hyperplasia | Erythroid hyperplasia | Hypoplasia Fatty infiltration | Hypercellular erythroblasts Giant metamyelocytes | As for $B_{12}$ deficiency |
| Normal | Abnormal | Abnormal | Normal | Normal | Normal |
| Normal/low | Normal/low | Normal/low | Normal | Normal | Low |
| Normal | Normal | Normal | Normal | Low | Normal |
| High | High | High | Low | Low | Low |
| Positive | Negative | Negative | Negative | Negative | Negative |
| Micro spherocytes Fragmented cells | Sickle cells Fragmented cells Target cells Poikilocytosis Anisochromia Howell-Jolly bodies | Fragmented cells Poikilocytosis Polychromasia Anisocytosis Anisochromia Normoblasts | Pancytopenia | Hyper-segmented neutrophils Macrocytes Poikilocytes Anisocytosis Leuko-erythroblastic picture | As for $B_{12}$ deficiency |
| High | Normal/high | Normal/high | Normal | High | High |
| High | Normal/high | Normal/high | Normal | High | High |
| Normal | Normal/low | Normal/low | Low | Normal/low | Normal/low |
| Normal | Normal/low | Normal/low | Low | Normal/low | Normal/low |
| High | Normal/high | Normal/high | Normal | High | High |
| High | Normal/high | Normal/high | Normal | High | High |
| Yes | Yes | Yes | No | No | No |
| Reduced | Reduced | Reduced | Normal | Normal | Normal |
| Yes | No | No | No | Yes/no | Yes/no |
| Yes | No | No | No | Yes/no | Yes/no |
| Yes | No | No | No | Yes/no | Yes/no |
| Yes | No | No | No | Yes/no | Yes/no |

tuberculosis
lymphoma
leukaemia
myeloma
- Hypersplenism: portal hypertension
  Felty's syndrome lipidoses
- Megaloblastic anaemia
- Myelosclerosis
- Paroxysmal nocturnal
  haemoglobinuria
- Osteopetrosis (marble bone disease)

# Megaloblastic anaemia

## Causes of megaloblastic anaemia
Vitamin B$_{12}$ deficiency
Folate deficiency

### Abnormalities of vitamin B$_{12}$ or folate metabolism
- Congenital: transcobalamin II
  deficiency
  Homocystinuria
  Methylmalonic aciduria
- Acquired: nitrous oxide
  Dihydrofolate reductase inhibitors
  (Methotrexate, Pyrimethamine,
  Trimethoprim)

### General defects in DNA synthesis
- Congenital: orotic aciduria
  Lesch–Nyhan syndrome
- Acquired: primary acquired
  sideroblastic anaemia
  Myeloid leukaemias
  Cytotoxic drugs (Mercaptopurine,
  Cytosine, Hydroxyurea, 5 fluorouracil)
  Alcohol

## Vitamin B$_{12}$ metabolism
- Naturally synthesised by micro-organisms
- Found in foods of animal origin. Not
  found in fruit or vegetables
- B$_{12}$ in food bound with intrinsic factor
  (IF) produced by gastric parietal cells
- This complex passes through the small

bowel to the terminal ileum, where
B$_{12}$ is absorbed
- Absorbed B$_{12}$ is bound to
  transcobalamin II (TCII) and
  transported to the bone marrow
- Most B$_{12}$ in the plasma is bound to
  transcobalamin I (TCI)
- Normal dietary intake is 7–30 µg/day
- Minimum daily requirement is 1–2 µg
- Maximum absorption is 2–3 µg/day
- Body stores are 2–3 mg (sufficient for
  2–4 years)

## Causes of B$_{12}$ deficiency
Malabsorption
- Pernicious anaemia
- Gastrectomy
- Congenital intrinsic factor deficiency
- Chronic tropical sprue
- Terminal ileal disease (Crohn's disease,
  ileal resection)
- Bacterial overgrowth
- Pancreatic disease
- Fish tapeworm
- Drugs: biguanides, anticonvulsants,
  neomycin, alcohol, colchicine
- Transcobalamin II deficiency
- Zollinger–Ellison syndrome
- Coeliac disease

### Dietary insufficiency
- Veganism

## Folate metabolism
- Humans are unable to synthesise folate
  de novo and require it from the diet
- Found in fruit and vegetables.
  (Destroyed by thorough cooking)
- Absorbed in the duodenum and
  jejunum
- When absorbed folate is converted to
  methyl tetrahydrofolate
- Mainly stored in the liver
- Normal dietary intake is 600–1000
  µg/day
- Minimum daily requirement is
  100–200 µg

- Maximum absorption is 300–800 µg/day
- Body stores are 10–12 mg (sufficient for 4 months)

## Causes of folate deficiency

### Dietary insufficiency
- Poverty
- Partial gastrectomy
- Scurvy
- Kwashiorkor
- Alcohol abuse

### Malabsorption
- Coeliac disease
- Tropical sprue
- Partial gastrectomy
- Jejunal resection
- Crohn's disease
- Congenital specific malabsorption
- Lymphoma
- Drugs: cholestyramine, sulphasalazine

### Increased requirements
- Pregnancy
- Lactation
- Prematurity
- Malignancy: carcinoma, lymphoma, myeloma, leukaemia
- Haemolytic anaemias
- Myelosclerosis
- Sideroblastic anaemia
- Homocystinuria
- Inflammatory diseases: Crohn's disease, tuberculosis, rheumatoid arthritis, psoriasis, erythroderma

### Excess urinary excretion
- Cardiac failure
- Acute liver disease
- Chronic renal dialysis

### Drugs
- Anticonvulsants

# Abnormalities of white cells

## Causes of neutrophilia

- Bacterial infection
- Inflammatory conditions: connective tissue diseases, vasculitis
- Tissue necrosis: myocardial infarction, pulmonary embolus, trauma
- Metabolic disorders: acidosis, eclampsia, gout
- Malignancy
- Haemolytic anaemia
- Acute haemorrhage
- Steroids
- Myeloproliferative disorders

## Causes of neutropenia

### Pancytopenia

### Drugs
- Anti-inflammatories
- Antibiotics (chloramphenicol, sulphonamides, cotrimoxazole)
- Anticonvulsants (phenytoin)
- Antithyroids (carbimazole)
- Hypoglycaemics (tolbutamide)
- Phenothiazines (chlorpromazine, promethazine)
- Miscellaneous (mepacrine, phenindione)

### Benign familial

### Cyclical

### Infections
- Viral
- Bacterial

### Miscellaneous
- Autoimmunity
- SLE
- Anaphylaxis

# Causes of monocytosis

- Chronic bacterial infection
- Protozoal diseases
- Chronic neutropenia
- Hodgkin's disease
- Myelomonocytic leukaemia
- Monocytic leukaemia

# Causes of eosinophilia

## Parasitic infection
- Amoebiasis
- Hookworm
- Ascariasis
- Tapeworms
- Filariasis
- Schistosomiasis

## Allergic diseases
- Bronchial asthma
- Hayfever
- Urticaria
- Food sensitivity

## Skin disease
- Psoriasis
- Pemphigus
- Dermatitis herpetiformis

## Miscellaneous
- Pulmonary eosinophilia
- Hypereosinophilic syndrome
- Drug sensitivity
- Polyarteritis nodosa
- Hodgkin's disease
- Eosinophilic leukaemia
- Post-acute sepsis

# Causes of basophilia

- Myeloproliferative disorders
- Hypothyroidism
- Smallpox infection
- Chickenpox infection

- Ulcerative colitis
- Tuberculosis
- Haemolytic anaemia
- Carcinoma
- Splenectomy

# Causes of lymphocytosis

## Infections
- Acute viral infection
- Chronic (tuberculosis, toxoplasmosis, brucellosis)

## Thyrotoxicosis

## CLL

# Causes of lymphopenia

- Bone marrow failure
- Normal
- Steroid therapy
- Immunosuppression
- Hodgkin's disease
- Radiation

# Causes of leukaemoid reaction

This is a reactive excessive leukocytosis characterised by the presence of immature cells in the peripheral blood, usually involving granulocytes.
- Severe infection
- Chronic infection
- Severe haemolysis
- Metastatic malignancy

# Causes of leuko-erythroblastic picture

This is characterised by the presence of immature red blood cells (erythroblasts), as well as immature white cells.

## Marrow infiltration

- Systemic malignancy
- Myelosclerosis
- Myeloid leukaemias
- Tuberculosis
- Lipidoses
- Marble-bone disease (osteopetrosis)

## Extramedullary haemopoeisis

- Severe haemorrhage
- Severe haemolysis
- Megaloblastic anaemia

# Leukaemia

Leukaemia is an accumulation of abnormal white cells in the bone marrow.

# Aetiology of leukaemia

## Viral infection

- EBV (Burkitt's lymphoma)
- HTLV (T-cell leukaemia)

## Radiation

**Table 7.4: Differentiation between leukaemoid reaction and chronic granulocytic leukaemia (CGL)**

| Leukaemoid reaction | CGL |
|---|---|
| Toxic granulation | Large proportion of myelocytes |
| Dohle bodies | Philadelphia chromosome |
| High neutrophil alkaline phosphatase | Low neutrophil alkaline phosphatase |

**Table 7.5: Differences between acute lymphoid leukaemia (ALL) and acute myeloid leukaemia (AML)**

| Feature | ALL | AML |
|---|---|---|
| Cell morphology | Undifferentiated blasts | Differentiation of blasts |
| Myeloperoxidase cytochemistry | – | + |
| Sudan black cytochemistry | – | + |
| Non-specific esterase cytochemistry | – | + |
| PAS cytochemistry | Coarse | Fine |
| Acid phosphatase cytochemistry | + (Thy ALL) | – |
| TdT enzyme test | + | – |
| Serum lysozyme | – | + |
| Anti-TdT | + | – |
| Rosettes with sheep RBC | + (Thy ALL) | – |
| Remission rate | 90% | 60–80% |
| Time to remission | + | ++ |
| Length of remission | ++ | + |
| Marrow failure | + | ++ |
| CNS prophylaxis | Yes | No |
| Bone marrow transplant | 2nd remission | 1st remission |
| Overall prognosis | Favourable | Poor |

# Lymphoma

## Histological classification of Hodgkin's disease

### *Lymphocyte predominant*
- Lymphocyte proliferation dominates
- Few Reed–Sternberg cells
- Nodular and diffuse patterns are recognised
- Associated with most favourable prognosis

### *Nodular sclerosis*
- Characterised by nodules of abnormal tissue
- Characteristic lacunar cell often found
- Cellular infiltrate may be lymphocyte predominant
- Mixed cellularity or lymphocyte depleted

### *Mixed cellularity*
- Numerous Reed–Sternberg cells
- Intermediate lymphocyte numbers

### *Lymphocyte depleted*
- Reticular pattern with predominant

## *Hereditary*
- Down's syndrome
- Fanconi's anaemia
- Bloom's syndrome
- Ataxia telangiectasia

## *Chemicals*
- Benzene
- Industrial solvents
- Cytotoxic drugs

Acute leukaemias are characterised by more than 50% blast cells in the marrow. AML-M3 is associated with disseminated intravascular coagulation (DIC).

**Table 7.6: Clinical staging of lymphomas**

|        | Clinical features |
|--------|-------------------|
| *Stage* |                  |
| 1      | Node involvement in one lymph node area |
| 2      | Involvement of two or more lymph node areas confined to one side of the diaphragm |
| 3      | Involvement of lymph nodes above and below the diaphragm and/or splenic involvement |
| 4      | Involvement outside the lymph node areas (includes infiltration of bone marrow, liver and other extranodal sites) |
| *Suffix* |                 |
| *a*:   | the absence of constitutional symptoms |
| *b*:   | the presence of constitutional symptoms |
| $_e$:  | denotes localised extranodal extension that does not advance the stage |
| $_s$:  | indicates splenic involvement |

Reed–Sternberg cells
- Sparse number of lymphocytes in a diffuse fibrotic pattern
- Associated with the worst prognosis

# Classification of non-Hodgkin's lymphoma

## Kiel classification
### Low-grade malignancy
- Lymphocytic
- Lymphoplasmacytoid
- Centrocytic

### High-grade malignancy
- Centroblastic
- Immunoblastic
- Lymphoblastic

## Rappaport classification
### Nodular lymphomas
- Lymphocytic poorly differentiated
- Mixed lymphocyte–histiocytic
- Histiocytic

### Diffuse lymphomas
- Lymphocytic well differentiated
- Lymphocytic poorly differentiated
- Mixed lymphocytic–histiocytic
- Histiocytic undifferentiated

# Causes of lymphadenopathy

## Infection
- Bacterial
- Viral
- Fungal
- Protozoal

## Inflammatory diseases
- Connective tissue diseases
- Sarcoidosis

## Malignancy
- Lymphoma
- Leukaemia
- Carcinoma
- Sarcoma
- Melanoma

## Immunological
- Angioimmunoblastic lymphadenopathy
- Hyperthyroidism
- Addison's disease

## Congenital
- Histiocytosis
- Lymphangioma
- Cystic hygroma

## Drugs
- Phenytoin
- Beryllium

# Myeloproliferative disorders

## Types of myeloproliferative disorder

- Polycythaemia rubra vera
- Essential thrombocythaemia
- Myelosclerosis

## Causes of polycythaemia

### Primary
- Polycythaemia rubra vera

### Secondary
#### Compensatory increase in erythropoietin
- Chronic pulmonary disease
- High altitude
- Congenital cyanotic heart disease

- Alveolar hypoventilation
- Familial polycythaemia
- Smoking
- Methaemoglobinaemia

### Inappropriate increase in erythropoietin
- Chronic renal disease
- Massive uterine fibromyomata
- Hepatocellular carcinoma
- Cerebellar haemangioblastoma
- Cushing's syndrome
- Phaeochromocytoma

### Relative
- Stress (spurious) polycythaemia
- Hypovolaemia

## Causes of thrombocythaemia

### Reactive
- <u>Haemorrhage</u>
- <u>Trauma</u>
- <u>Postoperative</u>
- Chronic iron deficiency
- Malignancy
- Chronic infections
- Connective tissue diseases
- Postsplenectomy with continuing haemolysis

### Endogenous
- Essential thrombocythaemia
- Polycythaemia rubra vera
- Myelosclerosis
- CGL

# Platelet disorders

## Causes of thrombocytopenia

### Increased destruction of platelets
**Acute immune thrombocytopenic purpura**
- Postviral infection

**Chronic autoimmune thrombocytopenic purpura**
- Idiopathic
- Post vaccination
- Measles
- Chickenpox
- Glandular fever

**Secondary immune thrombocytopenia**
- Post infection
- SLE
- CLL
- Lymphomas

**Drug-induced immune thrombocytopenia**
- Quinine
- Quinidine
- PAS
- Sulphonamides
- Rifampicin
- Digoxin
- Heparin

**Miscellaneous**
- Post-transfusion purpura
- Disseminated intravascular coagulation

### Failure of platelet production
- Drugs
- Chemicals
- Viral infection
- Pancytopenia

### Abnormal distribution of platelets
- Splenomegaly

# Causes of disseminated intravascular coagulation

## Sepsis
- Gram-negative septicaemia
- Meningococcal septicaemia
- Falciparum malaria

## Shock
- Hypovolaemia
- Anaphylaxis
- Severe burns
- Severe hypothermia

## Obstetric complications
- Amniotic fluid embolism
- Intrauterine death
- Abruptio placentae

## Tissue factor release
- Severe trauma
- Burns
- Promyelocytic leukaemia
- Haemolytic transfusion reactions
- Acute pancreatitis

## Miscellaneous
- Microangiopathic haemolytic anaemia
- Malignant hypertension
- Giant haemangiomas
- Pre-eclampsia
- Thrombotic thrombocytopenic purpura
- Snake bites
- Malignancy

# Disorders of platelet function

## Hereditary
- Thrombasthenia
- Bernard–Soulier syndrome
- Von Willebrand's disease
- Cyclo-oxygenase deficiency

## Acquired

- Aspirin
- Hyperglobulinaemia (multiple myeloma, Waldenström's macroglobulinaemia)
- Uraemia
- Liver disease
- Myeloproliferative disorders

# Blood coagulation

## Normal haemostatic response

### Vasoconstriction
- Injured vessels immediately vasoconstrict, slowing blood flow to the area of injury
- This prevents exsanguination and allows contact activation of platelets and coagulation factors

### Platelet reactions
- Platelets initially adhere to exposed connective tissue of an injured vessel
- Platelet adhesion is dependent on von Willebrand's factor
- Following adherence, the platelets release the contents of their granules

---

**Box 7.9: Tests of haemostatic function**

Full blood count
Blood film examination
Bleeding time (tests platelet function)
Prothrombin time (tests the instrinsic and common pathways of coagulation cascade)
Activated partial thromboplastin time (measures the intrinsic pathway of the coagulation cascade)
Fibrinogen levels
Thrombin time (assesses fibrinogen levels)
Specific coagulation factor assays
Fibrin degradation products (measure fibrinolysis)

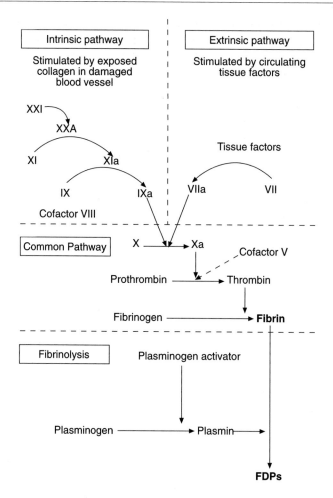

**Fig. 7.6: Coagulation cascade**

**Table 7.7: Features of coagulation disorders**

| Feature | Haemophilia A | Haemophilia B | Von Willebrand's disease |
|---|---|---|---|
| Inheritance | X-linked | X-linked | Autosomal dominant |
| Sites of haemorrhage | Muscle, joints | Muscle, joints | Mucous membranes |
| Platelet count | Normal | Normal | Normal |
| Bleeding time | Normal | Normal | Prolonged |
| PT | Normal | Normal | Normal |
| APPT | Prolonged | Prolonged | Normal/prolonged |
| Factor VIII:C | Low | Normal | Low |
| Factor VIII:AG | Normal | Normal | Low |
| Factor IX | Normal | Low | Normal |
| Ristocetin-induced platelet aggregation | Normal | Normal | Impaired |

(ADP, serotonin, fibrinogen, lysozomal enzymes, heparin and platelet-neutralising factor (platelet factor IV)
- Prostaglandin synthesis is also stimulated, leading to the production of thromboxane A2
- This substance potentiates platelet aggregation and has a powerful vasoconstrictive activity
- The aggregation of further platelets leads to the formation of a firm haemostatic plug
- This process is in theory self-perpetuating but is inhibited and controlled by prostacycline produced by endothelial and smooth muscle cells in the vessel wall

## Stabilisation of platelet plug
- Following formation of the haemostatic plug, coagulation pathways are activated (Fig. 7.6)
- This leads to the formation of fibrin
- Fibrin forms a mesh which anchors and extends the platelet plug

- After 24 hours the platelets autolyse and leave this fibrin mesh in place
- The production of fibrin is regulated by the process of fibrinolysis (Fig. 7.6)

# Anticoagulant Drugs

## Heparin
- An acidic mucopolysaccharide
- Not absorbed from the GI tract
- Inactivated by the liver and excreted in the urine
- Half-life 1 hour
- Potentiates antithrombin 3
- Effects of heparin reversed by protamine sulphate

## Warfarin
- Commonly used oral anticoagulant
- Well absorbed from the gut
- Acts as a vitamin K antagonist
- Decreases biological activity of vitamin K-dependent factors (2, 7, 9 and 10)

### Table 7.8: ABO blood group system

| Phenotype | Genotype | Antigens | Antibodies | Frequency in UK (%) |
|-----------|----------|----------|------------|---------------------|
| O | OO | O | Anti-A, B | 46 |
| A | AO or AO | A | Anti-B | 42 |
| B | BB or BO | B | Anti-A | 9 |
| AB | AB | AB | None | 3 |

### Table 7.9: Other blood products

| Product | Uses |
|---------|------|
| Granulocyte concentrates | Neutropenia |
| Platelet concentrates | Thrombocytopenia |
| Fresh frozen plasma (coagulation factors) | Haemophilia, massive haemorrhage, to counteract warfarin-induced haemorrhage |
| Human albumin infusions | Hypoalbuminaemia |
| Cryoprecipitate (factor VIII and fibrinogen) | Haemophilia A, von Willebrand's disease |
| Fibrinogen | Disseminated intravascular coagulation |
| Immunoglobulin | Hypogammaglobulinaemia |
| $C_1$ esterase inhibitor | $C_1$ esterase inhibitor deficiency |

- Actions of warfarin are reversed by fresh frozen plasma and vitamin K

### Thrombolytic agents
- These are enzymes which potentiate plasmin to enhance fibrinolysis

# Blood transfusion

## Red blood cells

- Approximately 400 blood group antigens have been described
- These are inherited in a simple Mendelian fashion
- They are stable characteristics and useful for paternity testing
- The most important blood group antigens are ABO (Table 7.8) and the rhesus groups

## Complications of blood transfusion

### Early
- Pyrogenic reactions due to plasma proteins or HLA antibodies
- Volume overload
- Immediate haemolysis
- Delayed haemolysis
- Reactions due to infected blood
- Allergic reactions to white cells platelets or proteins
- Air embolism
- Thrombophlebitis
- Citrate toxicity
- Hypokalaemia
- Clotting abnormalities (after massive transfusion)

### Late
- Transmission of viral disease
- Iron overload
- Immune sensitisation

# Spleen disorders

## Normal anatomy

The adult spleen is 8–13 cm in length and weighs 200–300 g.

## Functions of the spleen

- Haemopoieisis
- Red blood cell sequestration
- Red blood cell phagocytosis
- Cell-mediated immune competence
- Humoral immune competence
- Blood pool
- Control of plasma volume

## Causes of splenomegaly

### Infection
- Viral infection
- Tropical infection (malaria, kala-azar, schistosomiasis)
- Chronic bacterial infection (tuberculosis, brucellosis)

### Portal hypertension
- Hepatic or portal vein thrombosis
- Congestive cardiac failure
- Hepatic cirrhosis
- Biliary cirrhosis

### Haematological disorders
- Haemolytic anaemias
- Lymphoproliferative disorders
- Myeloproliferative disorders

### Miscellaneous
- Collagen vascular disease (Felty's syndrome, SLE)
- Metabolic storage disease (Niemann–Pick disease, Gaucher's disease, histiocytosis X)
- Sarcoidosis
- Amyloid

- Splenic tumours

## Causes of hyposplenism

- Splenectomy
- Sickle cell disease
- Coeliac disease
- Congenital absence
- SLE
- Senile atrophy
- Inflammatory bowel disease
- Essential thrombocythaemia
- Fanconi's anaemia
- Steroids
- Cytotoxic drugs

# Hypercoagulopathy

Term used for any situation which shows an increased risk of thromboembolism.

## Causes of hypercoagulopathy

### Circulatory stasis
- Prolonged immobility
- Pelvic tumours
- Pregnancy
- Cardiac failure
- Hypovolaemia
- Hyperviscosity

### Abnormalities of platelet–vessel wall interaction
- Essential thrombocythaemia
- Diabetes mellitus
- Thrombotic thrombocytopenic purpura

### Coagulation factor abnormalities
- Increased levels of factor VIII
- Factor V leiden

- Antithrombin III deficiency
- Lupus anticoagulant
- Protein C deficiency
- Protein S deficiency

## Causes of hyperviscosity

- Polycythaemia
- Paraproteinaemia (Waldenström's macroglobulinaemia, myeloma)
- Chronic myeloid leukaemia
- Acute leukaemia with high white cell count
- Iatrogenic

## Causes of paraproteinaemia

- Multiple myeloma
- Benign monoclonal gammopathy
- Waldenström's macroglobulinaemia
- Malignant lymphoma
- CLL
- Chronic cold haemagglutinin disease
- Carcinoma
- Heavy chain disease

# Bone marrow transplantation

## Indications for bone marrow transplantation

### Aplastic anaemia
- Persistent life-threatening agranulocytosis or thrombocytopenia

### Acute leukaemia
- ALL (second remission)

- AML (first remission)
- Blast crisis in CGL

## *Chronic granulocytic leukaemia (chronic phase)*

## *Congenital haematological disorders*
- Immunodeficiency

# Complications of bone marrow transplantation

## *Immediate*
- Effects of pancytopenia
- Drug toxicity (rashes, cardiomyopathy, parotitis, pancreatitis, gastrointestinal symptoms

## *Early (first few weeks)*
- Graft rejection
- Infection
- Acute graft-versus-host disease
- Interstitial pneumonitis
- Leukaemic relapse

## *Late (months)*
- Chronic graft-versus-host disease
- Leukaemic relapse
- Infection

## *Long term*
- Cataracts
- Sterility
- Growth retardation

# Section III

# Organ-based Diseases

# 8 Cardiology

## Contents

## Anatomy

- Normal heart weighs 250–300g
- Major cardiac cell is the myocyte
- Each myocyte is 100 μm long and 15 μm wide
- Each myocyte contains 150 myofibrils (1 μm in diameter)
- Each myofibril is made up of repeating contraction units called sarcomeres (2 μm in length) (Fig. 8.1)
- The A band is 1.5 μm in length and consists of thick filaments
- Each thick filament is comprised of 400 myosin molecules
- Each myosin molecule has a molecular weight of 460,000 daltons
- Interdigitating with the thick filaments are thin filaments
- Thin filaments are comprised of two chains of actin molecules forming a

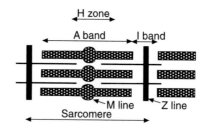

**Fig. 8.1: Diagrammatic interpretation of the relationship between thick and thin filaments in a sarcomere**

helical structure
- Each actin molecule has a molecular weight of 42,000 daltons
- On the actin chains are tropomyosin molecules (MW 68,000 daltons) and troponin complexes
- Each troponin complex consists of troponin C (MW 18,000 daltons), troponin I (MW 28,000 daltons) and

troponin T (MW 41,000 daltons)

## Conduction system of the heart

- Sinoatrial node located at the junction between the superior vena cava and right atrium
- Atrioventricular node found in the lower interatrial septum
- Nerve supply to the heart comes from (1) adrenergic nerves supplying atrial and ventricular muscle and nerve conduction system via $B_1$ receptors and (2) cholinergic nerves via the vagus nerve which supply the sinoatrial and atrioventricular nodes via $M_2$ muscarinic receptors

## Blood supply to the heart

- Blood supply to the heart comes from the coronary arteries
- Right coronary artery arises from the right coronary sinus and runs down the atrioventricular groove, giving vessels to the right atrium and right ventricle. It continues as the posterior descending coronary artery, running posteriorly in the intraventricular groove and supplying the posterior intraventricular septum and posterior left ventricular wall
- Left coronary artery arises from the left coronary sinus. Left main coronary artery divides into left anterior descending artery which runs in the anterior intraventricular groove supplying the anterior left ventricular wall. The circumflex artery runs along the left atrioventricular groove and gives branches to the left atrium and left ventricle (marginal branches)
- The sinus node is supplied by the right coronary artery in 60% of people
- The atrioventricular node is supplied by the right coronary artery in 90% of people
- Resting coronary blood flow is 0.8 ml/min/g
- Resting cardiac oxygen consumption is 27 ml/min

# Physiology

For normal cardiac pressure and saturations, see Table 8.1.

**Table 8.1: Normal cardiac pressure and saturations**

| Location | Pressure (mmHg) | | $O_2$ Saturation (%) |
|---|---|---|---|
| Right atrium | a | 2–10 | 74 |
| | v | 2–10 | |
| | Mean | 0–8 | |
| Right ventricle | Systolic | 15–30 | 74 |
| | End-diastolic | 0–8 | |
| Pulmonary artery | Systolic | 15–30 | 74 |
| | End-diastolic | 3–12 | |
| | Mean | 9–16 | |
| Pulmonary capillary wedge (left atrium) | a | 3–15 | 98 |
| | v | 3–12 | |
| | Mean | 1–10 | |
| Left ventricle | Systolic | 100–140 | 98 |
| | End-diastolic | 3–12 | |
| Aorta | Systolic | 100–140 | 98 |
| | End-diastolic | 60–90 | |

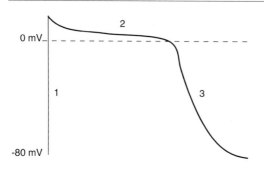

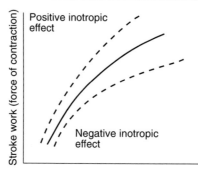

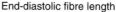

**Fig. 8.2: Myocardial cell action potential**

**Fig. 8.3: The relationship between end-diastolic fibre length and left ventricular stroke work**
*Shows displacement to the left with an increase in contractility and to the right with a reduction in contractility*

## Cardiac muscle contraction
- Calcium released from the sarco-plasmic reticulum binds to troponin C
- This complex inhibits troponin I, which usually prevents interaction between actin and myosin
- Inhibition of troponin I leads to actin–myosin interaction and shortening of the sarcomere
- Shortening of the sarcomere leads to muscle contraction
- Contraction ends when calcium is reabsorbed back into the sarcoplasmic reticulum

## Energy for contraction
- Major energy substrates for the heart are fatty acids, glucose and lactate
- In the resting state 60% of the total oxygen consumption of the heart comes from metabolism of fatty acids, 28% from glucose and 11% from lactate
- During exercise fatty acid metabolism increases
- During ischaemia or hypoxia the main substrate becomes glucose

## Action potential (Fig. 8.2)
> *Phase 1* caused by rapid sodium influx
> *Phase 2* caused by slow calcium and sodium influx (mainly calcium)
> *Phase 3* (repolarisation) caused by potassium efflux

## Myocardial mechanics
Myocardial contraction is dependent on inotropy, preload, afterload, rate and rhythm.

### Inotropy
- Inotropy refers to the force of muscle contraction and is mediated by changes in the amount of calcium released from the sarcoplasmic reticulum
- Increases in sympathetic discharge and circulating catecholamines are positively inotropic

### Preload
- Venous return to the heart is dependent on right atrial pressure, which is represented by the end-diastolic volume (EDV)
- Starling's law states that increases in end-diastolic volume lead to increases in contractility (Fig. 8.3)
- Negative inotropic effects shift the curve to the right
- Positive inotropic effects shift the curve to the left

### Afterload
- Afterload is a measure of the pulmonary and systemic vascular resistances that

ventricular pressures must exceed in order to produce a cardiac output
- Increasing afterload reduces cardiac output

### Rate and rhythm
- Increases in heart rate may improve contractile performance initially
- Too great an increase in heart rate reduces the time for ventricular filling and reduces cardiac output
- Increases in heart rate are mediated by circulating catecholamines and increases in sympathetic discharge
- Decreases in heart rate are mediated by effects on the sinoatrial and atrioventricular nodes

# Symptoms and signs

## Causes of chest pain

### Cardiac
- Angina pectoris
- Myocardial infarction
- Tachyarrhythmias
- Acute pericarditis
- Aortic stenosis
- Aneurysm of ascending aorta
- Dissecting aortic aneurysm
- Mitral valve prolapse
- Syndrome X
- Hypertrophic cardiomyopathy
- Prinzmetal's angina

### Pulmonary
- Pulmonary embolism
- Pneumonia
- Pulmonary hypertension
- Hyperventilation

### Gastrointestinal
- Gastro-oesophageal reflux
- Oesophagitis
- Oesophageal spasm

- Oesophageal rupture
- Peptic ulcer disease
- Gallbladder disease
- Pancreatic disease

### Musculoskeletal
- Muscular strain
- Costochondritis
- Rib metastases
- Thoracic spine pathology
- Bornholm's disease
- Rheumatoid arthritis
- Rib fractures
- Osteoarthritis

### Miscellaneous
- Varicella zoster
- Tabes dorsalis
- Da Costa's syndrome

## Characteristic features of chest pain

### Cardiac ischaemia
- Retrosternal tightness, radiating to neck, jaw, teeth and arms (usually left)
- Precipitated by exertion, particularly walking into a cold wind
- May occur after a large meal
- If unstable, may have rest and/or nocturnal pain
- Associated symptoms include nausea, vomiting, sweating and shortness of breath (SOB)
- Relieved by nitrates.

### Pericardial disease
- Similar to cardiac ischaemia
- Often has a pleuritic component and may be relieved by leaning forward
- Not relieved by nitrates

### Dissecting aneurysm
- Sudden, severe and tearing retrosternal pain, radiating through to the back and left shoulder

## Pulmonary disease

- Pleuritic pain, sharp in nature, well localised, worse on inspiration and on coughing
- May be aggravated by movement and associated with chest wall tenderness
- Dyspnoea more prominent than in cardiac ischaemia

## Gastro-oesophageal disease

- Retrosternal/upper abdominal pain, typically burning in nature but may mimic cardiac ischaemia
- Worse after eating (especially acidic or fatty food, hot liquids, alcohol) and in recumbent posture
- Oesophageal spasm may be exacerbated by exercise and relieved by nitrates
- Oesophageal rupture may mimic cardiac ischaemia.

## Gallbladder disease

- Intermittent episodes of severe colicky right upper quadrant (RUQ) pain radiating to tip of right shoulder blade
- May be associated with dyspepsia and vomiting
- Fatty food intolerance.

## Musculoskeletal problems

- Well localised with pinpoint tenderness
- Exacerbated by posture, movement, respiration and coughing
- No associated symptoms
- Relieved with simple analgesia

## Varicella zoster

- Localised to dermatome
- Hyperasthesia may precede rash.

## Da Costa's syndrome

- Intermittent, well localised left submammary stabbing pain lasting a few seconds at a time
- Associated with anxiety

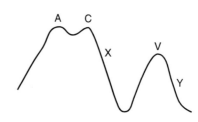

**Fig. 8.4:  Waveform of normal jugular venous pulse**

# Normal jugular venous pulse waveform (Fig. 8.4)

*A-wave*: represents atrial systole, occurs just before carotid pulse
*C-wave*: not visible with naked eye. Caused by tricuspid valve closure on atrial pressure
*X-descent*: represents fall in atrial pressure during ventricular systole
*V-wave*: represents atrial filling against closed tricuspid valve
*Y-descent*: represents diastolic collapse following opening of the tricuspid valve

# Abnormalities of jugular venous pulse

## Raised JVP with normal waveform

- Right heart failure
- Fluid overload
- Bradycardia

## Large a wave

- Tricuspid stenosis
- Pulmonary hypertension
- Pulmonary stenosis
- Left ventricular hypertrophy (Bernheim effect)
- Extrasystoles with atrioventricular conduction defects

- Fourth heart sound

### Cannon waves
- <u>Severe tricuspid stenosis</u>
- <u>Complete heart block</u>
- Nodal rhythms
- Ventricular extra systoles
- Ventricular tachycardia

### Absent A-wave
- Atrial fibrillation

### Large V-wave
- Tricuspid regurgitation

### Slow Y-descent
- <u>Tricuspid stenosis</u>
- Left ventricular hypertrophy

### Deep X- and Y-descents
- Constrictive pericarditis
- Pericardial tamponade

### Raised JVP with absent pulsation
- Superior vena cava (SVC) obstruction

## Causes of pulsus paradoxus

- <u>Severe acute asthma</u>
- <u>Constrictive pericarditis</u>
- <u>Pericardial tamponade</u>
- Hypovolaemia
- Massive pulmonary embolism

## Abnormalities of first heart sound

### Loud first heart sound
- <u>Mitral stenosis</u>
- Short PR interval
- Tachyarrhythmias

### Quiet first heart sound
- <u>Mitral regurgitation</u>
- <u>Pericardial effusion</u>
- Prolonged PR interval
- Heart block
- Aortic stenosis

### Variable intensity first heart sound
- Third-degree atrioventricular block
- Atrial fibrillation
- Nodal tachycardia
- Ventricular tachycardia

## Causes of third heart sound

- <u>Young age (normal)</u>
- <u>Severe non-rheumatic mitral regurgitation</u>
- <u>Left ventricular dilatation</u>
- Constrictive pericarditis
- Restrictive cardiomyopathy
- Hypertrophic cardiomyopathy
- Ventricular septal defect (VSD)
- Thyrotoxicosis

## Causes of fourth heart sound

- Left ventricular dilatation
- Left ventricular hypertrophy
- Post acute myocardial infarction

## Abnormalities of second heart sound

### Wide splitting of second heart sound
- <u>Pulmonary hypertension</u>
- <u>Pulmonary stenosis</u>
- Massive pulmonary embolus
- Right bundle branch block
- Deep inspiration

- Mitral regurgitation
- VSD

## Fixed splitting of second heart sound
- Atrial septal defect (ASD)

## Reverse splitting of second heart sound
- Systemic hypertension
- Aortic stenosis
- Left bundle branch block
- β-blockers (if pre-existing left ventricular disease)
- Patent ductus arteriosus
- Right ventricular pacing

## Loud A2
- Systolic hypertension
- Tachycardia
- Transposition

## Soft A2
- Aortic stenosis

## Loud P2
- Pulmonary hypertension

## Soft P2
- Pulmonary stenosis

# Causes of ejection systolic murmurs

- Aortic stenosis
- Aortic sclerosis
- Pulmonary stenosis
- Hyperdynamic circulation
- Closing VSD
- Functional due to increased flow, (ASD, total anomalous pulmonary venous drainage)
- Hypertrophic cardiomyopathy

# Causes of pansystolic murmurs

- Mitral regurgitation
- Tricuspid regurgitation
- Atrial myxoma
- VSD
- Mitral valve prolapse

# Causes of early diastolic murmurs

- Aortic regurgitation
- Pulmonary regurgitation
- Graham Steel murmur (mitral stenosis)

# Causes of mid-diastolic murmurs

- Mitral stenosis
- Tricuspid stenosis
- Atrial myxoma
- Austin Flint murmur (aortic regurgitation)
- Carey Coombs murmur (active rheumatic fever)
- Functional owing to increased flow (ASD, VSD, persistent ductus arteriosus, mitral valve prolapse)

# Causes of continuous machinery murmurs

- Prosthetic valve
- Persistent ductus arteriosus
- Venous hum
- Aorticopulmonary septal defect
- Pulmonary AV fistula
- Bronchial artery anastomosis in pulmonary atresia
- Artificial ductus (Blalock shunt)

# Electrocardiogram

## Normal ECG

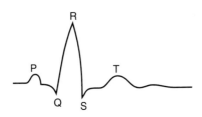

**Fig. 8.5: Normal electrocardiographic electrical complex**

- *P-wave*: represents atrial contraction
- *PR-interval*: represents time for depolarisation wave to reach atrio-ventricular node (AVN) (normally 0.12–0.2 s)
- *QRS-complex*: represents ventricular contraction (normally < 0.12 s)
- *QT-interval*: represents time for ventricular contraction and relaxation (normally 0.38–0.42 s)
- *ST-segment*: represents refractory period of absent electrical activity
- *T-wave*: represents repolarisation

## Causes of bundle branch block

### Right bundle branch block
- Young age (normal)
- Pulmonary embolism
- Pulmonary hytertension

- Ischaemic heart disease
- Isolated congenital lesion
- Congenital heart disease (ASD, Fallot's tetralogy)
- Pulmonary stenosis
- Hyperkalaemia

### Left bundle branch block
- Ischaemic heart disease
- Cardiomyopathy
- Left ventricular hypertrophy

## Abnormalities of QT-interval

### Short QT-interval
- Digoxin
- Tachycardia
- Hypercalcaemia
- Hyperthermia
- Hyperkalaemia

### Prolonged QT-interval
- Drugs:
  Class Ia and III agents
  Flecainide, terfenadine
  Tricyclic antidepressants
- Acute myocardial infarction
- Hypocalcaemia
- Acute myocarditis
- Cerebral injury
- Hypertrophic cardiomyopathy
- Hypothermia
- Torsades de pointes
- Jervel–Lange–Neilson syndrome
- Romano–Ward syndrome
- Hypokalaemia
- Organophosphate poisoning

---

**Box 8.1: Abnormalities of PR-interval**

**Short**
Tachycardia
Wolff–Parkinson–White syndrome
Lown–Ganong–Levine syndrome

**Prolonged**
AV block

# Congenital heart disease

## Incidence

Congenital heart disease occurs in approximately 8 per 1,000 live births.

## Complications of cyanotic congenital heart disease

- Polycythaemia
- Hyperuricaemia
- Skin sepsis
- Gingivitis
- Renal failure
- Hyperviscosity syndrome
- Anaemia
- Cerebral abscess
- Arthritis

## Causes of Eisenmenger's syndrome

- VSD
- ASD
- Patent ductus arteriosus
- Transposition of the great arteries
- Tricuspid atresia with large VSD
- Total anomalous pulmonary venous drainage

# Arrhythmias

## Causes of sinus bradycardia

- Normal in athletes and during sleep
- Ischaemic heart disease
- Myocardial infarction
- Drugs: digoxin, β-blockers, adenosine, verapamil
- Hypothermia
- Hypokalaemia
- Obstructive jaundice
- Uraemia
- Raised intercranial pressure
- Sick sinus syndrome
- Hypothyroidism

## Causes of sick sinus syndrome

- Ischaemic heart disease
- Sinus node degeneration/fibrosis
- Cardiomyopathy
- Myocarditis
- Amyloid
- Drugs: digoxin, quinidine, β-blockers
- Cardiac surgery

**Table 8.2: Types of congenital heart disease**

| Cyanotic | Acyanotic |
|---|---|
| Severe pulmonary stenosis | VSD |
| Fallot's tetralogy | Persistent ductus arteriosus |
| Transposition of the great arteries | Congenital aortic stenosis |
| Tricuspid atresia | Coarctation of the aorta |
| Pulmonary atresia | ASD |
| Ebstein's anomaly with ASD | |
| Hypoplastic left heart | |
| Total anomalous pulmonary venous drainage | |

**Table 8.3: Causes of congenital heart disease**

| Cause | Defects |
| --- | --- |
| Rubella | Persistent ductus arteriosus |
| | ASD |
| | Pulmonary stenosis |
| Alcohol | VSD |
| Lithium | Ebstein's anomaly |
| | Tricuspid atresia |
| Marfan's syndrome | Aortic dilatation and incompetence |
| | Mitral incompetence |
| Ehlers–Danlos | Mitral regurgitation |
| | Arterial dilatation |
| Mucopolysaccharidoses | Valve disease |
| | Cardiomyopathy |
| Homocystinuria | Aortic and pulmonary dilatation |
| Pompes' disease | Dilated cardiomyopathy |
| Down's syndrome | ASD |
| | VSD |
| | Fallot's tetralogy |
| Trisomies 13 and 18 | VSD |
| | Pulmonary stenosis |
| Turner's syndrome | Coarctation of the aorta |
| | Bicuspid aortic valve |
| | Pulmonary stenosis |
| | VSD |

# Causes of atrioventricular block

- Young age (1st degree, Wenkebach may be normal)
- Idiopathic fibrosis
- Ischaemic heart disease
- Myocardial infarction
- Aortic valve disease
- Cardiac surgery
- Infiltration (tumour)
- Syphilis
- Endocarditis
- Inflammation (ankylosing spondylitis)
- Reiter's syndrome
- Rheumatoid arthritis
- Sarcoidosis
- Rheumatic fever
- Dystrophia myotonica
- Diphtheria
- Chagas' disease
- Lymes' disease
- Scleroderma

# Causes of sinus tachycardia

- Anxiety
- Pain
- Fear
- Fever
- Exercise
- Drugs:
    adrenaline, atropine, salbutamol, aminophylline, caffeine
- Ischaemic heart disease

### Table 8.4: Antiarrhythmic drug classification

| Class | Action | Examples |
|-------|--------|----------|
| I | Impede transcellular sodium transport thereby reducing rate of rise of the action potential | |
| Ia | Increase duration of action potential | Quinidine, procainamide, disopyramide |
| Ib | Shorten duration of action potential | Lignocaine, mexiletine, propafenone |
| Ic | No effect on duration of action potential | Flecainide |
| II | Interfere with effects of sympathetic nervous system<br>Do not affect action potential | β-blockers, bretylium |
| III | Prolong duration of action potential and refractory period | Amiodarone, sotalol |
| IV | Impede transcellular calcium transport | Verapamil, diltiazem |

- Acute myocardial infarction
- Heart failure
- Pulmonary embolism
- Hypovolaemia
- Anaemia
- Hyperthyroidism

# Causes of atrial tachycardia

- Digoxin toxicity
- Ischaemic heart disease
- Rheumatic heart disease
- Cardiomyopathy
- Sick sinus syndrome

---

**Box 8.2: Differentiation between SVT and VT**

VT more likely if:
  broad QRS complexes > 0.14s (beware SVT with bundle branch block)
  bizarre QRS morphology (unlike bundle branch block)
  fusion and capture beats
  independent atrial activity
  marked axis deviation
  concordant chest lead pattern (all positive or all negative)
  complexes similar to ectopic beats

---

# Causes of atrial fibrillation

- Hypertension
- Ischaemic heart disease
- Alcohol
- Rheumatic mitral valve disease
- Sepsis (particularly older people)
- Atrial myxoma
- Hyperthyroidism
- Sick sinus syndrome
- Cardiomyopathy
- Atrial septal defect
- Pericarditis
- Myocarditis
- Pulmonary embolism
- Pneumonia
- Cardiac surgery
- Idiopathic
- Wolff–Parkinson–White syndrome

# Causes of ventricular tachycardia

- Acute myocardial infarction
- Ischaemic heart disease
- Proarrhythmic drugs
- Hypertrophic cardiomyopathy
- Dilated cardiomyopathy
- Mitral valve prolapse
- Myocarditis

- Congenital heart disease
- Idiopathic
- Electrolyte disturbance

## Causes of torsades de pointes

- <u>Drugs</u>: tricyclic antidepressants, erythromycin, quinidine, disopyramide
- Bradycardia due to sick sinus syndrome or AV block
- Romano–Ward syndrome
- Jervel–Lange–Neilson syndrome
- Hypokalaemia
- Hypomagnesaemia

# Ischaemic heart disease

## Management of acute myocardial infarction

- Urgent admission to coronary care unit and bed rest
- Oxygen, Aspirin 300 mg stat, analgesia and antiemetic (i.v. diamorphine and maxolon)
- *Thrombolysis*: ideally should be given within 1 hour of onset of symptoms. For major benefit must be given within 6 hours. No benefit after 24 hours
- *i.v. Heparin*: should be routinely given following rt-PA. Many centres routinely use it after any thrombolysis, but evidence for its benefits limited. Useful if continuing pain post infarct (unstable angina)
- *i.v. Insulin and Glucose*: as per sliding scale
- *i.v. β-blockers*: useful in patients with large anterolateral infarcts, tachycardia

and hypertension. Contraindicated if in cardiac failure
- *Nitrate infusion*: in conjunction with i.v. heparin, useful for patients with continuing pain. Also useful in patients with left ventricular failure or hypertension
- *Angiography*: can be used in the acute setting for patients with contra-indications to thrombolysis, or those with progressive infarction post thrombolysis. Depends on local availability
- *Treatment of complications*: anti-arrhythmics for arrhythmias
Diuretics for cardiac failure
Inotropes for cardiogenic shock
- *Subsequent treatment*: regular aspirin β-blockers (beware cardiac failure) ACE inhibitors particularly indicated in patients with large anterior infarctions, cardiac failure,

---

**Box 8.3: Risk factors for ischaemic heart disease**

<u>Increasing age</u>
<u>High total serum cholesterol</u>
<u>High total triglycerides</u>
<u>Low HDL cholesterol</u>
<u>Hypertension</u>
<u>Smoking</u>
<u>Glucose intolerance</u>
Male gender
Family history of premature ischaemic heart disease
Obesity
Lack of physical activity
High fibrinogen levels
Stress
Type A personality
Winter months
Soft water
Alcohol abuse
Chronic renal failure
Chronic obstructive pulmonary disease

diabetes mellitus
Lipid lowering agents
Antihypertensives and anti-
arrhythmics if indicated
Antianginals if postinfarct angina

# Indications for thrombolysis in acute myocardial infarction

- Patients with typical history of cardiac pain within the previous 24 hours
- ST elevation of at least 2 mm
- Typical history of cardiac pain plus left bundle branch block on ECG
- Particular benefit from thrombolysis is derived in the following groups of patients:
    anterior infarction; aged > 75 years; poor left ventricular function
- Patients whose pain began 24 hours previously should still receive thrombo-lysis if they continue to have pain.
- Patients with unstable angina should not receive thrombolysis

# Complications of acute myocardial infarction

- Sudden death
- Cardiac arrhythmia
- Cardiac failure
- Pericarditis
- Mural thrombus
- Systemic embolism
- Pulmonary embolism
- Pericardial tamponade
- Mitral regurgitation due to papillary muscle rupture
- Ventricular septal defect due to rupture of intraventricular septum
- Left ventricular aneurysm
- Shoulder–hand syndrome
- Depression

---

**Box 8.4: Contraindications to thrombolysis**

Recent stroke (in the last 6 months)
Recent gastrointestinal haemorrhage
Bleeding diathesis
Warfarin treatment
Recent surgery (within 1 month)
Pregnancy
Trauma
Prolonged cardiopulmonary resuscitation
Aortic dissection
Aortic aneurysm
Left ventricular aneurysm with thrombus
Liver disease
Renal disease
Menstrual bleeding
Active ulcerative colitis
Severe hypertension (> 200/l00)

---

# Cardiac failure

## Causes of cardiac failure

### *Low-output failure*
*Intrinsic heart muscle disease*
- Cardiomyopathy
- Ischaemia
- Infarction
- Hypertension
- Myocarditis
- Endocarditis

*Chronic excess afterload*
- Hypertension
- Aortic stenosis

*Chronic excess preload*
- Mitral regurgitation
- Restricted filling:
    constrictive pericarditis, pericardial tamponade, restrictive cardio-myopathy, bradycardia, negatively inotropic drugs, myocardial infarction

## High-output failure

- Anaemia
- Hyperthyroidism
- Paget's disease
- Arteriovenous malformation
- Pregnancy
- Thiamine deficiency (beri-beri)

# Management of acute pulmonary oedema

- Always look for underlying cause and treat accordingly
- Sit patient up
- Oxygen therapy
- Nebulised salbutamol: may provide some symptomatic relief, but beware tachycardia
- i.v. Diuretic: frusemide 40–80 mg stat
- i.v. Diamorphine 2.5 mg + maxolon 10 mg
- i.v. Nitrate infusion: particularly if coronary ischaemia or hypertension. Care if hypotension
- Inotropes: for cardiogenic shock
- i.v. Aminophylline: may be useful particularly if bronchospasm (cardiac asthma)
- Treat arryhthmias, hypertension and coronary ischaemia as indicated

# Cardiomyopathy

## Causes of cardiomyopathy

### Dilated
- Idiopathic
- Ischaemic heart disease
- Hypertension
- Alcohol
- Cobalt
- Haemochromatosis
- Uraemia
- Phaeochromocytoma

- Selenium deficiency (Keshan's disease)
- Sarcoid
- Myocarditis
- Amyloid
- Dermatomyositis
- Duchenne muscular dystrophy
- Dystrophia myotonica
- Facioscapulohumeral dystrophy
- Mitochondrial dystrophy
- Friedreich's ataxia
- Cytotoxic chemotherapy
- Postpartum
- Hypothyroidism
- Addison's disease
- Irradiation
- Glycogen storage diseases
- Acromegaly

### Restrictive
- Amyloid
- Carcinoid syndrome
- Sarcoid
- Haemochromatosis
- Hypereosinophilic syndrome
- Churg–Strauss syndrome
- Parasitic infection
- Filiariasis
- Schistosomiasis
- *Ascaris lumbricoides*
- Neoplastic infiltration
- Pseudoxanthoma elasticum
- Methysergide
- Hypertrophic cardiomyopathy
- Autosomal dominant inheritance
- Friedreich's ataxia
- Busulphan

# Valvular disease

## Causes of aortic stenosis

### Valvular
- Congenital (unicuspid or bicuspid)
- Senile calcification

**Box 8.5: Features suggestive of pathological murmur**

Symptoms
Cyanosis
Thrill
Cardiomegaly
Diastolic murmur
A loud murmur
ECG abnormalities

- Rheumatic fever
- Rheumatoid arthritis
- Hyperlipidaemia
- Infective endocarditis

### Supravalvular
- Williams' syndrome
- Hypercalcaemia
- Hypervitaminosis D
- Aortic valve regurgitation
- Mesenteric artery stenosis
- Thoracic aortic aneurysms
- Rubella

### Subvalvular
- Discrete fibromuscular ring
- Hypertrophic obstructive cardiomyopathy

# Causes of mitral stenosis

- Rheumatic fever
- Isolated congenital lesion
- Lutembacher's syndrome
- Senile calcification
- Infective endocarditis
- Rheumatoid arthritis
- SLE
- Mucopolysaccharidoses
- Endocardial fibroelastosis
- Malignant carcinoid syndrome

# Causes of aortic regurgitation

### Congenital
- Bicuspid aortic valve
- Supravalvular stenosis
- Discrete subvalvular fibromuscular ring
- Ventricular septal defect
- Ruptured sinus of Valsalva aneurysm

### Acquired
- Rheumatic fever
- Infective endocarditis
- Rheumatoid arthritis
- SLE
- Ankylosing spondylitis
- Reiter's syndrome
- Giant cell aortitis
- Relapsing polychondritis
- Pseudoxanthoma elasticum
- Mucopolysaccharidoses
- Aortic root dissection
- Syphilis
- Marfan's syndrome
- Ehlers–Danlos syndrome
- Osteogenesis imperfecta
- Psoriasis
- Hypertension
- Trauma
- Fallot's tetralogy

# Causes of mitral regurgitation

- Ischaemic heart disease
- Acute myocardial infarction
- Dilated cardiomyopathy
- Rheumatic fever
- Mitral valve prolapse
- Infective endocarditis
- Marfan's syndrome
- Ehlers–Danlos syndrome
- Pseudoxanthoma elasticum
- Osteogenesis imperfecta
- Thyrotoxicosis

- Endomyocardial fibrosis
- Mitral annular calcification
- Wolff–Parkinson–White syndrome
- Persistent ductus arteriosus
- Turner's syndrome
- Sarcoidosis
- Amyloidosis
- Mucopolysaccharidoses

## Causes of pulmonary stenosis

### Valvular
- Isolated congenital lesion
- Rheumatic fever
- Noonan's syndrome
- Fallot's tetralogy
- Rubella
- Carcinoid syndrome

### Supravalvular
- Isolated congenital lesion
- Ventricular septal defect
- Fallot's tetralogy
- Williams' syndrome

### Subvalvular
- Right-sided hypertrophic cardiomyopathy

## Causes of pulmonary regurgitation

- Pulmonary hypertension
- Mitral stenosis
- Rheumatic fever
- Carcinoid syndrome

## Causes of tricuspid stenosis

- Rheumatic fever
- Carcinoid syndrome
- Ebstein's anomaly
- Isolated congenital lesion

## Causes of tricuspid regurgitation

- Right heart failure
- Pulmonary hypertension
- Acute myocardial infarction
- Infective endocarditis
- Rheumatic fever
- Ebstein's anomaly
- Carcinoid syndrome
- Endomyocardial fibrosis
- Tricuspid valve prolapse

# Cardiac infections

## Causes of infective endocarditis

### Bacterial
- *Streptococcus viridans*
- *Enterococci*
- *Staphylococci (aureus, epidermidis)*
- *Haemophilus*
- *Bacteroides*
- *Escherichia coli*
- *Proteus*
- *Enterobacter*
- *Pseudomonas*
- *Seratia*
- *Listeria*
- *Brucella*
- *Legionella*
- *Fusobacterium*

### Rickettsiae
- *Coxiella burneti*
- *Chlamydia (psittaci, trachomatis)*

### Fungal
- *Candida*
- *Aspergillus*
- *Histoplasma*

**Box 8.6: Antibiotic prophylaxis against bacterial endocarditis**

1  Without anaesthetic or under local anaesthesia:
   Amoxycillin 3 g orally 1 hour before procedure.
   If allergic to penicillin, either clindamycin 600 mg 1 hour before procedure or erythromycin 1.5 g orally before procedure, plus 500 mg 6 hours later.
2  Under general anaesthetic:
   Amoxycillin 1 g intravenously with premedication plus 500 mg orally 6 hours later.
   If penicillin allergy, vancomycin 1 g i.v. over 30 min plus gentamicin 120 mg i.v. before induction or teicoplanin 400 mg i.v. and gentamicin 120 mg i.v. before induction or clindamycin 300 mg i.v. over 10 min before induction.
3  Special-risk patients, patients with prosthetic heart valves or history of previous infective endocarditis:
   Amoxycillin 1 g plus gentamicin 120 mg i.v. with premedication, plus amoxycillin 500 mg orally at 6 hours.
   If penicillin allergy, use regimen under (2) above.

# Infectious causes of myocarditis

## *Viruses*
- Enterovirus (Coxsackie A and B)
- Echo virus
- Polio
- Arbo virus (dengue fever, yellow fever)
- Influenza
- Herpes viruses (herpes simplex, varicella zoster, Epstein–Barr virus (EBV), cytomegalovirus (CMV) )
- Mumps
- Rabies

## *Bacteria*
- Diphtheria
- Streptococcus
- Meningococcus

## *Rickettsia*
- *Chlamydia*
- *Coxiella*
- Scrub typhus
- Rocky Mountain spotted fever

## *Spirochaetes*
- Leptospirosis

## *Protozoa*
- *Trypanosoma cruzi*

# Rheumatic fever

- Following acute rheumatic fever, 70% develop rheumatic valvular disease
- Diagnosis of acute rheumatic fever is supported by the presence of two major criteria or one major and two minor criteria

**Table 8.5: Features of rheumatic fever**

| Major | Minor |
| --- | --- |
| Polyarthritis | Fever |
| Carditis (pericarditis, myocarditis, endocarditis or pancarditis) | Arthralgia |
| | Prolonged PR interval on ECG |
| Subcutaneous nodules | Raised ESR |
| Sydenham's chorea (St Vitus' dance) | Raised white blood count |
| Erythema marginatum | Raised CRP |
| | Evidence of β-haemolytic streptococcus infection |

# Cardiac tumours

## Types of cardiac tumour

### Benign
* Atrial myxoma
* Lymphoma
* Fibroelastoma
* Rhabdomyoma

### Malignant
* Metastases
* Angiosarcoma
* Rhabdomyosarcoma

## Features of atrial myxomas

* Arise from the fossa ovalis
* 75% left-sided
* 75% women
* Presentation in late middle age
* Clinical presentation simulates mitral stenosis producing initially left heart failure and leading to subsequent pulmonary hypertension and additional right-sided heart failure
* There may be recurrent episodes of pulmonary oedema or syncope
* Sudden death may occur
* Other features include: fever
  anorexia
  weight loss
  myalgia
  arthralgia
  Raynaud's phenomenon
  clubbing
* Auscultation reveals a mid-diastolic murmur in 20% of patients and classically a tumour plop is heard instead of an opening snap
* More commonly mitral regurgitation is heard
* Systemic emboli may occur
* Investigations may show:
  normochromic normocytic anaemia
  raised ESR
  raised gammaglobulin

# Hypertension

## Causes of secondary hypertension

### Renal disease
* Renal artery stenosis/fibromuscular dysplasia
* Chronic renal disease

### Endocrine disorders
* Primary hyperaldosteronism
* Cushing's syndrome

---

**Box 8.7: Features suggesting secondary hypertension**

**History**
Known renal disease
Urinary symptoms
Abdominal trauma
Drug history

**Examination**
Femoral pulses delayed
Palpable kidneys
Enlarged bladder
Uraemic features
Oedema
Abdominal bruits
Features of Cushing's syndrome or acromegaly
Café au lait patches
Neurofibroma
Orthostatic hypotension

**Investigations**
Abnormalities of serum urea, creatinine or potassium
Proteinuria, haematuria, glycosuria

- Phaeochromocytoma
- Congenital adrenal hyperplasia
- Extrarenal renin-secreting tumours
- 11 β-Hydroxysteroid dehydrogenase deficiency
- Hyperparathyroidism
- Acromegaly
- Drugs: oral contraceptives, corticosteroids, carbenoxolone, liquorice, sympathomimetics, monoamine oxidase inhibitors, non-steroidal anti-inflammatory drugs (NSAIDs), alcohol

## *Miscellaneous*
- Coarctation of the aorta
- Pre-eclampsia
- Acute intermittent porphyria
- Acute lead poisoning
- Raised intracranial pressure
- Tetanus
- Poliomyelitis

# Management of malignant hypertension

## *Recognition*
- Severe headache, visual disturbance, vomiting and confusion progressing to encephalopathy with seizures and coma
- May present with acute left ventricular failure, acute renal failure
- Fundoscopy reveals grade 3 or 4 retinopathy with haemorrhages and exudates
- Urinalysis shows proteinuria and haematuria

## *Treatment*
- Bed rest. Main aim is smooth and gradual reduction in BP. If BP is lowered too rapidly, can lead to coronary and cerebral ischaemia
- *Oral nifedipine*: 10mg orally effective but once given cannot be reversed. Fine control of BP lowering therefore not as good as parenteral agents. Best avoided if tachycardia or cardiac failure
- *Sublingual nifedipine*: more rapid onset

**Table 8.6: Adverse effects of anti-hypertensive agents**

| Condition | Thiazide diuretic | β-blocker | ACE inhibitor | Calcium channel blocker | α-blocker |
|---|---|---|---|---|---|
| Diabetes mellitus | − | − | √ | + | + |
| Gout | − | + | + | + | + |
| Hyperlipidaemia | − | − | + | + | + |
| Ischaemic heart disease | + | √ | √ | √ | + |
| Heart failure | √ | +/− * | √ | +/− † | + |
| Asthma | + | − | + | + | + |
| Peripheral vascular disease | + | − | + | √ | + |
| Renal artery stenosis | + | − | − | + | + |

Key: − adverse effect; + no adverse effect; √ particularly indicated.

  * Some newer β-blockers may be beneficial.

  † Some calcium channel blockers (e.g. Amlodipine, Nicardipine) have positive inotropic effect, and are therefore safer.

of action than oral preparation. Often leads to too rapid a fall in BP. The higher the initial BP, the faster the fall. Little indication for its use

- *i.v. Nitrates*: particularly effective if coexistent cardiac failure or coronary ischaemia
- *i.v. Sodium nitroprusside* - very effective and for many the drug of choice, particularly if co-existent cardiac failure. Avoid in pre-eclampsia and protect from light to prevent cyanide production. Depends on local availability
- *i.v. Labetolol*: effective, but contraindicated if co-existent cardiac failure, heart block, asthma
- *i.v. Hydralazine*: effective and first choice in pregnancy. Avoid in ischaemic heart disease
- *i.v. Phentolamine*: primarily indicated in phaeochromocytoma

# Cardiac pacing

## Types of permanent pacemaker

Pacemaker codes contain three letters: the first indicates the chamber paced; the second indicates the chamber sensed; the third indicates the response to sensed impulses.

- AOO: single wire in right atrium. Asynchronous pacing. Used to overdrive atrial tachycardias
- AAI: single wire in right atrium inhibited by sensed atrial impulses, useful in patients with sick sinus syndrome and normal AV node function. Contraindicated in AV block, bifasicular block, atrial flutter, atrial fibrillation, carotid sinus syndrome
- VOO: single wire in right ventricle. Fixed-rate pacing. No sensing or

response, therefore pacemaker not inhibited by spontaneous ventricular impulses. This can lead to a R on T phenomenon and VT. Now rarely used

- VVI: single wire in right ventricle inhibited by sensed ventricular impulses. Unit of choice in patients with AV block and atrial fibrillation, sick sinus syndrome with intermittent AF or atrial paralysis. Contraindicated in patients with persistent sinus node function. Endless loop tachycardia may develop owing to retrograde conduction of ventricular impulses via an accessory pathway. Pacemaker syndrome may also develop in which atrial contractions against closed AV valves leads to a fall in cardiac output, hypotension and syncope
- VAT: Two wires, one in right atrium, one in right ventricle. Atrial impulses are sensed and stimulate ventricular pacing. As there is no ventricular sensing, there is a risk of R on T phenomenon. Useful in patients with AV block and normal

---

**Box 8.8:**
**Indications for temporary pacing following acute myocardial infarction**

Complete AV block
Wenckebach second-degree AV block (if anterior infarction or cardiogenic shock)
Mobitz type 2 AV block
Trifascicular block
Sinoatrial disease

**Indications for permanent pacing**

Chronic complete AV block ± Stokes-Adams attacks
Chronic Mobitz type 2 AV block
Post myocardial infarction (massive anterior infarction)
Symptomatic bi- or trifasicular block
Sick sinus syndrome
Carotid sinus syndrome

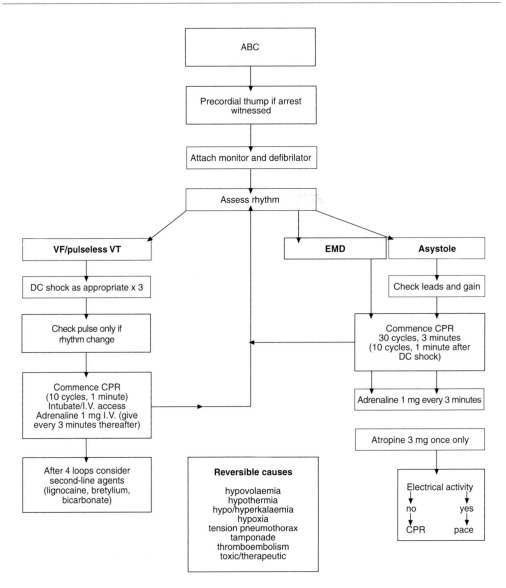

**Fig. 8.6: Cardiopulmonary resuscitation guidelines**
*Based on the recommendations of the UK Resuscitation Council*

sinus node function. Contraindicated in AF (atrial flutter)

- DVI: Two wires (right atrium and right ventricle). Ventricular impulses are sensed and stimulate atrial impulse followed shortly by a ventricular impulse. Useful in AV block. Contraindicated in AF

- DDD: Two wires, (right atrium and right ventricle). Dual-chamber sensing. Useful in sick sinus syndrome with additional AV nodal disease. If AF develops it reverts to VVI mode. Retrograde conduction may occur. Contraindicated in atrial tachy-arrythmias

# Pericardial disease

## Causes of acute pericarditis

- Idiopathic
- Viral infection
- Dressler's syndrome
- Rheumatic fever
- Bacterial infection
- Fungal infection
- Uraemia
- Trauma
- SLE
- Rheumatoid arthritis
- Scleroderma
- Polyarteritis nodosa
- Giant-cell arteritis
- Malignant disease
- Radiotherapy
- Hypothyroidism

## Causes of pericardial tamponade

- Myocardial infarction with rupture of ventricular wall
- Aortic dissection
- Post cardiac surgery
- Malignant disease
- Chest trauma
- Uraemic patients undergoing haemodialysis
- Radiotherapy
- Anticoagulant treatment in association with acute pericarditis
- Collagen vascular disease
- Dressler's syndrome
- Viral infection
- Bacterial infection
- Tuberculous pericarditis
- Chylo pericardium
- Hypothyroidism

# Causes of constrictive pericarditis

- Idiopathic
- Viral infection
- Tuberculosis
- Radiotherapy
- Malignancy
- Collagen vascular disease
- Bacterial infections
- Uraemia
- Trauma
- Drugs: procainamide, hydralazine

# Clinical case scenarios

## Mitral valve disease

### *Mitral stenosis*
- Patient may have a malar flush and left thoracotomy scar (previous valvotomy)
- Patient may be in atrial fibrillation
- Apex beat not displaced and tapping in nature
- The first heart sound is typically loud
- Murmur: opening snap followed by a mid-diastolic murmur heard at the apex and loudest with the patient in expiration in the left lateral position. Presystolic accentuation if the patient is in sinus rhythm (this does not occur if the patient is in atrial fibrillation)

- Other features to look for:
    Small volume pulse
    Slow rising pulse
    Pulmonary regurgitation (Graham Steel murmur)
    Neurological signs due to cerebral emboli
    Signs of cardiac failure or infective endocarditis

## Mitral regurgitation

- Patient may be in atrial fibrillation
- Apex beat displaced and thrusting in nature
- There may be a thrill and parasternal heave
- First heart sound may be soft
- Murmur: pansystolic. May be heard all over praecordium but typically loudest at the apex and axilla with the patient in expiration in the left lateral position

- Other features to look for:
  Collapsing pulse
  Left thoracotomy scar (previous mitral valvotomy)
  Signs of cardiac failure or infective endocarditis
  Blue sclerae (osteogenesis imperfecta)
  Features of Turner's syndrome, Marfan's syndrome
  Elastic skin (Ehlers–Danlos, pseudoxanthoma elasticum)

## Mitral valve prolapse

- Young female, usually in sinus rhythm
- Apex beat usually undisplaced and of normal quality
- There are no thrills or heaves and heart sounds are normal
- Murmur: mid-systolic click loudest at the left sternal edge
- Usually no cardiac failure if uncomplicated

- Other features to look for:
  Neurological signs due to cerebral emboli
  Signs of infective endocarditis

## Mixed mitral valve disease

- Mixed features with the murmurs of regurgitation and stenosis (Table 8.7)

**Table 8.7: Features indicating dominant mitral valve lesion**

| Feature | Mitral stenosis | Mitral regurgitation |
|---|---|---|
| Pulse | Small volume | Collapsing |
| Apex beat | Undisplaced, tapping | Displaced, thrusting |
| First heart sound | Loud | Soft |
| Third heart sound | Absent | Present |

# Aortic valve disease

## Aortic stenosis

- The pulse is small volume and slow rising (best assessed at the carotids)
- The BP has a small pulse pressure
- The apex beat is not displaced and is heaving in nature
- A double apical impulse may be felt
- There may be a palpable thrill
- Murmur: ejection systolic, left sternal edge, radiating to the carotids and loudest with the patient sitting forward in expiration
- The A2 component of the second heart sound is soft and delayed (may lead to reversed splitting of the second heart sound)

- Other features to look for:
  Signs of cardiac failure or infective endocarditis
  Fourth heart sound
  Flfin facies in a child (Williams' syndrome)

## Aortic regurgitation

- The pulse is large volume and collapsing (assessed at the wrist)
- The BP has a large pulse pressure
- The apex beat is displaced and thrusting
- Murmur: early diastolic, left sternal

edge, loudest with the patient sitting forward in expiration

- Other features to look for:
  Signs of cardiac failure or infective endocarditis
  Argyll Robertson pupils (syphilis) marfanoid appearance
  Vigorous arterial pulsations in neck (Corrigan's sign)
  Head nodding with arterial pulsation (De Musset's sign)
  Capillary pulsation of nailbed (Quincke's sign)
  Pistol-shot femoral pulses (Duroziez's sign)
  Mid-diastolic murmur (Austin Flint murmur)

## Mixed aortic valve disease
- Mixed features and murmurs of both regurgitation and stenosis (Table 8.8)

## Mixed aortic and mitral valve disease
- Patient may have mixed features as discussed above
- Use the criteria given in Tables 8.7 and 8.8 to determine which lesions are dominant
- Remember that if you hear one obvious murmur, do not fail to search for other less obvious ones

**Table 8.8: Features indicating dominant aortic valve lesion**

| Feature | Aortic stenosis | Aortic regurgitation |
|---|---|---|
| Pulse | Slow rising | Collapsing |
| Apex beat | Undisplaced, heaving | Displaced, thrusting |
| Systolic thrill | Present | Absent |
| Systolic murmur | Loud | Soft |
| Pulse pressure | Small | Large |

# Congenital heart disease

## Atrial septal defect
- Patient usually middle-aged
- Patient will have atrial fibrillation
- Apex beat not displaced
- Left parasternal heave
- There is wide fixed splitting of the second heart sound
- There may be pulmonary and tricuspid flow murmurs

- Other features to look for:
  Mitral stenosis (Lutembacher's syndrome)
  Signs of cardiac failure or infective endocarditis
  Signs of Eisenmenger's syndrome, features of Down's or Turner's syndromes

## Ventricular septal defect
- Patient may be young
- Patient usually in sinus rhythm
- Apex beat not displaced
- Left parasternal heave and systolic thrill
- Murmur: pansystolic at the lower left sternal edge, radiating to apex
- There may be a pulmonary flow murmur

- Other features to look for:
  Signs of cardiac failure or infective endocarditis
  Signs of Eisenmenger's syndrome, features of Down's or Turner's syndromes

## Patent ductus arteriosus
- Pulse is collapsing
- Apex beat is displaced and thrusting
- Left parasternal heave
- Murmur: continuous, machinery heard loudest below the left clavicle and radiating through to the back

- Other features to look for:
    Signs of cardiac failure or infective
        endocarditis
    Signs of Eisenmenger's syndrome

## Coarctation of the aorta
- Patient usually young
- Patient is in sinus ryhthm
- Carotid pulsations are vigorous, but radial pulse is not collapsing
- Femoral pulses are small volume and delayed
- Apex beat not displaced and is heaving
- Visible arterial pulsations may be seen around the scapulae, anterior axilla and left sternal border
- Thrills may be palpable and bruits audible over visible arterial pulsations
- Murmur: systolic murmur audible both anteriorly and posteriorly

- Other features to look for:
    Signs of cardiac failure or infective
        endocarditis
    Features of Turner's syndrome
    Aortic stenosis (associated bicuspid
        aortic valve)
    Third cranial nerve palsy (posterior
        communicating artery aneurysm)

## Fallot's tetralogy
- There is a thoracotomy scar (Blalock shunt)
- There is central cyanosis and clubbing
- Patient normally in sinus rhythm. Pulse weaker on left
- Prominent a-wave in JVP
- Apex beat not displaced
- Left parasternal heave and systolic thrill
- Murmur: pulmonary stenosis – ejection systolic murmur right sternal edge, loudest with the patient sitting forward in inspiration
- There is splitting of the second heart sound and the pulmonary component is soft

- Other features to look for:
    Signs of cardiac failure and infective
        endocarditis

## Eisenmenger's syndrome
- There is central cyanosis and clubbing
- Patient normally in sinus rhythm
- Prominent a-wave in JVP (pulmonary hypertension)
- Prominent v-wave in JVP (tricuspid regurgitation)
- Apex best not displaced
- Left parasternal heave and palpable thrill
- Pulmonary component of second heart sound is loud
- Fourth heart sound may be heard
- Murmurs: pulmonary regurgitation – early diastolic murmur right sternal edge loudest with the patient sitting forward in inspiration
- Triscupid regurgitation – pansystolic murmur right sternal edge loudest with the patient in the left lateral position in inspiration

- Other features to look for:
    Signs of cardiac failure or infective
        endocarditis (in particular look

**Table 8.9: Differentiation between Fallot's tetralogy and Eisenmenger's syndrome**

| Feature | Eisenmenger's | Fallot's |
|---|---|---|
| Pulmonary systolic thrill | Absent | Present |
| Pulmonary systolic murmur | Absent | Present |
| Right ventricle | Very hypertrophied | Hypertrophied |
| CXR | Pulmonary plethora, large small pulmonary arteries | Pulmonary oligaemia, pulmonary arteries |

for pulsatile hepatomegaly indicative of tricuspid regurgitation)

*(NB: murmurs due to underlying causes of Eisenmenger's syndrome usually disappear as a result of equalisation of right and left cardiac pressures.)*

## Miscellaneous conditions

### Hypertrophic cardiomyopathy
- Patient may be young and athletic
- Patient usually in sinus rhythm
- Pulse character may be normal or jerky in nature (not slow-rising as in aortic stenosis)
- Apex beat displaced and forceful with presystolic lift which may give a double apical impulse
- Third and fourth heart sounds may be heard
- Murmur: ejection systolic, radiates to apex and axilla. May be associated mitral regurgitation

### Prosthetic valves
- Artificial first heart sound indicative of prosthetic mitral valve
- Artificial second heart sound indicative of prosthetic aortic valve
- There is usually a flow murmur across the artificial valves (mid-diastolic in mitral valve replacement and ejection systolic in aortic valve replacement)
- The artificial valves may also be leaking, leading to regurgitant murmurs (pansystolic in mitral valve replacement and early diastolic in aortic valve replacement)
- Do not forget that there may be other murmurs across unreplaced valves
- The artificial clicks of the opening and closing of artificial valves only occurs in metal valves

- Other features to look for:
  Signs of cardiac failure or infective endocarditis
  Neurological signs due to cerebral emboli

### Dextrocardia
- The apex beat is not palpable on the left side, but is felt on the right. May be associated with bronchiectasis and situs inversus (liver on left side)

# Landmark cardiology studies

## Hyperlipidaemia

**Scandinavian Simvastatin Survival Study Group**
Randomised trial of cholesterol lowering in 4,444 patients with coronary heart disease: the Scandanavian Simvastatin Survival Study Group (4S).
*Lancet* 1994; 344: 1383–9

**West of Scotland Coronary Prevention Study Group (WOSCOP)**
Prevention of coronary heart disease with pravastatin in men with hypercholesterolaemia.
*N Engl J Med* 1995; 333: 1301–7

**Sacks FM, Pfeffer MA, Moye LA et al, for the Cholesterol and Recurrent Events trial investigation (CARE)**
The effect of pravastatin on coronary events after myocardial infarction in patients with average cholesterol levels.
*N Engl J Med* 1996; 335: 1001–9

**The Long Term Intervention with Pravastatin in Ischaemic Disease (LIPID) study group**
Prevention of cardiovascular events and

death with pravastatin in patients with coronary heart disease and a broad range of cholesterol levels.
*N Engl J Med* 1998; 339: 1349–57

*The above trials examined the effects of cholesterol-lowering drugs in patients with coronary heart disease (4S, WOSCOPS, LIPID) or without coronary heart disease (CARE). They showed that cholesterol lowering reduces the risk of coronary events and death both from coronary heart disease and from any cause.*

# Ischaemic heart disease

## Antiplatelet Trialists Collaboration
Collaborative overview of randomised trials of anti-platelet therapy: prevention of death, myocardial infarction and stroke by prolonged anti-platelet therapy in various categories of patients.
*BMJ* 1994; 308: 81–106

*Meta-analysis of trials examining the benefit of aspirin therapy in secondary prevention. The results show that aspirin therapy post myocardial infarction reduces the risk of further coronary events, the risk of stroke and the risk of death both from coronary heart disease and from any cause.*

## ISIS-2 (Second International Study of Infarct Survival) Collaborative Group
Randomised trial of intravenous streptokinase, oral aspirin, both, or neither among 17,187 cases of suspected acute myocardial infarction.
*Lancet* 1988; ii: 349–60

*Established the benefits of aspirin and thrombolysis in acute myocardial infarction.*

## Fibrinolytic Therapy Trialists (FTT) Collaborative Group
Indications for fibrinolytic therapy in suspected acute myocardial infarction: a collaborative overview of early mortality and major morbidity results from all randomised trials of more than 1,000 patients.
*Lancet* 1994; 343: 311–22
*Meta-analysis of major thrombolysis trials confirming the benefits of thrombolysis in acute myocardial infarction.*

## ISIS-4 (Fourth International Study of Infarct Survival) Collaborative Group
A randomised factorial trial assessing early oral captopril, oral mononitrate and intravenous magnesium sulphate in 58,050 patients with suspected acute myocardial infarction.
*Lancet* 1995; 345: 669–85

## CONSENSUS-II Study Group
Effects of the early administration of enalapril on mortality in patients with acute myocardial infarction.
*N Engl J Med* 1992; 327: 678–84

## The Acute Infarction Ramipril Efficacy (AIRE) Study Investigators
Effect of ramipril on mortality and morbidity of survivors of acute myocardial infarction with clinical evidence of heart failure.
*Lancet* 1993; 342: 821–8

## GISSI-3
Effects of lisinopril and transdermal glyceryl trinitrate singly and together on 6 week mortality and ventricular function after acute myocardial infarction.
*Lancet* 1994; 343: 1115–22

*The above trials examined the benefit of various ACE inhibitors post myocardial infarction. They showed that early treatment with ACE inhibitors post myocardial infarction reduces the risk of further coronary events and mortality. The benefits are particularly great in patients with left ventricular impairment or overt heart failure post infarction.*

## Malmberg K, Ryden L, Efendic S et al

Randomised trial of insulin–glucose infusion followed by subcutaneous insulin treatment in diabetic patients with acute myocardial infarction (DIGAMI study).
*J Am Coll Cardiol* 1995; 26: 57–65

*This study has established the benefit of tight glycaemic control on the long-term outcome of diabetic patients following acute myocardial infarction.*

# Hypertension

## Amery A, Birkenhager W, Brixko P et al

Mortality and morbidity results from the European Working Party on High Blood Pressure in the Elderly trial
*Lancet* 1985; i: 1349–54

## SHEP Cooperative Research Group

Prevention of stroke by antihypertensive drug treatment in older persons with isolated systolic hypertension
*JAMA* 1991; 265: 3255–64

## Dahlof B, Lindholm LH, Hannson L et al

Morbidity and mortality in the Swedish trial in old patients with hypertension
*Lancet* 1991; 338: 1281–5

*The above trials have established the particular benefit derived from treating hypertension in older people.*

# 9 Respiratory medicine

## Contents

## Anatomy

### Trachea

- The trachea commences at the lower border of the cricoid cartilage (C6) and bifurcates into left and right main bronchi at the sternal angle (T4)
- The trachea is l0 cm in length and its cross section is D-shaped with a curved anterior portion containing horseshoe-shaped cartilage rings

### Bronchi

- The main bronchi are similar in structure to the trachea
- Both bronchi run to the lung hila
- The right main bronchus is 2.5 cm long and enters the hilum at T5
- It is more vertical than the left main bronchus, which is 5 cm long and enters the hilum at T6

### Bronchopulmonary segments

- At the hilum the right main bronchus divides into three lobar bronchi, which supply each of the three lobes of the right lung (upper, middle, lower)
- The left main bronchus divides into two lobar bronchi (upper and lower)
- These five lobar bronchi divide into segmental bronchi which supply the bronchopulmonary segments of each lung
- Each lung has 10 bronchopulmonary segments (see Fig. 9.1 and Table 9.1)

### Bronchioles

- Further division of the segmental bronchi eventually leads to the production of bronchioles
- These are airways with no cartilage or mucous glands in their walls
- Further division leads to the terminal bronchiole, respiratory bronchiole, and finally the acinus

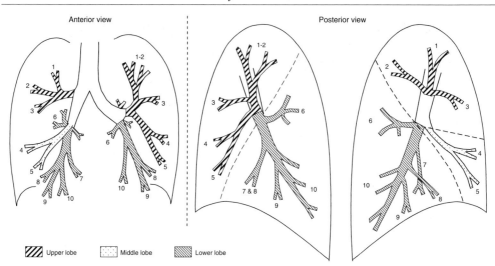

**Fig. 9.1: Diagram of lobar and segmental bronchial tree anatomy**

**Table 9.1: The bronchopulmonary segments of the lungs**

| **Right lung** | Upper lobe | Middle lobe | Lower lobe |
|---|---|---|---|
| | 1 Apical | 4 Lateral | 6 Apical |
| | 2 Posterior | 5 Medial | 7 Medial basal |
| | 3 Anterior | | 8 Anterior basal |
| | | | 9 Lateral basal |
| | | | 10 Posterior basal |
| **Left Lung** | Upper lobe | Lower lobe | |
| | 1 & 2 Apicoposterior | 6 Apical | |
| | 3 Anterior | 7 & 8 Anteromedial basal | |
| | 4 Superior lingula | 9 Lateral basal | |
| | 5 Inferior lingula | 10 Posterior basal | |

# Cells of the respiratory tract

## *Epithelium*

The airways are lined with pseudostratified columnar epithelium, which is several layers thick in the trachea and main bronchi but becomes progressively thinned as the airways become smaller, until at the terminal bronchiole level it is only one cell thick.

## *Ciliated cells*

• These are found from the trachea to the terminal bronchiole
• The cilia are composed of a central pair of microtubules surrounded by a matrix containing nine similar pairs of microtubules
• One of each pair of the outer microtubules is larger and contains a protein strand (dynein arm)
• Defects of the dynein arm lead to cilia immotility

## Feyrter cells (K cells)

- These cells are part of the amine precursor uptake and decarboxylation (APUD) system
- They are most numerous in the small bronchi
- Bronchial carcinoids and oat cell tumours are derived from these cells

## Goblet cells

- These are responsible for producing the mucus that lines the airways
- They are found from the trachea to the terminal bronchiole
- They are less numerous than ciliated cells

## Clara cells

- These are most numerous in the bronchioles and are concerned with the secretion of surfactant

## Alveolar cells

*Type 1 pneumocytes*: provide the main barrier to gaseous exchange

*Type 2 pneumocytes*: are concerned with the production of surfactant and also act as progenitors of type 1 pneumocytes

*Type 3 pneumocytes*: are involved in chemoreception and fluid absorption

- Alveolar macrophages are vital for immune defence
- These in particular may be damaged and inhibited by inhaled smoke

# Physiology

## Ventilatory pump

- In normal subjects resting tidal ventilation equals 5–6 l/min
- During strenuous exercise this may increase to 80 l/min

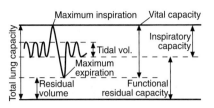

**Fig. 9.2: The subdivision of lung volumes**

- The maximum ventilatory capacity is l00 l/min
- At rest normal inspiration is mainly achieved by downward movement of the diaphragm and outward expansion of the inspiratory intercostal muscles
- Expiration is usually a passive process produced by the elastic recoil of lung tissue
- Inspiratory intercostal muscles play a part during early expiration to break the recoil
- During exercise there is increased diaphragmatic and inspiratory intercostal muscular activity
- There is also associated use of accessory muscles (sternomastoid)
- During expiration there is increased activity of expiratory intercostal muscles with the additional use of abdominal muscles

## Airway mechanics

In order to inflate lungs two forces need to be overcome:

### 1. Elastic resistance

- This is given by the elasticity of lung tissue and the surface tension produced by surfactant
- Elasticity is also referred to as compliance

  *Compliance*: defined as the change in volume produced by a unit change of pressure difference

*Static compliance*: reflects the elastic recoil of the lungs and expansibility of the thoracic cage
*Dynamic compliance*: refers to the compliance during respiration
- This is greatest during expiration
It is influenced by airway obstruction and is nonlinear, being greatest at mid lung volumes and lowest at the extremes of lung volume

### 2. Non-elastic resistance (airways resistance)
- 80% of airways resistance occurs in the extrathoracic and large intrathoracic airways
- This resistance is increased during nasal breathing
- Bronchioles have an enormous surface area and therefore provide little resistance to air flow
- Airways resistance is greatest during expiration, and is increased by parasympathetic activity

## Gas exchange

- At rest tidal inspiration equals 350–500 ml
- Air inspired at the end of inspiration makes no contribution to pulmonary gas exchange and is exhaled unchanged
- Only two-thirds of the inspired air mixes completely with alveolar gas
- Partial pressure of oxygen falls progressively as the inspired air passes through the small airways

Alveolar $P_{O_2}$ =
    inspired $P_{O_2}$ – alveolar $P_{CO_2}$ / R
R = respiratory exchange ratio
    (VQ ratio)
Alveolar $P_{CO_2}$ = arterial $P_{CO_2}$
    (normally 5.3 kPa)

Inspired $P_{O_2}$ at sea level = 20 kPa
Alveolar $P_{O_2}$ is therefore normally
    13.3 kPa
If pulmonary gas exchange is perfect, arterial $P_{O_2}$ = alveolar $P_{O_2}$

## Pulmonary circulation

- The mean pulmonary artery pressure is 12–15 mmHg
- Left atrial pressure is 5 mmHg
- There is therefore a pressure gradient across the lungs of 7–10 mmHg
- The vascular resistance of the pulmonary circulation is one-tenth that of the systemic circulation
- In an upright posture, blood flow is greatest at the lung bases
- During exercise, blood flow distribution becomes more even
- Similarly, ventilation is normally greatest at the bases, but there is a less dramatic difference than with blood distribution
- If V equals the volume of air entering alveoli (normally 4 l/min) and Q equals blood flow through lungs (normally 5 l/min):
    normal VQ ratio equals 0.8
    normal apical VQ ratio 3.3 (more V)
    basal VQ ratio 0.63 (more Q)

## Control of ventilation

### Central chemoreceptors
- Situated in the medulla
- Respond primarily to changes in $P_{CO_2}$ levels and also to changes in hydrogen ion levels and $P_{O_2}$ levels

### Peripheral chemoreceptors
- These are situated in the carotid and aortic bodies
- They respond primarily to changes in $P_{O_2}$ but also to changes in $P_{CO_2}$ and

hydrogen ion concentration
- Carotid bodies also respond to reduced blood flow
- $CO_2$ is the most important variable regulating ventilation
- Maximal increases in $Pco_2$ lead to a tenfold increase in ventilation
- Maximal falls in $Po_2$ lead to a two-thirds increase in ventilation
- Maximal increases in hydrogen ion concentrations lead to a fivefold increase in ventilation

## Mechanoreceptors
- These are situated in the large airways and lung parenchyma
- They are responsible for the Herring–Bruer reflex (distension of the lung leads to slowing of the respiratory rate), which is mediated by the vagus nerve
- Irritant receptors are stimulated by noxious inhaled agents
- J (juxta) capillary receptors are stimulated by stretching of the pulmonary microvasculature

# Symptoms and signs

## Causes of dyspnoea

### Pulmonary disease
- Pulmonary embolism
- Pulmonary oedema

**Table 9.2: Causes of cough**

| Characteristic | Condition |
| --- | --- |
| Dry, hacking, non-productive | Pharyngitis |
| | Tracheobronchitis |
| | Laryngitis |
| | Whooping cough |
| Bovine | Vocal cord paralysis due to left recurrent laryngeal nerve lesion: |
| |     Carcinoma of bronchus |
| |     Carcinoma of oesophagus |
| |     Lymphadenopathy |
| |     Aortic aneurysm |
| Aphonic and weak | Complete paralysis of both vocal cords: |
| |     Polyneuritis |
| |     Muscular dystrophy |
| |     Guillain–Barré syndrome |
| |     Neurotoxins |
| |     Myasthenia gravis |
| Nocturnal | Asthma |
| Early morning cough with expectoration | Chronic obstructive pulmonary disease |
| Coughing after food or in recumbent position | Aspiration |
| Cough precipitated by postural change | Bronchiectasis |
| Chronic dry cough | Carcinoma of bronchus |
| | Psychogenic |

### 3–4 mm
- Sarcoid
- Bronchial pneumonia
- Secondary deposits
- Tuberculosis

### Calcified nodules
- Previous varicella pneumonia
- Histoplasmosis
- Microlithiasis (mitral stenosis)
- Stony lung disease

## Causes of solitary pulmonary nodules

- Carcinoma of the bronchus
- Bronchial adenoma
- Bronchial hamartoma
- Bronchial carcinoid
- Bronchogenic cyst
- Neurogenic tumours
- Tuberculoma
- Secondary deposits
- Granuloma
- Localised pneumonia
- Pulmonary infarct
- Hydatid cyst
- Rheumatoid nodule
- Lipoid pneumonia
- AV fistula
- Pneumoconiotic nodule

## Causes of cavitating lesions

- Bullae
- Bronchiectasis
- Lung abscess
- Bacterial pneumonia
- Tuberculosis
- Tumour
- Infarction
- Pneumoconiotic nodule
- Granuloma
- Fungal infection

## Causes of bilateral hilar lymphadenopathy

- Sarcoid
- Carcinoma
- Metastases
- Pulmonary artery enlargement
- Lymphoma
- Leukaemia
- Tuberculosis
- Silicosis
- Berylliosis
- Agammaglobulinaemia
- Histoplasmosis
- Coccidioidomycosis
- Glandular fever

## Causes of mediastinal masses

### Anterior
- Goitre
- Lymphadenopathy
- Aortic aneurysm
- Thymus

**Table 9.5: Indications for bronchoscopy**

| Diagnostic | Treatment |
| --- | --- |
| Suspected carcinoma | Removal of foreign bodies |
| Unexplained haemoptysis | Endobronchial surgery |
| Unexplained chest x-ray abnormality | Laser treatment |
| Unexplained respiratory symptoms | |
| For bronchoscopic bronchogram | |
| Microbiological sampling | |

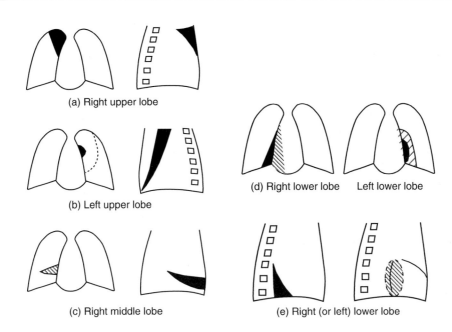

(a) Right upper lobe

(b) Left upper lobe

(c) Right middle lobe

(d) Right lower lobe    Left lower lobe

(e) Right (or left) lower lobe

**Fig. 9.3: Features of chest X-ray collapse**

- Teratoma
- Dermoid cyst
- Bronchogenic cyst
- Pericardial cyst

*Posterior*
- Neurogenic tumours
- Aortic aneurysm
- Paravertebral abscess
- Hiatus hernia

# Respiratory infections

## Causes of coryza

- Rhinovirus
- Coronavirus
- Influenza viruses
- Parainfluenza virus
- Respiratory syncytial virus
- Adenovirus

- Echovirus
- Coxsackie viruses

## Causes of acute laryngitis/ pharyngitis

- Viral (as for coryza + Epstein–Barr virus)
- *Streptococcus pyogenes*
- *Streptococcus pneumoniae*
- *Haemophilus influenzae*
- Diphtheria
- *Fusobacterium*
- *Neisseria gonorrhoea*
- Candidiasis

## Causes of acute tracheobronchitis

- Parainfluenza virus
- Respiratory syncytial virus
- Adenovirus
- Coronavirus

- Influenza virus
- Enteroviruses
- *Streptococcus pneumoniae*
- *Haemophilus influenzae*
- *Mycoplasma pneumonia*
- *Chlamydia psittaci*

# Causes of acute bronchitis (with pre-existing chronic bronchitis)

- *Haemophilus influenzae*
- *Streptococcus pneumoniae*
- Viruses
- *Mycoplasma pneumoniae*

# Causes of community-acquired pneumonia

- *Streptococcus pneumoniae*
- *Haemophilus influenzae*
- *Staphylococcus aureus*
- *Legionella pneumoniae*
- *Mycoplasma pneumoniae*
- *Neisseria meningitidis*
- *Branhamella catarrhalis*
- *Chlamydia psittaci*
- *Coxiella burneti*
- *Mycobacterium tuberculosis*
- Viruses (respiratory syncytial virus, influenza, parainfluenza, rhinovirus, adeno virus, CMV, measles, varicella zoster)

# Causes of nosocomial pneumonia

## Gram-negative bacteria
- *Pseudomonas*
- *Klebsiella*
- *Escherichia coli*
- *Proteus*
- *Serratia*

- *Bacteroides*
- *Fusobacterium*
- *Legionella*

## Gram-positive bacteria
- *Streptococcus pneumoniae*
- *Staphylococcus aureus*
- *Clostridium*
- Gram-positive cocci

# Factors predisposing to aspiration pneumonia

## Reduced consciousness
- Drug overdose
- Anaesthesia
- Epilepsy
- Stroke

## Dysphagia

## Artificial enteral feeding

## CNS disorder
- Pseudobulbar palsy
- Motor neuron disease
- Multiple sclerosis
- Idiopathic Parkinson's disease

## Miscellaneous
- Dental sepsis
- Upper respiratory tract infection
- Terminal illness

# Rare causes of pneumonia

## Bacterial
- *Salmonella typhi*
- *Salmonella paratyphi*
- *Brucella abortus*
- *Pasteurella pestis*
- *Pasteurella tularaesis*
- *Bacillus anthracis*
- *Leptospira icterohaemorrhagica*
- Actinomycosis

## Viral
- Herpes zoster virus
- Epstein–Barr virus

## Rickettsial
- Typhus

## Fungal
- Coccidiodomycosis
- Cystoplasmosis

# Causes of pneumonia in immunocompromised patients

## Gram-negative bacteria
- *Klebsiella*
- *Escherichia coli*
- *Pseudomonas*
- *Legionella*
- *Enterobacter*
- *Serratia*

## Gram-positive bacteria
- *Staphylococcus*
- *Streptococcus pneumoniae*
- *Nocardia*
- *Mycobacterium tuberculosis*
- *Mycobacterium avium intracellulare*

## Fungi
- *Aspergillus*
- *Cryptococcus*

## Protozoa
- *Pneumocystis carinii*
- *Toxoplasma gondii*

## Helminths
- *Strongyloides*

## Viruses
- CMV
- Varicella zoster virus
- Herpes simplex virus

---

**Box 9.2: Indicators of severe pneumonia**

Age > 60 years
Respiratory rate > 30/min
Diastolic blood pressure < 60 mmHg
Atrial fibrillation
Confusion
Immunosuppression
Raised urea
Low or very high white blood count
Hypoalbuminaemia
$Po_2$ < 8 kPa

---

# Causes of other infections

## Acute epiglottitis
- *Haemophilus influenzae*

## Bronchiolitis
- Respiratory syncytial virus

## Bronchiectasis
- *Haemophilus influenzae*
- *Pseudomonas*

## Causes of lung abscesses
- Aspiration
- *Staphylococcus aureus*
- *Klebsiella*
- Tuberculosis
- *Pseudomonas*
- Anaerobic bacteria
- Bronchial obstruction
- Septicaemia
- Right-sided bacterial endocarditis
- Infected intravenous cannulae
- Intravenous drug abuse
- Extension of subphrenic abscess
- Extension of hepatic abscess
- Actinomycosis
- Fungi
- *Entamoeba histolytica*
- Pulmonary infarction
- Infected bullae
- Cavitating lung tumour
- Wegener's granulomatosis

- Pneumoconiosis

### Causes of empyema
- Pulmonary infection (pneumonia, lung abscess, bronchiectasis)
- Septicaemia
- Thoracic surgery
- Penetrating chest wounds
- Extension from subphrenic abscess
- Extension from hepatic abscess
- Pulmonary infarction
- Oesophageal perforation

# Pulmonary manifestations of HIV infection

### Infection
- *Pneumocystis carinii*
- CMV
- Atypical *Mycobacterium*
- Tuberculosis
- *Cryptococcus neoformans*
- Nocardia
- Fungi
- *Toxoplasma gondii*

### Malignancy
- Kaposi's sarcoma
- Lymphoma

### Miscellaneous
- Lymphocytic interstitial pneumonitis

# Obstructive airways disease

## Asthma

### Triggers of acute asthma
#### Industrial causes
- Toluene (polyurethane)
- Soldering flux (electrical engineering)
- Cotton dust (byssinosis/textile)

- Animal dander (veterinary, agriculture)
- Flour, grain (bakers and millers)
- Wood dust (carpenters)
- Sulphur dioxide, ozone, chloride (chemical industry)

### Others
- Respiratory tract infections
- Exercise
- Cold air
- Laughter
- Smoke
- Chemical fumes
- Stress
- Drugs: cholinergic agents, cholinesterase inhibitors, β-blockers, non steroidal anti-inflammatories, tartrazine, carbamazepine, parenteral penicillin, parenteral iron, parenteral *N*-acetylcysteine, inhaled ampicillin, inhaled benzylpenicillin, inhaled cephalosporins, inhaled α-methyldopa, inhaled cimetidine, inhaled piperazine, inhaled pancreatic extract

### Treatment of acute asthma attack
- This is an acute medical emergency
- Patient requires urgent attention
- Main objectives of treatment are to provide oxygen and restore airway

> **Box 9.3: Indicators of severe asthma attack**
>
> Peak expiratory flow rate (PEFR) < 50% normal
> Use of accessory muscles for respiration
> Heart rate > 130 beats/min
> Pulsus paradoxus > 10 mmHg
> $Po_2$ < 8 kPa
> $Pco_2$ > 5.5 kPa
> Hyperinflation of the lungs
> Cyanosis
> Reduced conscious level
> Silent chest
> ECG abnormalities
> Pneumothorax

## Guidelines for the treatment of chronic asthma in adults
*Based on the guidelines of the British Thoracic Society*

STEP 1
Occasional use of relief bronchodilators (short-acting inhaled β-agonists)
*If they are needed more than daily, move to step 2, but ensure adequate inhaler technique before doing so*

STEP 2
Addition of regular low-dose inhaled corticosteroid

STEP 3
Addition of high-dose inhaled steroid
*or* long-acting inhaled β-agonist
*or* oral theophylline

STEP 4
Addition of high-dose inhaled steroid
*plus*
long-acting inhaled β-agonist *or* oral theophylline *or* inhaled ipratropium *or* long-acting oral β-agonist

STEP 5
Addition of regular oral steroids

*Good practice*
Patients should start treatment at the step most appropriate to the initial severity
A rescue course of prednisolone may be needed at any time and at any step
Prescribe a peak flow meter and monitor response to treatment

*Good control, indicated by:*
Minimal (ideally nil) chronic symptoms
Minimal (infrequent) exacerbations
Minimal need for relieving bronchodilators
No limitation of activities
Circadian variation in PEFR < 20%
PEFR 80% of predicted or best
Minimal (or no) side effects from treatment

patency
- Patient should receive l00% oxygen (there is little risk of $CO_2$ retention)
- Patient should also receive salbutamol nebuliser 2.5–5 mg
- Intravenous hydrocortisone 200 mg stat
- If there is no response, intravenous aminophylline or intravenous salbutamol may be tried
- Sedation should be avoided
- Antibiotics should be given if there are signs of infection

- Ultimately artificial ventilation may be required if patient becomes acidotic, hypercapnic and hypoxic without responding to treatment, or if they become extremely tired

# Emphysema

## *Pathogenesis of emphysema*
- Cigarette smoking increases the number of alveolar macrophages
- Macrophages release neutrophil chemotactic factor
- Attracted neutrophils are damaged by the smoke and release proteolytic enzymes (elastase)
- Elastase attacks the interstitial lung matrix (elastin, basement membranes, collagen)
- Elastase normally inhibited by $\alpha_1$-antitrypsin
- Smoke impairs the effectiveness of this enzyme leading to unchecked damage

## *Causes of emphysema*
- Cigarette smoking
- Occupational dust
- Atmospheric pollution
- Macleod's syndrome
- Chronic asthma
- $\alpha_1$-antitrypsin deficiency
- Cadmium

# Bronchiectasis

## *Causes of bronchiectasis*

### *Idiopathic*

### *Post infective*
- Bronchiolitis
- Measles
- Pertussis
- Tuberculosis
- Any other cause of pneumonia

- Macleod's's syndrome

### *Mechanical bronchial obstruction*
- Foreign bodies
- Bronchial neoplasms
- Mucus plugging
- Lymphadenopathy
- Thymoma

### *Abnormal ciliary action*
- Kartagener's syndrome

### *Cystic fibrosis*

### *Neuropathic disorders*
- Riley–Day syndrome
- Chagas' disease

### *Immunological*
- Hypogammaglobulinaemia
- IgA deficiency
- IgG deficiencies (especially $IgG_2$)
- Allergic bronchopulmonary aspergillosis

# Restrictive lung disease

## Causes of pulmonary fibrosis

### *Lung disease*
- Idiopathic (cryptogenic fibrosing alveolitis)
- Infection
- Pneumoconiosis
- Extrinsic allergic alveolitis
- Collagen vascular disease
- Sarcoid
- Aspiration

### *Malignancy*
- Alveolar cell carcinoma

* Lymphangitis carcinomatosis

## Drugs
* Cytotoxics (bleomycin, mitomycin c, busulphan, chlorambucil, melphalan, cyclophosphamide)
* Hexamethonium
* Oxygen
* Nitrofurantoin
* Amiodarone

## Chemicals
* Nitrogen dioxide
* Chlorine
* Paraquat

## Miscellaneous
* Niemann–Pick's disease
* Gaucher's disease
* Tuberous sclerosis
* Neurofibromatosis
* Agammaglobulinaemia
* Biliary cirrhosis
* Radiation
* Ankylosing spondylitis
* Histiocytosis X

# Causes of upper zone fibrosis

* Tuberculosis
* Sarcoid
* Ankylosing spondylitis
* Extrinsic allergic alveolitis
* Aspergillosis
* Silicosis
* Radiation

# Causes of extrinsic allergic alveolitis

## Micro-organisms
* Farmer's lung
* Wood-pulp worker's lung
* Malt worker's lung
* Doghouse disease
* Sequoiosis
* Sewage worker's lung
* Summer-type hypersensitivity pneumonitis
* Maple bark stripper's lung
* Lycoperdenosis
* Paprika-splitter's lung
* Cheese-washer's lung
* Suberosis
* Mushroom worker's lung
* Bagassosis
* Byssinosis
* Humidifier lung
* Sauna taker's lung

## Animals
* Bird-fancier's lung
* Fishmeal worker's lung
* Pituitary snuff-taker's lung
* Furrier's lung
* Rodent handler's lung

**Table 9.6: Causes of pneumoconiosis**

| Type | Causative agent |
| --- | --- |
| Coal-worker's pneumoconiosis | Coal dust |
| Silicosis | Silica |
| Asbestosis | Asbestos |
| Talc pneumoconiosis | Magnesium silicate |
| Kaolin pneumoconiosis | Kaolin |
| Fuller's earth pneumoconiosis | Fuller's earth |
| Mica pneumoconiosis | Ground mica |
| Fibrous erionite | Aluminium silicate |
| Berylliosis | Beryllium |
| Haematite lung | Iron ore |
| Siderosis | Iron oxide |
| Baritosis | Barium |
| Stannosis | Tin oxide |
| Shaver's disease | Aluminium oxide |
| Hard metal disease | Tungsten carbide |

## Vegetation
- Woodworker's lung

## Chemicals
- Vineyard sprayer's lung

# Features of sarcoid

## Pulmonary
- Bilateral hilar lymphadenopathy
- Pulmonary infiltrates
- Pulmonary fibrosis

## Cardiac
- Cardiomyopathy

## Neurological
- Myopathy
- Neuropathy

## Dermatological
- Erythema nodosum
- Lupus pernio

## Ophthalmological
- Uveitis
- Conjunctivitis
- Sjögren's syndrome

## Bone
- Arthralgia
- Bone cysts

## Splenomegaly

## Metabolic
- Hypercalciuria
- Hypercalcaemia

- Raised serum ACE

## Staging of thoracic sarcoid
Stage 1: normal CXR
Stage 2: bilateral hilar lymphadenopathy
Stage 3: bilateral hilar lymphadenopathy and pulmonary infiltrates
Stage 4: pulmonary infiltrates and pulmonary fibrosis

# Pulmonary vascular disease

## Causes of pulmonary hypertension

### Chronic hypoxia

### Cardiac disease
- Atrial septal defect
- Ventricular septal defect
- Patent ductus arteriosus
- Mitral stenosis
- Left ventricular failure

### Collagen vascular disease
- Polyarteritis nodosa
- SLE
- Scleroderma

---

**Box 9.4: Effects of asbestos**

Pleural plaques
Pleural effusion
Asbestosis
Mesothelioma
Carcinoma of the lung

---

**Box 9.5: Indications for steroids in sarcoid**

Eye involvement
Pulmonary infiltrates
Pulmonary fibrosis
Hypercalcaemia
Hypercalciuria
Severe skin involvement
Cardiomyopathy
Neurological involvement
Salivary gland involvement

## Drugs

- Combined oral contraceptive pill
- Amphetamines
- Fenfluramine
- Phenformin

## Miscellaneous

- Pulmonary embolus
- Hyperviscosity syndrome
- Schistosomiasis
- Primary pulmonary hypertension
- Chest wall deformity

# Causes of pulmonary haemorrhage

### Chronic pulmonary venous congestion

- Mitral stenosis
- Left ventricular failure
- Pulmonary veno-occlusive disease

### Miscellaneous

- Goodpasture's syndrome
- Idiopathic pulmonary haemosiderosis
- Pulmonary vasculitis

# Causes of pulmonary vasculitis and granulomatosis

## Vasculitis

- Wegener's granulomatosis
- Henloch–Schönlein purpura
- Polyarteritis nodosa

## Infection

- Tuberculosis
- Syphilis
- Brucellosis
- Cat scratch bacillus
- Leprosy
- Fungi

## Miscellaneous

- Lymphomatoid granulomatosis
- Necrotising sarcoid granulomatosis
- Essential mixed cryoglobulinaemia
- Behçet's syndrome
- Hughes Stovin syndrome
- Histiocytosis X
- Berylliosis
- Agammaglobulinaemia
- Foreign body
- Crohn's disease

## Collagen vascular disease

- Rheumatoid disease
- SLE

### Table 9.7: Clinical presentation of pulmonary embolus

| History | Examination | Investigations |
| --- | --- | --- |
| Dyspnoea of sudden onset | Hyperventilation | Arterial hypoxia |
| Pleuritic chest pain | Pleural rub (not always heard) | CXR usually normal |
| Haemoptysis | Pleural effusion | ECG usually normal or sinus |
| Collapse | Evidence of deep vein | tachycardia (may show right |
| Dizziness on upright posture | thrombosis (DVT) (not | bundle branch block, right |
| (indicative of massive | always present) | axis deviation, S1Q3T3) |
| pulmonary embolus) | Tachycardia | |
| | Cardiac failure | |
| | Hypotension | |
| | Fever | |

- Systemic sclerosis
- Dermatopolymyositis
- Mixed connective tissue disease

### *Malignancy*
- Lymphoma
- Carcinoma

## Management of acute pulmonary embolus

- Have a high index of suspicion
- Give high-flow oxygen therapy
- Avoid venodilators (morphine)
- Avoid hypovolaemia (diuretics)
- Anticoagulate with heparin initially and Warfarin later
- Inotropic support may be needed for massive pulmonary emboli
- Thrombolysis or embolectomy may be required for massive pulmonary emboli

# Malignancy

## Aetiology of bronchial carcinoma

- Tobacco
- Asbestos
- Radioactive isotopes (uranium, radon)
- Polycyclic aromatic hydrocarbons
- Nickel exposure
- Chromate exposure
- Arsenic exposure
- Air pollution

## Contraindications to surgery for bronchial carcinoma

- Coexisting premorbid conditions (especially ischaemic heart disease)

- Contraindications to general anaesthetic
- $FEV_1 < 1.5$ l
- Oat cell carcinoma
- Tumour within 2 cm of carina
- Pulmonary hypertension
- Recurrent laryngeal nerve palsy
- Malignant pleural effusion
- Chest wall involvement
- SVC obstruction
- Pericardial involvement
- Mediastinal lymphadenopathy
- Distant metastases

---

**Box 9.6: Non-metastatic manifestations of bronchial carcinoma**

**Invasion of adjacent structures**
Horner's syndrome
Vocal cord paralysis
Superior vena cava (SVC) obstruction
Dysphagia
Phrenic nerve palsy
Pericardial effusion
Cardiac arrhythmias
Rib involvement
Spontaneous pneumothorax

**Endocrine and metabolic manifestations**
Syndrome of inappropriate ADH secretion (SIADH)
Cushing's syndrome
Hypercalcaemia
Gynaecomastia
Hyperthyroidism
Spontaneous hypoglycaemia
Carcinoid syndromes
Excess pigmentation
Myopathies
Neuropathies
Eton Lambert's syndrome
Hypertrophic pulmonary osteoarthropathy

# Miscellaneous pulmonary conditions

## Causes of obstructive sleep apnoea

- Obesity
- Pharyngeal obstruction
- Enlarged tonsils
- Enlarged adenoids
- Acromegaly
- Mucopolysaccharidoses
- Superior vena caval obstruction
- Myxoedema
- Rhinitis
- Drugs that depress respiration (alcohol, sedatives, opiates)
- Shy–Drager syndrome

---

**Box 9.7: Symptoms of obstructive sleep apnoea syndrome**

Heavy snoring
Restless sleep
Nocturnal apnoeic pauses
Daytime somnolence
Hypertension
Poor concentration
Morning headaches
Impotence
Deterioration in personality
Cognitive impairment
Nocturnal enuresis
Cor pulmonale
Respiratory failure
Cardiac failure
Ischaemic heart disease
Sudden death
Polycythaemia

---

# Causes of pneumothorax

## *Spontaneous*
- Idiopathic
- Chronic obstructive pulmonary disease
- Pulmonary fibrosis
- Asthma
- Cystic fibrosis
- Bronchiectasis
- Tuberculosis
- Marfan's syndrome
- Ehlers–Danlos syndrome
- Congenital cysts
- Catamenial
- Endometriosis
- Eosinophilic granuloma
- Tuberous sclerosis
- Lung abscess
- Malignancy
- Hydatid cyst
- Pseudoxanthoma elasticum

## *Non-spontaneous*
- Chest trauma
- Mechanical ventilation
- Oesophageal rupture

# Causes of ARDS

- Hypovolaemic shock
- Infection (pulmonary/extra pulmonary)
- Trauma
- Fat embolism
- Air/amniotic fluid embolism
- Inhalation (toxic gases, oxygen, gastric juice, fresh and saltwater)
- Disseminated intravascular coagulation
- Massive blood transfusion
- Diabetic ketoacidosis
- Uraemia
- Neurogenic (cerebral oedema, intracranial haemorrhage)
- Drugs: hydrochlorothiazide, salicylates, naloxone, heroin, cocaine
- Acute pancreatitis

> **Box 9.8: Indications for lung transplantation**
>
> Bronchiectasis
> Emphysema
> Pulmonary vascular disease
> Severe and progressive disease with a poor prognosis of < 2 years
> Age < 50 years (for heart–lung transplant), < 60 years (for lung transplant)
> No significant comorbidity
> Psychologically stable

> **Box 9.9: Indications for long-term oxygen therapy**
>
> Patients with stable chronic obstructive airways disease and:
> $FEV1 < 1.5$ l
> $FVC < 2$ l
> $Po_2 < 7.3$ kPa
> $Pco_2 > 6$ kPa
> Other patients with chronic obstructive airways disease with similar spirometry and hypoxia but no hypercapnia
> Patients with severe hypoxia due to advanced pulmonary fibrosis and other lung infiltrations

- High altitude
- Eclampsia
- Neurogenic pulmonary oedema

# Known causes of pulmonary eosinophilia

### Allergic bronchopulmonary mycoses
- *Aspergillus*
- *Candida*

### Helminth infections
- *Ascaris lumbricoides*
- *Strongyloides*
- Filiariasis
- *Ancylostoma*
- Schistosomiasis
- *Toxocara*

### Granulomatous disease
- Wegener's granulomatosis
- Churg–Strauss syndrome

### Drugs
- Sulphonamides
- Penicillins
- Tetracycline
- Aspirin
- Naproxen
- Sulphasalazine
- Chlorpropramide
- Chlorpromazine
- Imipramine
- Carbamazepine
- Phenytoin
- Nitrofurantoin
- Methotrexate
- Gold
- Penicillamine

### Miscellaneous
- Asthma
- Lymphangiography
- Blood transfusion

# Unknown causes of pulmonary eosinophilia

- Simple pulmonary eosinophilia (Loeffler's syndrome)
- Prolonged pulmonary eosinophilia (eosinophilic pneumonia)

# Pulmonary manifestations of connective tissue disorders

### SLE
- Pleurisy
- Lupus pneumonitis

- Atelectasis
- Pulmonary oedema
- Fibrosing alveolitis
- Pneumonia
- Pleural effusions
- Vanishing lung syndrome

## Systemic sclerosis
- Fibrosing alveolitis
- Aspiration pneumonia
- Bronchiectasis
- Pleural effusion
- Scleroderma of the chest wall

## Rheumatoid arthritis
- Pleural effusions
- Obliterative bronchiolitis
- Pneumonia
- Fibrosing alveolitis
- Pulmonary nodules
- Bronchiectasis

## Dermatomyositis
- Bronchial neoplasm
- Aspiration pneumonia
- Myositis

## Ankylosing spondylitis
- Fusion of costovertebral joints
- Upper lobe pulmonary fibrosis

# Clinical case scenarios

## Pleural effusion

- The trachea is usually central and expansion normal
- The effusion is characterised by a stony dull percussion note, reduced breath sounds, reduced tactile vocal fremitus and reduced vocal resonance

- Other features to look for:
  Signs of carcinoma of the bronchus
  Butterfly rash (SLE)
  Peripheral oedema (nephrotic syndrome)
  Signs of chronic liver disease
  Signs of cardiac failure
  Abdominal scars (peritoneal dialysis)
  Yellow nails (yellow nail syndrome)

**Table 9.8: Signs of chest abnormalities**

| Abnormality | Consolidation | Collapse | Pleural effusion | Pneumo-thorax | Pleural thickening |
|---|---|---|---|---|---|
| Mediastinal shift | No | Towards collapse | Away from effusion | Away if tension | No |
| Chest wall movements | Normal or reduced | Reduced | Reduced | Normal or reduced | Reduced |
| Breath sounds | Increased (bronchial) | Reduced | Reduced | Reduced | Reduced |
| Added sounds | Crepitations | No | No | Occasional click | No |
| Percussion note | Normal or reduced | Reduced | Reduced | Increased | Reduced |
| Tactile fremitus/ vocal resonance | Increased | Reduced | Reduced | Reduced | Reduced |

Hepatomegaly (raised right
  hemidiaphragm)
Thyroid status
Hands (rheumatoid arthritis)
Signs of consolidation or collapse
  (superimposed pneumonia)

# Cryptogenic fibrosing alveolitis

- The patient is usually clubbed and
  there is central cyanosis
- On auscultation there are fine end-
  inspiratory basal crepitations

- Other features to look for:
  Signs of other autoimmune
    conditions
  Other causes of fibrosis
  Erythema nodosum (sarcoid)
  Subcutaneous coal dust
    (coalworker's pneumoconiosis)

# Chronic obstructive pulmonary disease

- Patients may fall into one of the two
  classical cases, namely 'blue bloaters'
  or 'pink puffers'
- Often patients will have mixed signs
  rather than falling at one end of the
  spectrum

- Certain features are common to both
  conditions:
  Nicotine-stained fingers
  Hyperinflated lungs
  Use of accessory muscles during
    respiration
  In-drawing of intercostal muscles
  Reduced suprasternal notch–cricoid
    distance
  Tracheal tug during respiration
  Reduced chest expansion
- If patients do fall at one end of the
  spectrum there are certain differences
  between the two cases, as illustrated
  earlier in the chapter (Table 9.9)

- Other features to look for:
  Signs of respiratory failure (flapping
    tremor, collapsing pulse)
  Signs of cor pulmonale (right heart
    failure)
  Collapse
  Consolidation
  Signs of bronchial carcinoma

# Bronchiectasis

- The patient may be underweight,
  breathless and cyanosed
- There may be clubbing
- The patient may have a frequent
  productive cough (if there is a sputum
  pot, look in it)

**Table 9.9: Distinctions between emphysema and chronic bronchitis**

| Feature | Emphysema | Chronic bronchitis |
| --- | --- | --- |
| Course | Relentless, progressive dyspnoea | Intermittent with exacerbations |
| Sputum | Scanty | Profuse |
| Cor pulmonale | Infrequent | Frequent |
| Polycythaemia | Uncommon | Common |
| CXR | Attenuated peripheral vessels | Normal peripheral vessels |
| Arterial $P_{CO_2}$ | Normal | Raised |
| Alveolar gas transfer | Reduced | Normal |
| Nocturnal hypoxia | Mild | Profound |

- Coarse crepitations and rhonchi are heard throughout both lung fields, or may be localised in localised disease
- Breath sounds are normal and are not bronchial unless there is active superimposed infection

- Other features to look for:
  Right-sided cardiac apex
  (Kartagener's syndrome)
  Young, thin patient (cystic fibrosis)
  Signs of sarcoid
  Old tuberculosis

## SVC obstruction

- There may be stridor
- Face and upper extremities are oedematous and cyanosed (may be a clear line of demarcation)
- The eyes are suffused
- The superficial veins of the upper thorax are dilated and prominent
- The neck veins are engorged, fixed and non-pulsatile

- Other features to look for:
  Radiation burns
  Signs of bronchial carcinoma
  Goitre
  Pulsatile neck mass (aortic aneurysm)
  Lymphadenopathy

## Carcinoma of the bronchus

- Patient may be cachectic and clubbed
- There will be nicotine staining of the fingers
- There may be supraclavicular lymph nodes and axillary lymph nodes
- In the lungs there may be signs of effusion, collapse and consolidation
- With apical tumours there may be:

Horner's syndrome
Wasting of the small muscles of the hand
Sensory loss indicative of a T1 lesion

- Other features to look for:
  Radiation burns indicating previous radiotherapy
  Signs of SVC obstruction
  Gynaecomastia
  Acanthosis nigricans
  Thoracotomy scar from previous surgery
  Cushingoid appearance due to ectopic ACTH production
  Myopathy which may be fatiguable in Eton–Lambert syndrome
  Peripheral neuropathy
  Cerebellar signs
  Hypertrophic pulmonary Osteoarthropathy (pain and swelling of wrists and/or ankles + clubbing + new bone formation on X-ray)

## Cor pulmonale

- This is the presence of right-sided heart failure, secondary to chronic pulmonary disease
- Look for evidence of chronic obstructive pulmonary disease or bronchiectasis, with signs of superimposed right heart failure

# 10 Renal medicine

## Contents

## Anatomy

- Each kidney is 10–12 cm in length
- Each kidney weighs 150 g
- Kidneys are situated retroperitoneally and lie between T12 and L3
- Right kidney is 1.5 cm lower than left
- Both kidneys move 3 cm during respiration
- Each kidney contains about one million nephrons
- Nerve supply to kidneys and ureters derived from T10–L1
- Blood supply to kidneys is derived from renal arteries and drained via renal veins
- Renal blood flow = 25% of resting cardiac output (1300 ml)
- Renal plasma flow = 70 ml/min
- 25% of renal plasma flow is ultrafiltered at the glomeruli

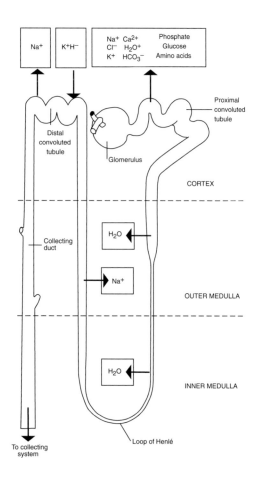

**Fig. 10.1: Histological and functional anatomy of renal tubular system**

**Table 10.1:  Waste product excretion**

| Substance | Filtered load (mmol per 24h) | Urinary excretion (mmol per 24h) | Reabsorbed (%) | Site of reabsorption | Secreted |
|---|---|---|---|---|---|
| Water | 180 litres | 0.75–2.5 litres | 98–99.6 | Distal tubule Collecting ducts | No |
| Sodium | 25000 | 100–250 | 99–99.6 | Proximal tubule (50–75%) Ascending loop of Henlé (25–50%) | No |
| Potassium | 720 | 60–120 | 80–90 | Proximal tubule (75%) Ascending loop of Henlé (25%) | Distal tubule |
| Calcium | 234 | 5 | 98 | Proximal tubule (50%) Ascending loop of Henlé (50%) | No |
| Bicarbonate | 4300 | 5 | 99.9 | Proximal tubule (80–90%) Distal tubule (10–20%) | No |
| Hydrogen | n/a | n/a | n/a | n/a | Proximal and distal tubules |
| Glucose | 10 | 1 | 99.9 | Proximal tubule | No |

- Normal glomerular filtration rate = 120 ml/min (180 l/day)
- Ultrafiltration pressure (10 mmHg) = capillary pressure (45 mmHg) – pressure within Bowman's space (10 mmHg) + plasma oncotic pressure (25 mmHg))

# Physiology

## Excretion of waste products (Table 10.1)

- Urine = (glomerular filtrate + tubular secretion) – tubular reabsorption

# Water and salt homeostasis

- Normal body water = 50% of adult weight (50 l)
- Total body water = interstitial (10.5 l) + plasma (3.5 l) + intracellular (36 l)
- Body water content controlled mainly by antidiuretic hormone (ADH: vasopressin)
- ADH produced in hypothalamus
- ADH stored in posterior pituitary
- ADH release stimulated by: stimulation of hypothalamic osmoreceptors
    Stimulation of left atrial osmoreceptors

**Table 10.2: Endocrine functions**

| Hormone | Synthesised in kidney | Action on kidney |
| --- | --- | --- |
| Calcitriol | Yes | Increases calcium reabsorption |
| Renin/angiotensin | Yes | Autoregulation of renal blood flow |
| Prostaglandins (E2, I2) | Yes | Autoregulation of renal blood flow |
| | | Increase renin release |
| | | Affect sodium and water handling |
| Erythropoietin | Yes | None |
| Kallikrein | Yes | Autoregulation of renal blood flow |
| | | Affects sodium and water handling |
| Parathyroid hormone (PTH) | No | Phosphaturia |
| | | Bicarbonaturia |
| | | Increases calcium reabsorption |
| | | Increases calcitriol synthesis |
| Vasopressin (ADH) | No | Increases antidiuresis |
| Aldosterone | No | Increases sodium reabsorption |
| | | Increases hydrogen and potassium secretion |
| Catecholamines | No | Increase renin release |
| Atrial natriuretic peptide | No | Increases sodium and water excretion |

(atrial natriuretic peptide production)
Angiotensin II
Catecholamines
Endogenous opiates
- ADH acts on distal tubules and collecting ducts
- ADH increases permeability to water and increases water reabsorption
- Typical rate of water excretion 0.75–2.5 l/day (can range from 0.5–25 l/day)

# Acid–base homoeostasis

- 15 000–20 000 mmol of $CO_2$ produced per day
- Virtually all $CO_2$ excreted via lungs
- Small amounts of carbonic acid produced
- Major urinary buffers: bicarbonate, ammonia, phosphate

# Assessment of renal function

## Measurement of creatinine clearance

- Empty bladder at beginning of collection period and note time
- Collect all urine voided over the next 24 hours and measure total volume (V) and creatinine concentration (U)
- During collection period, take one blood sample for serum creatinine concentration (P)
- Creatinine clearance = UV / P $\times$ 100

# Changes in urea and creatinine

### Serum urea raised out of proportion to serum creatinine
- Sodium and water depletion

## Table 10.3: Measures of glomerular filtration rate (GFR)

| Measure | Advantages | Disadvantages |
|---|---|---|
| Inulin clearance | Physiologically suitable (completely filtered, not secreted or reabsorbed by tubules, stable in urine) Traditional 'gold standard' No radiation | Poor solubility Activates complement Time-consuming |
| Creatinine clearance | Simple Cheap No radiation (pregnancy, children) | Requires patient cooperation Overestimates GFR in advanced disease (increased tubular secretion) Reduced by cimetidine, trimethoprim, spironolactone, amiloride (reduced tubular secretion) |
| Serum creatinine | Similar to creatinine clearance No urine collection needed | Affected by diet Less accurate if renal function normal and in advanced disease |
| $^{51}$Cr EDTA clearance | Similar to inulin No urine collection needed | Underestimates GFR Less accurate in advanced disease Radiation exposure |
| $^{125}$I sodium iothalamic acid | Similar to inulin No urine collection needed | Similar to $^{51}$Cr EDTA |
| $^{99}$Tc-SN-DTPA | Short half-life (lower radiation dose) No urine collection needed | Less accurate in advanced disease Not yet available for clinical use |
| B$_2$ microglobulin | Useful for nephrotoxic drug monitoring and early detection of transplant rejection, diabetic nephropathy and for patients on regular haemodialysis and with advanced disease | Expensive Time-consuming Increased in immunological diseases, malignancy, liver disease |
| Serum urea | Simple Cheap No radiation No urine collection needed | Affected by diet Diurnal variation Dependent on urinary flow rate |

(predominant water depletion)
• Pure water depletion
• Cardiac failure
• Gastrointestinal haemorrhage
• High protein intake in the presence of

renal disease
• Protein catabolism:
    Corticosteroid therapy
    Tetracycline (overdose or in the presence of renal disease)

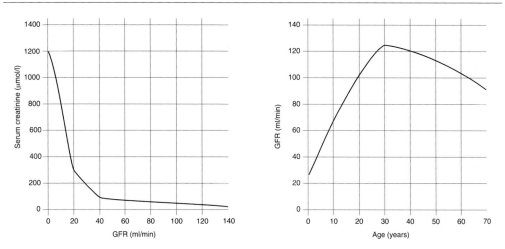

**Fig. 10.2: Glomerular filtration rate (GFR)**

Trauma
Acute illness

### Serum creatinine raised out of proportion to serum urea
- Rhabdomyolysis
- Drugs: aspirin, cotrimoxazole, penacemide

### Serum urea depressed out of proportion to serum creatinine
- Pregnancy
- Liver disease
- High fluid intake
- Low-protein diet

### Serum urea and creatinine raised in parallel
- Established acute renal failure
- Chronic renal failure

# Renal biopsy

## Indications
- Nephrotic syndrome
- Unexplained renal failure with normal-sized kidneys
- Failure to recover from assumed reversible acute renal failure

- Diagnosis of systemic diseases with renal involvement (sarcoid, amyloid)
- Assessment of transplanted kidney

## Contraindications
- Uncooperative patient
- Single kidney
- Small kidneys
- Bleeding diathesis
- Gross obesity
- Ascites
- Uncontrolled hypertension
- Renal cystic disease

## Complications
- Macroscopic haematuria
- Loin pain
- Perirenal haematoma
- AV malformation
- Sepsis
- Mortality (0.1%)

---

**Box 10.1: Measures of renal plasma flow**

Para-aminohippurate clearance
Hippurate clearance
Colour flow Doppler ultrasound (in experienced hands)

# Urine abnormalities

## Causes of proteinuria

- Urinary tract infection
- Nephrotic syndrome
- Postural
- Malignant hypertension
- Pre-eclampsia
- Diabetic nephropathy
- Fanconi's syndrome
- Balkan nephropathy
- Myeloma
- Waldenström's macroglobulinaemia
- Essential cryoglobulinaemia
- Fever (young children)
- Congestive cardiac failure
- Reflux nephropathy
- Analgesic nephropathy
- Polycystic kidney disease
- Haemolytic uraemic syndrome
- Postpartum renal failure
- Thrombotic thrombocytopenic purpura
- Congenital cyanotic heart disease
- Gross obesity
- Obstructive nephropathy

## Causes of aminoaciduria

### Normal
- Glycine
- Glutamine
- Alanine
- Serine
- Histidine

### Inherited metabolic disorder
- Phenylketonuria
- Maple syrup urine disease

### Severe chronic liver disease

### Selective failure of tubular reabsorption

---

**Box 10.2: Positive clinitest reaction**

**Tests for reducing sugars**
*Positive test turns blue to orange*
Glucose
Lactose
Pentose
Fructose
Galactose
Homogentisic acid
Salicylates
Isoniazid
L-Dopa
Vitamin C
Nalidixic acid
Tetracycline

---

- Cystinuria
- Hartnup's disease

### General tubular damage
- Fanconi's syndrome

## Causes of glycosuria

- Diabetes mellitus
- Pregnancy
- Phaeochromocytoma
- Anxiety
- Strenuous exercise
- Cerebral trauma
- Cerebral haemorrhage
- Liver disease
- Sepsis

## Causes of haematuria

- Neoplasia
- Infection
- Calculi
- Glomerulonephritis
- Drugs: anticoagulants
- Malignant hypertension
- Subacute bacterial endocarditis

> **Box 10.3: Pathological findings in urinary sediment**
>
> **White cell casts**
> Pyelonephritis
> Glomerulonephritis
>
> **Red blood cells**
> Glomerular damage
>
> **Large broad hyaline casts**
> Advanced chronic renal disease
>
> **Epithelial cell casts and coarse granular casts**
> Acute tubular necrosis

- Papillary necrosis
- Polycystic disease
- Renal trauma
- Bleeding diathesis
- Familial benign haematuria
- Analgesic nephropathy
- Sickle cell disease
- Congenital cyanotic heart disease

## Causes of abnormal urine colour other than haematuria

- Porphyria
- Haemoglobinuria
- Myoglobinuria
- Beetroot consumption
- Rifampicin
- Para-aminosalicylic acid
- Alkaptonuria
- Obstructive jaundice
- L-Dopa

## Causes of sterile pyuria

- Antibiotic therapy prior to urine collection
- Specimen contaminated with antiseptic
- Inappropriate culture conditions
- Renal tuberculosis
- Chlamydia infection
- Calculi
- Analgesic nephropathy
- Cyclophosphamide
- Acute glomerulonephritis
- Polycystic disease
- Vaginal discharge
- Bladder tumour
- Appendicitis
- Chronic renal disease
- Interstitial nephritis
- Interstitial cystitis
- Papillary necrosis

# Sodium metabolism

## Causes of hyponatraemia

### *Sodium depletion*
**Excessive loss**
- from kidneys
  Recovery phase of acute tubular necrosis
  After relief of bilateral ureteric obstruction
  Excessive diuretic therapy
  Medullary cystic disease
  Analgesic nephropathy
  Pyelonephritis
  Polycystic kidney disease
  Hyperglycaemia
  Adrenocortical insufficiency
- from gastrointestinal tract
  Vomiting
  Diarrhoea
  Paralytic ileus
  Fistulae
  Intestinal obstruction
- from skin
  Burns
  Cystic fibrosis

*Inadequate intake*
- Only if excessive loss

## Water excess
### Increased intake
- Excessive parenteral dextrose
- Polydipsia
- Beer drinker's potomania

### Decreased excretion
- SIADH
- Renal failure (acute/chronic)
- Cirrhosis of liver
- Nephrotic syndrome
- Cardiac failure
- Adrenocortical insufficiency
- Pregnancy
- Hypothyroidism

## Pseudohyponatraemia
- Hyperlipidaemia
- Paraproteinaemia

## Miscellaneous
- Sick cell syndrome


# Causes of hypernatraemia

## Water depletion
### Excessive loss
- from kidneys
  Diabetes insipidus
  Solute diuresis: Hyperglycaemia
    Uraemia
    Mannitol
    Hypercatabolic states
- from gastrointestinal tract
  Vomiting
  Diarrhoea
- from skin
  Sweating
  Burns
  Erythroderma
- from lungs
  Hyperventilation

*Inadequate intake*
- Infancy
- Elderly
- Confusion
- Impaired consciousness
- Dysphagia
- Iatrogenic

## Sodium excess
### Increased intake
- Iatrogenic
  Excessive parenteral saline
  Saline enemas
  Saline emetics
  Dialysate solutions

### Decreased excretion
- Primary aldosteronism
- Cushing's syndrome


# Potassium metabolism

## Causes of hypokalaemia

### Decreased intake
- Oral
- Parenteral
- Malabsorption

### Excessive loss
- from kidneys
  Diuretic therapy
  Alkalosis
  Solute diuresis: Glucose
    Urea
    Mannitol
    Saline
    Carbenicillin
    Penicillin
  Aldosteronism: Primary
    Secondary
    Renin-secreting tumours
  Bartter's syndrome

Liddle's disease
Magnesium depletion
Renal tubular acidosis (types 1 and 2)
Gentamicin
Amikacin
Acute myeloid leukaemia
- from gastrointestinal tract
Diarrhoea
Vomiting
Ileostomy
Ureteroenterostomy
Villous adenoma of rectum
Fistulae
VIPoma (Verner–Morrison syndrome)
Calcium resonium

### Intracellular shifts
- Alkalosis
- High-dose insulin
- $\beta_2$ adrenergic stimulation
- Theophylline overdose
- Hypokalaemic periodic paralysis

## Causes of hyperkalaemia

### Increased intake
- Oral
- Parenteral
- Stored blood

### Decreased loss
- from kidneys
  Acute renal failure
  Chronic renal failure
  Potassium-sparing diuretics
  Renal tubular acidosis (type 4)
  Treatment with ACE inhibitors

### Intracellular shifts
- Acidosis
- Crush injuries
- Burns
- Rhabdomyolysis
- Massive death of tumour cells
- Hyperkalaemic periodic paralysis
- Succinyl choline

- Digoxin poisoning
- Familial hyperkalaemic acidosis

### Pseudohyperkalaemia
- Haemolysed blood sample
- Leukaemia with very high white cell count
- Familial pseudohyperkalaemia
- Myeloproliferative disorders with very high white cell count

# Vasopressin metabolism
## Causes of SIADH

### Ectopic excretion
#### Malignant disease
- Carcinoma: lung (oat cell), pancreas, duodenum, thymus, prostate, adrenal, ureter, colon, nasopharynx
- Lymphoma: Hodgkin's, non-Hodgkin's
- Acute myeloid leukaemia

### Inappropriate excretion
#### Cerebral disease
- Intracranial sepsis
- Stroke
- Intracranial haemorrhage
- Head injury
- Post-transsphenoidal surgery
- Cerebral tumours
- Histiocytosis X
- Vasculitis
- Guillain–Barré syndrome
- Central pontine myelinosis

#### Pulmonary disease
- Sepsis
- Aspergillosis
- Cystic fibrosis
- Intermittent positive-pressure ventilation
- Pneumothorax

### Psychiatric disease

- Schizophrenia
- Acute psychoses

### Metabolic disease

- Acute intermittent porphyria
- Hypothyroidism
- Trauma
- Pain

### Drugs

- Chlorpropramide, carbamazepine, cyclophosphamide, vincristine, amitriptyline, tranylcypromine, fluphenazine, indomethacin, opiates, barbiturates, oxytocin, bromocriptine, nicotine, clofibrate

# Causes of diabetes insipidus

## Cranial (inadequate ADH production)

### Primary

- Idiopathic
- Familial
- DIDMOAD syndrome (diabetes insipidus, diabetes mellitus, optic atrophy, deafness)

### Secondary

- Head injury
- Iatrogenic
- Pituitary surgery
- Pituitary irradiation
- Malignancy
  Primary pituitary
  Secondary carcinoma (lung, breast)
  Lymphoma
  Leukaemia
  Teratoma
  Ectopic pinealoma
  Craniopharyngioma
- Granuloma
  Sarcoid

  Eosinophilic granuloma
  Tuberculosis
  Brucellosis
  Syphilis
  Histiocytosis X
- Infection
  Pyogenic abscess
  Meningitis
  Encephalitis
- Vascular
  Haemorrhage
  Thrombosis

---

### Box 10.4: Water deprivation test

Allow fluids overnight before test
On the morning of the test give a light breakfast with no fluid and prevent patient from smoking
Weigh patient at start of test and allow no fluids for 8 hours
Patient must be kept under constant supervision during this period
Every hour thereafter, for 8 hours: weigh patient (stop test if weight falls by > 3%) Measure urinary volume and osmolality
Collect blood samples for serum osmolality at 30 minutes, 4, 7 and 8 hours (stop test if osmolality exceeds 300 mol/kg)
After 8 hours, allow patient to drink and give 20 μg of desmopressin intranasally
Collect urine hourly for further 4 hours

**Findings**
*Diabetes insipidus*
Weight loss > 3% initial body weight
Serum osmolality > 300 mmol/kg
Urine:serum osmolality ratio < 1.9 (provided serum osmolality > 285 mmol/kg)

*Nephrogenic diabetes insipidus*
Urine does not concentrate within 4 hours of desmopressin

*Psychogenic polydipsia*
Urine concentrates during period of fluid deprivation

**Table 10.4: Distinctions between psychogenic polydipsia and diabetes insipidus**

| Psychogenic polydipsia | Diabetes insipidus |
|---|---|
| Erratic drinking pattern | Regular drinking pattern |
| No nocturnal polyuria | Nocturnal polyuria |
| Serum osmolality 265–280 mmol/kg | Serum osmolality 290–295 mmol/kg |
| Hyponatraemia | Hypernatraemia |
| Normal urine concentrating ability | Failure to concentrate urine after water deprivation |
| Other psychiatric conditions | |

Sheehan's syndrome
Sickle cell disease

## Nephrogenic (renal resistance to ADH)
- Familial
- Metabolic: hypercalcaemia, hypokalaemia
- Chronic renal disease: pyelonephritis, polycystic disease, amyloid
- Drugs: lithium, amphotericin B, glibenclamide, gentamicin, demeclocycline

# Causes of polyuria

## Deficient ADH
- Cranial diabetes insipidus

## Renal resistance to ADH
- Nephrogenic diabetes insipidus

## Drinking abnormalities
- Psychogenic polydipsia
- Hypothalamic polydipsia:
  Sarcoid
  Eosinophilic granuloma
  Hydrocephalus
  Encephalitis
- Drug induced:
  phenothiazines
  lithium
  amitriptyline

## Renal disease
- Postobstructive nephropathy

- Fanconi's syndrome
- Medullary cystic disease
- Analgesic nephropathy
- Hyperglobulinaemia
- Myeloma
- Sarcoid
- Sjögren's syndrome
- Amyloid
- SLE
- Sickle cell disease

## Solute diuresis
- Diabetes mellitus
- Uraemia
- High protein intake
- Hypertonic enemas
- Mannitol

**Box 10.5: Renal calculi**

| Types | Causes |
|---|---|
| Calcium (oxalate/ phosphate) (radio-opaque) | Hypercalciuria |
| Magnesium ammonium phosphate (radio-opaque) | Proteus infection Alkalotic urine |
| Urate (radiolucent) | Hyperuricaemia Acidic urine |
| Cysteine (radio-opaque) | Hereditary cystinuria Acidic urine |
| Xanthine (radiolucent) | Hereditary xanthinuria |

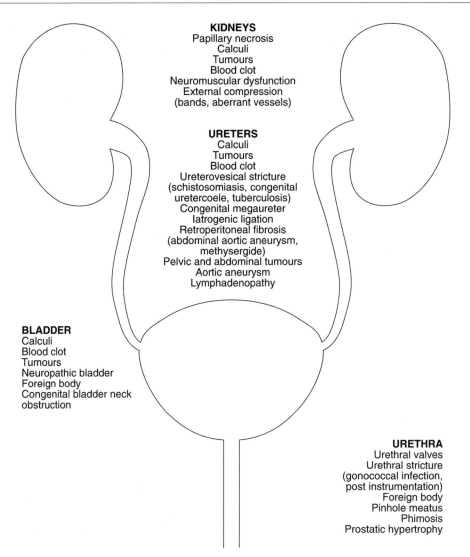

**KIDNEYS**
Papillary necrosis
Calculi
Tumours
Blood clot
Neuromuscular dysfunction
External compression
(bands, aberrant vessels)

**URETERS**
Calculi
Tumours
Blood clot
Ureterovesical stricture
(schistosomiasis, congenital
uretercoele, tuberculosis)
Congenital megaureter
Iatrogenic ligation
Retroperitoneal fibrosis
(abdominal aortic aneurysm,
methysergide)
Pelvic and abdominal tumours
Aortic aneurysm
Lymphadenopathy

**BLADDER**
Calculi
Blood clot
Tumours
Neuropathic bladder
Foreign body
Congenital bladder neck
obstruction

**URETHRA**
Urethral valves
Urethral stricture
(gonococcal infection,
post instrumentation)
Foreign body
Pinhole meatus
Phimosis
Prostatic hypertrophy

**Fig. 10.3: Common causes of obstructive nephropathy at different sites in the renal tract**

# Renal calculi

## Causes of hypercalciuria

### *Hypercalcaemia*

### *Normal serum calcium*
- Idiopathic hypercalciuria
- Hyperoxaluria (idiopathic, excess spinach, excess tea, Crohn's disease, vitamin C deficiency)
- Renal tubular acidosis (distal)
- Chronic cadmium poisoning
- Chronic berylliosis
- Wilson's disease
- Medullary sponge kidney
- Analgesic nephropathy

# Obstructive nephropathy

## Important clinical features

- Acute obstruction usually associated with pain
- Slowly progressive obstruction may be painfree
- Renal failure implies bilateral obstruction or obstruction of solitary functioning kidney
- Complete obstruction leads to anuria
- Partial obstruction may be associated with normal or increased urinary volumes
- Obstructive nephropathy should be considered in all presentations of renal impairment
- Recurrent/resistant urinary infections should raise the suspicion of obstructive nephropathy
- The most important investigation in a male with renal failure is a rectal examination

# Glomerulonephritis

## Causes of glomerulonephritis

### Acute glomerulonephritis
- Infection (usually respiratory)

### Membranous nephropathy
- Idiopathic
- Heavy metal intoxication (gold, mercury)
- Drugs (penicillamine, captopril)
- Infection (hepatitis B, malaria, syphilis)
- Carcinoma (bronchus, stomach, colon, pancreas, ovary, uterus)
- Leukaemia, lymphoma

- Connective tissue disease (Sjögren's syndrome, SLE)
- Rheumatoid arthiritis
- Kartagener's syndrome

### Minimal change nephropathy
- Idiopathic

### Focal glomerulosclerosis
- Idiopathic
- Heroin abuse
- AIDS
- Charcot–Marie–Tooth disease
- Mitochondrial cytopathy
- Diabetes mellitus

### Mesangiocapillary glomerulonephritis
- Shunt nephritis (*Staphylococcus epidermidis*)
- Post-streptococcal nephritis
- Neoplasia
- Sickle cell disease
- $\alpha_1$-Antitrypsin deficiency
- SLE
- Partial lipodystrophy
- Rheumatoid arthritis
- Kartagener's syndrome

### Focal proliferative glomerulonephritis
- Idiopathic
- Subacute infective endocarditis
- SLE
- Sjögren's syndrome
- Anti-glomerular basement membrane (anti-GBM) nephritis
- Polyarteritis nodosa
- Wegener's granulomatosis
- IgA nephropathy
- Henloch–Schönlein purpura

### Crescenteric glomerulonephritis
- Anti-GBM nephritis
- Henloch–Schönlein purpura
- Mixed cryoglobulinaemia
- Polyarteritis nodosa

## Table 10.5: Presentation of glomerulonephritis

| Type | Typical age | Typical presentation | Prognosis |
|---|---|---|---|
| Acute glomerulonephritis | Children | Acute nephrotic syndrome | Good |
| Membranous nephropathy | Adults | Asymptomatic proteinuria Nephrotic syndrome | Good |
| Minimal change nephropathy | Children | Nephrotic syndrome | Good |
| Focal glomerulosclerosis | Children Adults | Children: nephrotic syndrome Adults: asymptomatic proteinuria, hypertension | Poor |
| Mesangiocapillary glomerulonephritis | Young adults | Nephrotic syndrome Acute nephrotic syndrome Hypertension Asymptomatic proteinuria Asymptomatic haematuria | 50% develop renal failure |
| Crescenteric glomerulonephritis | Adults | Acute nephrotic syndrome Acute renal failure | Poor |
| IgA nephropathy | Young men | Asymptomatic haematuria | Good |
| Henloch–Schönlein purpura | Children Young adults | Purpura (extensor surfaces) Arthralgia Acute nephrotic syndrome Abdominal pain | Good |

- Wegener's granulomatosis
- Post-streptococcal nephritis
- Systemic sclerosis

### IgA nephropathy
- Cirrhosis
- Wiskott–Aldrich syndrome

### Henloch–Schönlein purpura
- Infection (usually respiratory)
- Sulphonamides
- Penicillins

### Hereditary glomerulonephritis
- Alport's syndrome
- Fabry's disease
- Cockayne syndrome

### Anti-GBM nephritis
- Infection
- Hydrocarbons
- Goodpasture's syndrome

# Immune complex involvement in glomerulonephritis

### Probable
- Postinfective acute glomerulonephritis
- Infective endocarditis
- Shunt nephritis
- Malaria
- Syphilis
- Hepatitis B, C
- SLE

### Possible
- Henloch–Schönlein purpura
- IgA nephropathy
- Mesangiocapillary glomerulonephritis
- Idiopathic rapidly progressive glomerulonephritis
- Focal segmental glomerulonephritis

# Tumours of the renal tract

## Presentation of renal cell adenocarcinoma

### Local effects
- Haematuria (50%)
- Loin pain
- Abdominal mass

### Metastases
- Bone pain
- Cough
- Dyspnoea

### Paraneoplastic effects
- Night sweats
- Fever
- Hypercalcaemia
- Polycythaemia
- Raised ESR

---

**Box 10.6: Tumours of the renal tract**

| Types | Associations |
|---|---|
| **Benign** | |
| Adenomata | |
| Hamartoma | Tuberous sclerosis |
| Fibromata | |
| Leiomyomata | |
| Neurogenic | |
| Juxtaglomerular cell (renin secreting) | |
| | |
| **Primary malignant** | |
| Renal cell adenocarcinoma (hypernephroma, Grawitz) | Smoking Von Hippel–Lindau syndrome |
| | |
| Transitional cell | Smoking Schistosomiasis haematobium Cystic kidney disease Aniline dyes Rubber Analgesic nephropathy Papillary necrosis Chronic calculus disease Chronic cystitis Cyclophosphamide |
| | |
| Wilms' tumour | |
| | |
| Sarcoma | Hamartoma |
| | |
| Metastatic | Lung, breast, stomach, melanoma, sarcoma, lymphoma |

# Infections of the renal tract

## Causes of urinary tract infection

- *Escherichia coli*
- Enterococci
- *Proteus*
- *Enterobacter*
- *Pseudomonas*
- Staphylococci
- *Klebsiella*
- *Candida*
- *Myobacterium tuberculosis*

## Infectious agents in human nephritis

### Bacteria
- *Streptococcus pyogenes*
- *Streptococcus viridans*
- *Streptococcus pneumoniae*
- *Staphylococcus aureus*
- *Staphylococcus epidermidis*
- *Meningococcus*
- *Salmonella typhi*
- *Mycobacterium tuberculosis*
- *Mycobacterium leprae*
- *Treponema pallidum*
- *Brucella*
- *Yersinia enterocolitica*
- *Leptospira*
- *Mycoplasma pneumoniae*

### Viruses
- Hepatitis B
- Epstein–Barr
- Mumps
- Measles
- Rubella
- CMV
- Coxsackie
- Variola
- Varicella
- Vaccinia
- HIV

### Rickettsiae
- *Coxiella*

### Fungi
- *Candida albicans*
- *Coccidioides immidis*

### Parasites
- *Plasmodium malariae*
- *Plasmodium falciparum*
- *Schistosoma mansoni*
- *Schistosoma haematobium*
- *Toxoplasma*
- *Wucheria bancrofti (filariae)*
- *Loa-loa*

# Nephrotic syndrome

Nephrotic syndrome is characterised by:
- proteinuria > 3 g/day,
- Hypoalbuminaemia
- Oedema

## Causes of nephrotic syndrome

### Glomerulonephritis
- Minimal change
- Membranous
- Mesangiocapillary
- Crescenteric
- Focal glomerulosclerosis
- Henloch–Schönlein purpura

### Infection
- Malaria
- CMV
- Syphilis
- Leprosy
- Staphylococcal septicaemia

## Box 10.7: Complications of nephrotic syndrome

Massive oedema
Pleural effusion
Ascites
Pericardial effusion
Hypovolaemia
Protein malnutrition
Growth retardation
Poor wound healing
Osteoporosis
Reduced immune competence
Hyperlipidaemia
Hyperviscosity
Sepsis

- Subacute bacterial endocarditis
- Hepatitis B

### Allergies
- Penicillin
- Bee sting
- Pollen
- Foods
- Ivy

### Miscellaneous
- Gross obesity
- Smallpox vaccination
- i.v. Drug abuse

### Vascular
- Renal artery stenosis
- Renal vein thrombosis
- Constrictive pericarditis
- Congenital cyanotic heart disease

### Malignancy
- Myeloma
- Hodgkin's disease

### Drugs
- Ethosuximide
- Propranolol
- Oral contraceptives
- Bismuth
- Phenindione
- Tolbutamide
- Phenylbutazone
- Gold

### Metabolic
- Amyloid
- Hypothyroidism

### Haematological
- Waldenström's macroglobulinaemia

# Interstitial nephritis

## Causes of interstitial nephritis

### Diseases
- Alport's syndrome
- Medullary cystic disease
- Sjögren's syndrome
- Kidney graft rejection
- Hypokalaemia
- Reflux nephropathy
- Balkan nephropathy
- Diabetes mellitus
- Sickle cell disease
- Chronic pyelonephritis
- SLE
- Hyperuricaemia
- Nephrocalcinosis

### Toxins
- Aniline
- Arsenic
- Bismuth
- Cadmium
- Copper
- Lead
- Mercury
- Platinum
- Silver
- Uranium

- Ethylene glycol
- Petroleum
- Mercury
- Thallium
- Carbon tetrachloride
- Insecticides
- Phenol
- Sodium chlorate
- Toluene
- Radiocontrast media
- Radiation
- Paraquat

## Drugs
### Antimicrobials
- Penicillins
- Cephalosporins
- Erythromycin
- Sulphonamides
- Cotrimoxazole
- Rifampicin
- Gentamicin
- Kanamycin
- Minocycline
- Isoniazid
- Para-aminosalicylic acid

### Analgesics
- NSAIDs
- Paracetamol

### Diuretics
- Loop diuretics
- Thiazides

### Metals
- Gold
- Lithium

### Anticonvulsants
- Phenytoin
- Carbamazepine
- Phenobarbitone

### Miscellaneous
- Allopurinol
- Amphotericin B

- Azathioprine
- Cimetidine
- Clofibrate
- Cyclosporin
- Phenindione
- Propranolol
- Interferon
- Iron

# Renal failure

## Causes of renal failure

### Acute
#### Pre-renal
- <u>Hypovolaemia</u>
- <u>Cardiogenic shock</u>
- <u>Septic shock</u>
- Renal artery stenosis

#### Renal
- *Acute tubular necrosis*
- *Acute interstitial nephritis*
- Acute cortical necrosis
- Hepatic failure (hepatorenal syndrome)
- Acute pyelonephritis
- Acute glomerulonephritis
- Hypercalcaemia
- Malignant hypertension
- Haemolytic uraemic syndrome
- Thrombotic thrombocytopenic purpura
- Postpartum renal failure
- Renal graft rejection

#### Post-renal
- Bilateral obstructive nephropathy
- Renal vein thrombosis

### Chronic
- <u>Idiopathic</u>
- <u>Chronic glomerulonephritis</u>
- <u>Chronic pyelonephritis</u>
- <u>Renal vascular disease</u>

### Table 10.6: Biochemical changes in renal failure

| Acute | Chronic |
|---|---|
| Raised urea | *As for acute renal failure, plus:* |
| Raised creatinine | |
| Hyperkalaemia | Low erythropoietin |
| Hyperphosphataemia | Raised parathormone (PTH) |
| Hypermagnesaemia | Hyperreninaemia |
| Hyperuricaemia | Hyperaldosteronism |
| Hyponatraemia | Raised VLDL, LDL |
| Hypocalcaemia | Low HDL |
| Metabolic acidosis | Low follicle-stimulating hormone (FSH) |
| | Low testosterone |
| | Raised growth hormone (GH) |
| | Raised luteinising hormone (LH) |
| | Hyperprolactinaemia |
| | Raised gastrin |
| | Raised glucagon |
| | Raised melanocyte-stimulating hormone (MSH) |

### Table 10.7: Distinctions between pre-renal failure and acute tubular necrosis (ATN)

| Pre-renal failure | ATN |
|---|---|
| Urinary sodium < 20 mmol/l | Urinary sodium > 40 mmol/l |
| Urine:serum urea concentration > 10:1 | Urine:serum urea concentration < 3:1 |
| Urine:serum creatinine concentration > 40:1 | Urine:serum creatinine concentration < 20:1 |
| Urine osmolality > 500 mmol/kg | Urine osmolality < 400 mmol/kg |
| Urine:serum osmolality > 1.5:1 | Urine:serum osmolality < 1.1:1 |
| Fractional sodium excretion < 1% | Fractional sodium excretion > 1% |
| Renal failure index < 1 | Renal failure index > 1 |

\* Osmolality = (2 × sodium) + urea + glucose

- Diabetes mellitus
- Hypertension
- Chronic interstitial nephritis
- Chronic obstructive nephropathy
- Drugs
- Cystic kidney disease
- Cystinosis
- Oxalosis
- Myeloma
- Amyloid
- Malignancy
- Trauma
- Rheumatoid arthritis

# Management of renal failure

## *Correct life-threatening biochemical abnormalities*

Hyperkalaemia should be treated immediately with 10 ml 10% i.v. calcium gluconate and 15 U Actrapid insulin i.v. with 50 ml 50% glucose. Following this, serum potassium should be maintained within the normal range by a continuous intravenous infusion of Actrapid insulin and glucose and calcium resonium 15 g orally or rectally. Acidosis usually recovers when the underlying cause has been treated, but occasionally sodium bicarbonate may be needed.

## Identify the underlying cause

A good history and examination may allow the identification of prerenal failure and obstructive nephropathy (symptoms and signs of fluid depletion, signs of fluid overload, symptoms and signs of prostatic enlargement). CVP measurements and biochemical urinalysis may be helpful. A renal ultrasound should be routinely done in all patients presenting with renal failure to exclude obstructive nephropathy as should a prostate-specific antigen (PSA) measurement in men. Other investigations aimed at identifying the cause of acute tubular necrosis include FBC, LFT, serum calcium, ESR, CRP, autoantibodies, ASO titre, blood cultures, urine microsopy and culture. A detailed drug history is vital. Hepatitis B status should be determined before dialysis. A renal biopsy may be indicated in some circumstances.

## Maintain fluid balance

Hypovolaemia should be corrected with fluid replacement and fluid overload should be treated with diuretics and fluid restriction. Inotropic support may be needed to maintain cardiovascular competence and aid renal blood flow. Careful monitoring of fluid balance is essential. The patient should be catheterised and weighed daily. Serial CVP readings may be helpful and postural hypotension is often the first sign of hypovolaemia. Fluid balance should be maintained so that input = previous day's urine output + 500 ml (to account for insensible losses). Particular care should be taken during the polyuric phase of renal failure or post relief of obstructive nephropathy, when significant polyuria can develop. Dialysis may be required in some cases.

## Other points to note

Acute renal failure is associated with a marked catabolic reaction and patients should be given nutritional supplements as carbohydrate or fat to prevent malnutrition. At the same time, protein intake

---

**Box 10.8: Sequelae of chronic renal failure**

**Haematological**
Normochromic normocytic anaemia
   (decreased production of erythropoietin;
   bone marrow suppression by uraemic
   toxins; shortened RBC survival)

**Cardiovascular**
Hypertension
Cardiac failure
Ischaemic heart disease
Cerebrovascular disease
Pericarditis
Pericardial effusion

**Skeletal**
Hyperparathyroidism
Osteomalacia
Osteosclerosis

**Gastrointestinal**
Peptic ulcer disease
Angiodysplasia

**CNS**
Cognitive impairment
Tremor
Myoclonus
Seizures
Nausea
Vomiting
Dementia
Encephalopathy
Peripheral neuropathy

**Metabolic**
Insulin resistance leading to
   hyperglycaemia

should be lowered to reduce the urea load on the kidneys

Patients with acute renal failure are susceptible to infection, and regular monitoring and sepsis screens should be undertaken. Infections should be treated promptly – initially with broad-spectrum antibiotics – but care should be taken with potentially nephrotoxic drugs.

Acute renal failure leads to impairment of platelet function, which can lead to bleeding, especially from the gastrointestinal tract. Stress ulceration of the gastrointestinal tract can exacerbate this problem and prophylactic cover with antiulcer medication should be considered.

# Dialysis and transplantation

## Complications of dialysis

### Haemodialysis
#### Cardiovascular
- Hypotension, hypertension
- Haemorrhage
- Thrombosis/aneurysm of AV fistula
- Raised cardiac output
- Vascular steal syndromes

#### Metabolic
- Hypernatraemia, hyponatraemia
- Hyperkalaemia, hypokalaemia
- Hard water syndrome (hypercalcaemia, hypermagnesaemia)
- Dialysis dementia (aluminium intoxication)
- Fluorosis
- Thiamine deficiency
- Tertiary hyperparathyroidism

#### Infective
- Sepsis
- Pyrogenic reactions

---

**Box 10.9: Indications for dialysis**

**Neurological**
Lowered conscious level
Encephalopathy
Confusion
Fits
Myoclonus
Peripheral neuropathy

**Cardiovascular/Pulmonary**
Pericarditis
Pleurisy
Volume overload (non-responsive)

**Dermatological**
Unremitting pruritus

**Gastrointestinal**
Unremitting nausea, vomiting, diarrhoea

**Metabolic**
Unremitting acidosis (pH < 7.15)

**Biochemical**
Serum urea > 40 mmol/l (despite low-protein diet)
Serum creatinine > 1200 mmol/l
Creatinine clearance < 5 ml/min
Unresponsive hyperkalaemia (> 7 mmol/l)

---

#### Haematological
- Haemolysis
- Complement–leukocyte-induced pulmonary dysfunction
- Leukopenia
- Thrombocytopenia
- Anaemia
- Priapism

#### Neurological
- Disequilibrium syndrome (raised CSF pressure)
- Carpal tunnel syndrome
- Air embolism
- Stroke
- Impotence

*Dermatological*
• Skin erosions
• Dermatitis

*Peritoneal dialysis*
• Sepsis
• Peritonitis
• Catheter obstruction
• Loss of peritoneal ultrafiltration
• Obesity
• Pleural effusion
• Abdominal wall hernias
• Haemorrhoids
• Low back pain
• Hypoproteinaemia
• Hyperglycaemia

# Acid–base balance

• Anion gap = (sodium + potassium) – (chloride + bicarbonate)
• Normal anion gap: 10 to 18

## Causes of metabolic acidosis

### High anion gap
*Ketoacidosis*
• Diabetes mellitus
• Alcohol
• Starvation

*Lactic acidosis*
• Biguanides
• Alcohol
• Severe liver disease
• Paracetamol poisoning
• Post-epileptic seizure
• Shock: septic, cardiogenic, haemorrhagic
• Traumatic
• Severe hypoxia
• Exercise
• Leukaemia
• Thiamine deficiency
• Fructose-1,6-diphosphate deficiency
• Pyruvate carboxylase deficiency
• Hereditary lactic acidosis
• Methanol poisoning
• Ethylene glycol

*Miscellaneous*
• Uraemia
• Salicylate poisoning
• Paraldehyde
• Reye's syndrome
• Ackee poisoning

### Normal anion gap
• Gastrointestinal bicarbonate loss (diarrhoea, pancreatic fistula)
• Renal tubular acidosis

- Ureteroenterostomy
- Ammonium chloride
- Carbonic anhydrase inhibitors
- Hyperkalaemia
- Hypoaldosteronism

# Causes of metabolic alkalosis

## Loss of unbuffered hydrogen ions
### Gastrointestinal
- Gastric aspiration
- Pyloric stenosis
- Congenital chloride-losing diarrhoea
- Anorexia nervosa

### Renal
- Hyperaldosteronism
- Non-potassium sparing diuretics
- Hypokalaemia
- Hypochloraemia

## Administration of alkali
### Iatrogenic
- Overtreated acidosis
- Forced alkaline diuresis

# Causes of respiratory acidosis

## Pulmonary disease
- Chronic obstructive pulmonary disease
- Bronchospasm
- Aspiration
- Upper respiratory tract obstruction
- Pulmonary fibrosis
- Severe pneumonia

## Depression of respiratory centre
- Drugs: (anaesthetics, barbiturates, benzodiazepines, opiates)
- Cerebral trauma
- Cerebral tumour

## Neuromuscular disease
- Guillain–Barré syndrome
- Motor neuron disease
- Myasthenia gravis
- Poliomyelitis
- Tetanus
- Neurotoxins
- Muscular dystrophy
- Acute porphyria

## Extrapulmonary disease
- Ankylosing spondylitis
- Traumatic flail chest
- Kyphoscoliosis
- Muscle relaxants
- Obstructive sleep apnoea (Pickwickian syndrome)

# Causes of respiratory alkalosis

## Hyperventilation
- Pulmonary oedema
- Pulmonary embolus
- Pneumothorax
- Mechanical overventilation
- Psychogenic

## Stimulation of respiratory centre
- Hypoxia
- High altitude
- Severe anaemia
- Respiratory stimulants (salicylates)
- Raised intracranial pressure
- Cerebral tumours
- Cerebral trauma
- Meningitis
- Encephalitis
- Gram-negative septicaemia
- CO poisoning
- Acute liver failure
- During recovery from metabolic acidosis

# Causes of renal tubular acidosis

## Proximal (type 2) (impaired bicarbonate reabsorption)

- Fanconi's syndrome
- Familial autosomal dominant
- Acetazolamide
- Renal transplant rejection

## Distal (type 1) (impaired hydrogen ion excretion)

- Sjögren's syndrome
- SLE
- Primary biliary cirrhosis
- Fibrosing alveolitis
- Hereditary autosomal dominant
- Carbonic anhydrase deficiency
- Hypergammaglobulinaemia
- Nephrocalcinosis
- Pyelonephritis
- Papillary necrosis
- Chronic obstructive nephropathy
- Medullary sponge kidney
- Sickle cell disease
- Analgesic nephropathy
- Amphotericin B
- Cryoglobulinaemia
- Lithium
- Renal transplant rejection
- Hyperparathyroidism

## Hyperkalaemic (type 4) (impaired potassium and hydrogen ion excretion)

- Hyporeninaemic hypoaldosteronism
- Diabetes mellitus
- Aldosterone antagonists
- Chronic pyelonephritis
- NSAIDs
- Cyclosporin

# Miscellaneous renal conditions

## Renal manifestations of HIV infection

### Glomerular damage
- Focal glomerulosclerosis
- Proteinuria

### Acute renal failure
- Acute tubular necrosis
- Pentamidine
- Aminoglycosides
- Amphotericin B

### Hyponatraemia
- Gut losses
- SIADH (if pulmonary, CNS involvement)

### Malignancy
- Non-Hodgkin's lymphoma

# Causes of papillary necrosis

- Diabetes mellitus
- Phaeochromocytoma
- Sickle cell disease
- Hyperviscosity syndromes
- Acute pyelonephritis
- Obstructive nephropathy
- Renal tuberculosis
- Dysproteinaemia
- Drugs: L-Dopa
  Lithium
  Amphetamines
  Antidepressants
  Alcohol withdrawal
  Caffeine
  Steroids
  Analgesics (especially phenacetin)

# Clinical case scenarios

## Polycystic kidneys

- Bilateral masses in the flanks which are bimanually ballottable
- Able to get above and below masses
- Masses move up and down during respiration

- Other features to look for:
  Uraemic facies
  Raised blood pressure
  Arteriovenous fistula for haemodialysis
  Palpable transplant kidney in the groin
  Hepatomegaly secondary to liver involvement
  Third-nerve palsy (posterior communicating artery aneurysm)
  Abdominal scars secondary to peritoneal dialysis

- Differential diagnosis of bilateral renal enlargement: polycystic disease bilateral hydronephrosis amyloidosis

## Nephrotic syndrome

- Main finding of extensive oedema affecting ankles, lower legs, periorbital region
- May also be pleural effusion and ascites
- Patient may be young
- Look out for characteristic butterfly rash of SLE
- Look out for evidence of rheumatoid arthritis (renal amyloid)
- If asked to examine the fundi, consider diabetic nephropathy
- Look out for purpura (Henloch–Schönlein purpura)
- Xanthelasma or xanthomata may be present, indicating hyperlipidaemia
- Commonest cause is glomerulonephritis

# 11 Gastroenterology

## Contents

# Anatomy

## Oesophagus

- Continuous with the lower end of the pharynx
- Extends from the lower end of the cricoid cartilage (C6) to the cardia of the stomach (T10)
- Upper third consists of striated muscle
- Lower two-thirds consist of smooth muscle
- Arterial supply: inferior thyroid branch of the thyrocervical trunk
  Thoracic aorta
  Bronchial arteries
  Left gastric artery
  Inferior phrenic artery
- Venous drainage: upper third – superior vena cava
  Middle third – azygous vein
  Lower third – portal venous system

## Stomach

- Continuous with the oesophagus at the gastro-oesophageal junction
- Extends from the gastro-oesophageal sphincter to the pyloric sphincter (pylorus)
- Divided into three parts: fundus, body and antrum
- Fundus and body contain parietal cells, which make hydrochloric acid and secrete intrinsic factor
- Antrum contains G cells which synthesise gastrin, and chief cells which secrete pepsinogens
- Arterial supply: coeliac trunk
- Venous drainage: via the portal venous system
- Nerve supply: parasympathetics via vagus, providing motor and secretory fibres
  Sympathetics via Auerbach's and Meissner's plexuses

**Table 11.1: Gut hormones**

| Hormone | Produced by | Stimulus of secretion | Inhibition of secretion | Actions |
|---------|-------------|----------------------|------------------------|---------|
| Gastrin | Gastric antrum (G cells) | Insulin, hypoglycaemia<br>Peptides, amino acids<br>Antral distension<br>Vagal stimulation, vagotomy<br>Zollinger–Ellison syndrome<br>Achlorhydria<br>Hypercalcaemia, renal failure<br>H₂ blockers, proton pump inhibitors | Gastric acid<br>Peptic ulcer<br>Fasting<br>Secretin<br>GIP<br>VIP | Increased small bowel motility<br>Increased bile bicarbonate<br>Gastric acid secretion<br>Pepsin secretion<br>Intrinsic factor secretion<br>Increased gastric motility<br>Increased pancreatic bicarbonate<br>Increased secretin secretion |
| Secretin | Duodenum<br>Jejunum | Intraluminal acid | | Increased pancreatic bicarbonate secretion<br>Increased bile bicarbonate<br>Reduced gastrin secretion<br>Reduced pepsin secretion<br>Delayed gastric emptying |
| Cholecystokinin-pancreozymin (CCK-PZ) | Duodenum<br>Jejunum | Intraluminal acid<br>Fat<br>Amino acids<br>Peptides<br>Calcium<br>Magnesium | | Increased pancreatic bicarbonate secretion<br>Increased pancreatic enzyme secretion<br>Increased gallbladder contraction<br>Reduced gastric acid<br>Relaxation of sphincter of Oddi<br>Delayed gastric emptying<br>Reduced small bowel motility<br>Reduced large bowel motility |
| Motilin | Duodenum<br>Jejunum | Postprandial | | Increased gastric motility<br>Increased intestinal motility |

**Table 11.1 continued**

| Hormone | Produced by | Stimulus of secretion | Inhibition of secretion | Actions |
|---|---|---|---|---|
| Gastric inhibitory polypeptide (GIP) | Duodenum Jejunum | Postprandial Glucose Amino acids Fat | | Reduced gastrin secretion Reduced gastric motility Increased postprandial insulin |
| Vasoactive intestinal polypeptide (VIP) | Pancreas Small bowel | VIPoma (Verner–Morrison syndrome) | | Reduced gastrin secretion Reduced pepsin secretion Increased pancreatic secretion Increased intestinal secretion |
| Pancreatic polypeptide (PP) | Pancreas | Protein | Atropine | Reduced pancreatic enzyme secretion Relaxation of gallbladder Reduced biliary secretion |
| Neurotensin | Terminal ileum | Postprandial | | Reduced gastric emptying |
| Somatostatin | Pancreas Entire GI tract | | | Reduced hormonal secretion Reduced intestinal secretions |
| Enteroglucagon | Terminal ileum Colon | Postprandial | | Reduced gastric emptying Trophic effects on gastric mucosa |

# Small intestine

- Continuous with the stomach at the pylorus
- Extends from the pylorus to the ileocaecal valve
- Comprised of the duodenum, jejunum and ileum
- Duodenum is composed of four parts
- Second part of the duodenum receives pancreatic and common bile ducts via the ampulla of Vater
- Duodenum also contains Brunner's glands, which secrete bicarbonate
- Arterial supply: duodenum–coeliac axis
  jejunum and ileum–superior mesenteric artery

# Large intestine

- Continuous with the ileum at the ileocaecal valve
- Extends from the ileocaecal valve to the anus
- Comprised of the caecum, ascending colon, transverse colon, descending colon and rectum
- Arterial supply: caecum to mid transverse colon – superior mesenteric artery
  Mid-transverse colon to rectum – inferior mesenteric artery

# Physiology

## Intestinal digestion and absorption

### Mouth
- Digestion begins with mastication of food by teeth and lubrication with salivary gland secretion

---

**Box 11.1: Control of gastric emptying**

**Increased**
Post gastrectomy
Motilin
Gastrin
Gastric distension
Cold
Emotion
Domperidone
Maxolon

**Reduced**
Carcinoma of the stomach
Pyloric stenosis
Post gastrectomy
Post vagotomy
Autonomic neuropathy
Enteroglucagon
Neurotensin
Secretin
CCK-PZ
GIP
Fatty acids
Polypeptides
Amino acids
Heat
Duodenal acid

---

- Saliva contains amylase and lipase, which begin chemical digestion of carbohydrate and fat

### Oesophagus
- Main function is transport of food bolus from mouth to stomach via peristaltic muscular activity
- Has little digestive function

### Stomach
- Relaxation of the lower oesophageal sphincter allows entry of food into stomach
- When food enters stomach the lower oesophageal sphincter closes to prevent reflux

- Main function of the stomach is the production of hydrochloric acid, controlled by gastrin
- Normal gastric pH is around 2
- Gastric acid production has two phases:
  *Cephalic*: anticipation of food, taste and smell of food stimulate acid production
  *Gastric*: gastric secretions stimulated by presence of food in stomach
  Hydrochloric acid begins protein digestion by converting pepsinogen into pepsin
- Other functions of the stomach:
  Reservoir for food until it passes into duodenum
  Mechanical digestion (churning)
  Secretion of intrinsic factor
  Secretion of pepsinogen (chief cells)
  Control of rate of passage through to the duodenum

## Small bowel
- Prime site of nutrient digestion and absorption

---

**Box 11.2: Control of gastric acid secretion**

**Increased**
Gastrin
Vagal stimulation
Histamine
Increased gastric pH
Duodenal ulcer

**Reduced**
Nausea
Fear
Lowered gastric pH
CCK-PZ
Secretin
GIP
Somatostatin
$H_2$ blockers
Proton pump inhibitors
Vagotomy

---

**Box 11.3: Control of intestinal secretions**

**Increased**
Vagal stimulation
CCK-PZ
Secretin
VIP

**Reduced**
Sympathetic stimulation
Somatostatin

---

- Also the site of water and electrolyte secretion

## Functions of small bowel
### Digestion
- Lipids (bile acids/lipase)
- Proteins (pepsin, trypsin, brush border peptidases)
- Carbohydrates (pancreatic amylase, brush border disaccharidases)

### Absorption
- Calcium
- Iron
- Amino acids
- Saccharides
- Fatty acids
- Trace elements
- Folate (duodenum and upper jejunum)
- $B_{12}$, bile acids (terminal ileum)

## Causes of change in small bowel motility
### Increased
- Vagal stimulation
- Cholinergic agents
- Gastrin
- CCK-PZ
- Motilin
- Prostaglandins
- Serotonin
- Irritable bowel syndrome
- Post bowel resection

*Reduced*
- Sympathetic stimulation
- Adrenergic agents
- Secretin
- Tumours
- Inflammatory strictures
- Diabetes mellitus
- Systemic sclerosis

## Large bowel
- Main function is to reabsorb salt and water from luminal contents to produce formed stools
- Also responsible for secretion of potassium and bicarbonate into lumen
- Normally absorbs 1–2 litres of fluid per day
- Experimentally may cope with up to 4–5 litres per day

## Causes of change in large bowel motility
*Increased*
- Vagal stimulation
- Cholinergic agents
- Bowel distension
- Emotion
- CCK-PZ
- Stimulant laxatives
- Post bowel resection
- Irritable bowel syndrome

*Reduced*
- Sympathetic stimulation
- Anticholinergic agents
- Inflammatory strictures
- Emotion
- Tumours
- Ischaemia
- Hirschsprung's disease
- Chagas' disease
- Irritable bowel syndrome
- Idiopathic

# Symptoms of gastrointestinal disease

## Diarrhoea

### Causes of diarrhoea
*Acute*
- Dietary indiscretion
- Drugs
- Gastrointestinal infection
- Allergy
- Psychogenic

*Chronic*
- Irritable bowel syndrome
- Diverticular disease
- Inflammatory bowel disease
- Neoplasm
- Malabsorption
- Autonomic neuropathy
- Overflow (constipation)
- Thyrotoxicosis
- Medullary carcinoma thyroid
- Pellagra
- Gut endocrine tumours (VIPoma, gastrinoma, carcinoid, glucagonoma, somatostatinoma)

### Infectious causes of diarrhoea
*Viral*
- Rotavirus
- Echovirus
- Norwalk agent
- Adenovirus

*Bacterial*
- *Salmonella*
- *Campylobacter*
- *Clostridium dificile*
- *Shigella*
- *Enterobacter*
- *Staphylococcus aureus*
- *Clostridium perfringens*
- *Escherichia coli*

- *Bacillus cereus*
- *Vibrio cholerae*
- *Yersinia enterocolitica*

**Protozoal**
- *Giardia lamblia*
- *Amoeba*
- *Cryptosporidium*

**Tapeworm**

# Dysentery

## Causes of dysentery
- *Shigella*
- *Amoeba*
- *Campylobacter*
- *Salmonella*
- *Escherichia coli*
- *Yersinia enterocolitica*
- *Clostridium dificile*

# Constipation

## Causes of constipation
**Colonic obstruction**
- Tumours
- Hernias
- Volvulus

**Abnormal muscle function**
- Advanced age
- Irritable bowel syndrome
- Diverticular disease
- Inflammatory bowel disease
- Ischaemic colitis
- Scleroderma
- Hirschsprung's disease
- Paralytic ileus

**Anorectal problems**
- Proctitis
- Fissure
- Prolapse
- Haemorrhoids

**Neuropsychiatric**
- Depression
- Spinal cord injury
- Corda equina lesions
- Multiple sclerosis
- Idiopathic Parkinson's disease
- Space-occupying lesion
- Stroke
- Anorexia
- Angio-oedema
- Rectal dyschezia (habitual neglect of call to stool)
- Chagas' disease

**Endocrine**
- Pregnancy
- Diabetes mellitus
- Hypothyroidism
- Hypopituitarism
- Phaeochromocytoma

**Metabolic**
- Dehydration
- Renal failure
- Hypokalaemia
- Porphyria
- Lead poisoning
- Hypercalcaemia

**Drugs**
- Anticholinergics
- Iron
- Diuretics
- Opiates
- Purgative abuse
- Antidepressants
- Anticonvulsants
- Aluminium salts
- Calcium salts
- Cholestyramine

# Abdominal pain

## Causes of abdominal pain
**Intra-abdominal disease**
- Peritonitis

- Motility disorders
- Bowel ischaemia
- Peptic ulcer disease
- Inflammatory bowel disease
- Oesophageal disease
- Renal disease
- Pancreatic disease
- Angio-oedema
- Biliary tract disease
- Hepatic disease
- Aortic dissection
- Gynaecological disease

*Extra-abdominal disease*
- Pleurisy
- Ischaemic heart disease
- Herpes zoster virus
- Spinal disease
- Acute intermittent porphyria
- Addison's disease
- Lead poisoning
- Strychnine poisoning
- Diabetic ketoacidosis
- Tabes dorsalis
- Migraine
- Epilepsy
- Sickle cell crises

# Vomiting

## Causes of vomiting
**Gastrointestinal disease**
- Dietary indiscretion
- Peptic ulcers
- Gastritis
- Gastroenteritis
- Bowel or biliary obstruction
- Achalasia
- Hepatitis
- Pancreatitis
- Peritonitis

**Endocrine**
- Pregnancy
- Diabetic ketoacidosis
- Renal failure

---

**Box 11.4: Causes of pruritus ani**

**Idiopathic**

**Anorectal disease**
Fissures
Haemorrhoids
Rectal carcinoma
Faecal soiling

**Infection**
Candida
Threadworm

**Skin disease**
Psoriasis
Dermatitis

**Psychogenic**
Depression
Anxiety

---

- Addison's disease

*Neurological*
- Drugs
- Motion sickness
- Psychological
- Migraine
- Pain
- Raised intracranial pressure
- Ménière's disease
- Labyrinthitis

*Miscellaneous*
- Sepsis
- Acute myocardial infarction
- Cyclical vomiting
- Anorexia
- Bulimia
- Radiation
- Angio-oedema

## Physiology of vomiting
**Nausea**
- Reduced motor activity of the stomach
- Increased motor activity of duodenum

and jejunum leads to reflux of duodenal contents into stomach

## Retching
- Contraction of chest wall and abdominal muscles and diaphragm against closed glottis leads to reflux of gastric contents into lower oesophagus

## Emesis
- Powerful sustained contraction of abdominal musculature and descent of the diaphragm lead to raised intra-abdominal pressure and emesis

## Neurophysiology of vomiting
- Afferent stimuli from stomach, intestine, gallbladder, biliary tract, peritoneum and heart.
  These afferent stimuli are carried by the vagus nerve
- Other afferents come from the nose (olfactory nerve) and inner ear (vestibular nerve)
- All afferents relay to the chemoreceptor trigger zone in the floor of the fourth ventricle within the area postrema, where there is no blood–brain barrier
- Many drugs act directly on this area
- From here signals are relayed to vomiting centre in the lateral reticular formation of the medulla
- Efferents pass from the vomiting centre via somatic nerves to the pharynx, respiratory and abdominal muscles, diaphragm and gastrointestinal tract
- Autonomic efferent signals induce hypersalivation, pallor and sweating

# Diseases of the mouth

## Causes of aphthous ulcers

- Idiopathic
- Behçet's syndrome
- Reiter's syndrome
- Wegener's granulomatosis
- SLE
- Tuberculosis
- Syphilis
- Epstein–Barr Virus (EBV)
- Agranulocytosis
- Drugs: gold, penicillamine, cytotoxics
- Crohn's disease
- Erythema multiforme
- Pemphigus vulgaris
- Lichen planus
- Coeliac disease

## Causes of glossitis

- Geographic tongue
- Iron deficiency
- Folate deficiency
- $B_{12}$ deficiency

## Causes of macroglossia

- Hypothyroidism
- Acromegaly
- Amyloid

## Causes of xerostomia

### Drugs
- Antihistamines
- Phenothiazines
- Tricyclic antidepressants
- Diuretics
- Anticholinergic agents

---

**Box 11.5: Aetiology of oral carcinoma**

Smoking (pipe, cigar)
Alcohol abuse
Syphilis
*Candida*
Herpes simplex virus
Leukoplakia

- Bullous pemphigoid
- Lichen planus

## Drugs
- Cytotoxics
- Mercury
- Bismuth
- Gold
- Arsenic
- Antibiotics

## Miscellaneous
- Advanced age
- Dehydration
- Anxiety
- Radiation
- Sjögren's syndrome
- Anaemia
- Salivary gland calculi
- *Candida*

## Miscellaneous
- Leukoplakia
- Neoplasm
- Allergy: dentures, denture medicaments, caustics
- Trauma: cheek biting
- Smoking
- Alcohol abuse
- Aphthous ulceration

# Causes of gingivostomatitis

## Infection
- Viral: herpes simplex virus, herpangina, Coxsackie A16
- Bacteria: *Borrelia vincente*, *Fusobacterium fuseformis*, TB, syphilis, *Bacteroides*
- Fungal: *Candida*, actinomycosis
- Parasites: malaria

## Systemic disease
- Behçet's syndrome
- Reiter's syndrome
- Erythema multiforme
- Neutropenia
- Crohn's disease
- Iron deficiency
- $B_{12}$ deficiency
- Folate deficiency
- Malnutrition
- Thrombocytopenia
- Scurvy

## Skin disease
- Pemphigus vulgaris

# Causes of gingival hypertrophy

- Pregnancy
- Phenytoin
- Combined oral contraceptive pill
- Leukaemia
- Phenobarbitone
- Primidone
- Acute leukaemia
- Amyloid
- Scurvy
- Mercury
- Arsenic
- Cyclosporin

# Causes of leukoplakia

- Idiopathic
- HIV
- Syphilis
- *Candida*
- Herpes simplex virus
- Smoking

- Friction
- Congenital

## Causes of parotid gland enlargement

### Systemic disease
- Sjögren's syndrome
- Sarcoid
- Cirrhosis
- Cystic fibrosis
- Hyperlipidaemia
- Malnutrition
- Diabetes mellitus
- Acromegaly
- Malignancy

### Infection
- Mumps
- Cytomegalovirus (CMV)
- Bacteria

### Drugs
- Iodide
- Thiouracil
- Phenylbutazone
- Lead
- Alcohol abuse

### Miscellaneous
- Gland calculi
- Pregnancy

# Oesophageal disease

## Causes of dysphagia

### Oropharyngeal
- Stomatitis
- Pharyngeal pouch
- Glossitis
- Oropharyngeal tumours
- Quinsy
- Retropharangeal abscess

- Pharyngeal web (Plummer–Vinson syndrome)

### Extrinsic oesophageal compression
- Thyroid enlargement
- Lymphadenopathy
- Carcinoma of the bronchus
- Aortic aneurysm
- Left atrial hypertrophy
- Pericardial effusion

### Intrinsic disease
- Oesophagitis
- Benign peptic stricture
- Carcinoma of the oesophagus
- Neuromuscular dysmotility
- Achalasia
- Schatski ring
- Scleroderma
- Chagas' disease
- Oesophageal diverticulum

### Neurological
- Stroke
- Pseudobulbar palsy
- Idiopathic Parkinson's disease
- Bulbar palsy
- Muscular dystrophy
- Motor neuron disease
- Myasthenia gravis
- Multiple sclerosis
- Huntington's chorea
- Dystrophia myotonica
- Diabetes mellitus

### Miscellaneous
- Foreign body
- Globus hystericus

## Causes of gastro-oesophageal reflux

### Disordered anatomy
- Hiatus hernia
- Obesity
- Post achalasia treatment

| Box 11.6:  Types of oesophageal neoplasm | Box 11.7:  Aetiology of oesophageal carcinoma |
|---|---|
| **Benign**<br>Leiomyoma<br>Adenoma<br>Cysts<br><br>**Malignant** *(usually found in the lower two-thirds of the oesophagus)*<br>Squamous Cell Carcinoma<br>Adenocarcinoma (Barrett's)<br>Melanoma<br>Sarcoma | Smoking<br>Alcohol abuse<br>Coeliac disease<br>Radiation<br>Achalasia<br>Acid or alkaline ingestion<br>Chronic reflux oesophagitis (Barrett's)<br>Plummer–Vinson syndrome<br>Tylosis<br>Absence of *Helicobacter pylori* |

- Artificial enteral feeding tubes
- Systemic sclerosis

## Chemical
- Acidic food
- Fatty food
- Coffee
- Tea
- Alcohol
- Milk
- Calcium antagonists
- β-agonists

## Miscellaneous
- Pregnancy
- Smoking
- Recumbent posture
- Large meals

# Investigation of oesophageal disease

## Dysphagia
- Oesophago-gastro-duodenoscopy (OGD) under direct vision is the investigation of choice
- Care needs to be taken in potential cases of pharyngeal pouch but if intubation is performed under direct vision this is usually not a problem
- Barium swallow is a second-line investigation for obstructive lesions, but is a better investigation for neuromuscular problems
- Videofluoroscopy is indicated for assessment of the oropharyngeal phase of swallowing
- A standardised swallow assessment is a useful clinical bedside tool for the detection of dysphagia

## Gastro-oesophageal reflux
- OGD is needed to exclude serious pathology
- A barium swallow may demonstrate some reflux
- The "gold standard" test is 24-hour oesophageal pH monitoring

## Motility
- OGD usually not helpful and is normal in achalasia
- Occasionally abnormal contractions may be seen down the endoscope
- A barium swallow is more helpful in demonstrating neuromuscular incoordination and may show a typical corkscrew oesophagus or tertiary spasms
- A barium swallow is also abnormal in achalasia, showing failure of relaxation of the lower oesophageal sphincter and proximal oesophageal

dilatation
- The "gold standard" test is 24-hour oesophageal manometry

# Diseases of the stomach

## Causes of hypochlorhydria

- Pernicious anaemia
- Vagotomy
- Partial gastrectomy
- Gastric ulcer
- Gastric carcinoma
- Gastric polyposis
- Iron deficiency
- Pregnancy
- Advanced age
- Radiation
- Pellagra
- Chronic atrophic gastritis

## Investigation of gastric pathology

OGD is preferred to barium swallow in view of the ability to obtain tissue samples and perform intervention if needed.

## Complications of gastrectomy

- Recurrence of ulcer
- Bile gastritis
- Dumping syndrome (rapid transit of hyperosmolar contents into jejunum leads to drawing of water into lumen, which causes sweating, palpitations, dizziness and reduction of the plasma compartment)
- Reactive hypoglycaemia (late dumping)

---

**Box 11.8: Aetiology of stomach disease**

**Peptic ulcer disease**
*Helicobacter pylori*
NSAIDs
Smoking
Steroids
Zollinger–Ellison syndrome
Stress
Burns
Blood group O (duodenal ulcer)
Positive family history

**Gastritis**
Infections
NSAIDs
Alcohol
*Helicobacter pylori (chronic atrophic gastritis)*
Iron
Renal failure

**Carcinoma of the stomach**
Pernicious anaemia
*Helicobacter pylori*
Achlorhydria
Partial gastrectomy
Smoking
Gastric adenomatous polyps
Nitrosamines
Japanese origin
Blood group A

---

- Malabsorption
- Steatorrhoea
- Iron deficiency
- $B_{12}$ deficiency
- Hypocalcaemia
- Vitamin D deficiency
- Carcinoma of the stomach

# Small bowel disease

## Causes of small bowel disease

- Coeliac disease
- Crohns disease
- *Giardia lamblia*
- Bacterial overgrowth
- *Strongyloides stercoralis*
- Fish tapeworm
- Tropical sprue
- Cow's milk intolerance
- HIV
- Terminal ileal disease
- Tuberculosis
- Radiation enteritis
- Whipple's disease
- Lymphangectasia
- Lymphoma
- Systemic sclerosis
- Abetalipoproteinaemia
- Amyloidosis
- α-Chain disease
- Systemic mastocytosis

### Table 11.2: Causes of malabsorption

| Mechanism | Causes | Steatorrhoea |
| --- | --- | --- |
| *Small bowel disease* | See page 236 | + |
| Osmotic diarrhoea | Disaccharidase deficiency | − |
| | Magnesium salts | |
| | Lactulose | |
| Secretory diarrhoea | Cholera | − |
| | VIPoma | |
| | Carcinoid syndrome | |
| | Medullary carcinoma of thyroid | |
| | Zollinger–Ellison syndrome | |
| | Bile salt deficiency | |
| | *Escherichia coli* | |
| | *Staphylococcus aureus* | |
| | *Clostridium dificile* | |
| | *Clostridium perfringens* | |
| | Phenolphthalein | |
| Other drugs | Neomycin | + |
| | Methyldopa | |
| | Alcohol | |
| | Cholestyramine | |
| | Liquid paraffin | |
| | Colchicine | |
| Endocrine disease | Somatostatinoma | + |
| | Addison's disease | |
| | Hypoparathyroidism | |
| Exocrine pancreatic disease | See page 245 | + |
| Rapid transit | Post gastrectomy | + |
| | Hyperthyroidism | |
| | Irritable bowel syndrome | |
| | Short bowel syndrome | |
| | Fistulae | |

- Mesenteric ischaemia
- Chronic venous congestion
- Dermatogenic enteropathy (erythroderma)
- Acrodermatitis enteropathica

# Causes of bacterial overgrowth

- Small bowel diverticuli
- Achlorhydria
- Partial gastrectomy
- Small bowel stricture
- Scleroderma
- Diabetic neuropathy
- Vagotomy
- Autonomic neuropathy
- Adhesions
- Fistulae
- Blind loops
- Advanced age

# Differences between secretory and osmotic diarrhoea

## Secretory
- Measured stool osmolality equals calculated stool osmolality
- After a 24-hour fast the diarrhoea continues unabated

## Osmotic
- Measured stool osmolality is greater than the calculated stool osmolality
- After a 24-hour fast there is some resolution of the diarrhoea

# Investigation of small bowel disease

## OGD
- Allows visualisation to the third part of the duodenum
- Duodenal biopsies allow for the diagnosis of coeliac disease
- Duodenal aspiration allows for the diagnosis of *Giardia* infection

## Enteroscopy
- Allows visualisation further down than normal OGD

## Barium studies
- Small bowel follow-through suitable for the diagnosis of diffuse mucosal disorders
- Small bowel enema required for the diagnosis of anatomical lesions and for visualisation of the terminal ileum
- Barium enema can sometimes allow visualisation of the terminal ileum

## Xylose absorption test
- Test of carbohydrate absorption
- Fast patient overnight
- Empty bladder before test
- Give 5 g of xylose in water
- Patient should drink at least 500 ml of water in the next 2 hours
- Collect all urine for 5 hours and measure urinary xylose
- At 1 hour measure serum xylose

Normal results: 1-hour serum
xylose > 1.3 mmol/l
5-hour urinary xylose > 7 mmol/l

- This test can be normal in patients with isolated terminal ileal disease or pancreatic disease
- False positive results may occur in renal failure, advanced age, delayed gastric emptying, oedema, obesity and bacterial overgrowth

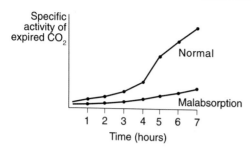

**Fig. 11.1: Typical patterns of $^{14}CO_2$ excretion in $^{14}C$ triolein breath test**

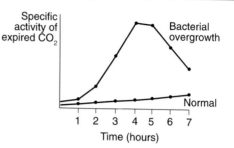

**Fig. 11.2: Typical patterns of $^{14}CO_2$ excretion in $^{14}C$ glycocholic breath test**

## Faecal fats

- Little used now owing to the unpleasant nature of the test
- All stools passed should be collected over 3–5 consecutive days
- Accurate collection is often a problem
- The patient should also eat at least 90–100 g of fat per day for 48 hours before and during the test
- Increases in faecal fat levels occur in pancreatic insufficiency

## Carbon 14 ($^{14}C$) triolein breath test

A useful test to examine fat malabsorption.
- Fast patient overnight
- Collect basal sample of expired $CO_2$
- Give $^{14}C$ triolein in 60g of a fat meal
- Collect 1 mmol samples of expired $CO_2$ every hour for 7 hours
- Measure the radioactivity of the $CO_2$ samples
- This test is not reliable in patients with diabetes mellitus, obesity, thyroid disease or chronic respiratory in-sufficiency, and is not suitable for use in pregnancy because of the radioactivity

## $^{14}C$ glycocholic acid breath test

A useful test for assessing bacterial over-growth.
- Fast patient overnight
- Collect basal sample of expired $CO_2$
- Give $^{14}C$ glycocholic acid in a test meal
- Collect 1 mmol samples of expired

$CO_2$ hourly for 7 h
- Measure the radioactivity of the $CO_2$ samples

# Large bowel disease

## Tumours of the large bowel

### Benign (no malignant potential)
- Metaplastic (hyperplastic)
- Lipomas
- Fibromas
- Leiomyomas
- Inflammatory polyps
- Hamartomas

### Benign (malignant potential)
- Adenomas (tubular, villous, tubulovillous)
- Familial adenomatous polyposis
- Gardner's syndrome

---

**Box 11.9: Aetiology of carcinoma of the large bowel**

High animal fat diet
Western lifestyle
Familial adenomatous polyposis
Gardner's syndrome
Inflammatory bowel disease
Adenomatous polyps

- Carcinoid

## Malignant
- <u>Adenocarcinoma</u>
- Carcinoid
- Lymphoma
- Leiomyosarcomas
- Fibrosarcomas
- Melanomas

# Complications of inflammatory bowel disease

## Gastrointestinal
- Aphthous ulceration
- Glossitis
- Stomatitis
- Fistulae
- Toxic dilatation
- Intestinal obstruction
- Abscesses
- Perforation
- Haemorrhage

- Stricture
- Carcinoma
- Perianal disease

## Nutritional
- <u>Iron deficiency anaemia</u>
- $B_{12}$ deficiency
- Folate deficiency
- Hypokalaemia
- Hypoproteinaemia
- Hypocalcaemia
- Hypomagnesaemia
- Vitamin deficiencies

## Skin
- Erythema nodosum
- Erythema multiforme
- Pyoderma gangrenosum
- Psoriasis
- Dermatitis
- Clubbing
- Vasculitis

## Hepatic
- Primary sclerosing cholangitis
- Cholangiocarcinoma

**Table 11.3: Duke's staging of carcinoma of the colon**

| Stage | Features | 5-year survival (%) |
|-------|----------|---------------------|
| A | Mucosa and submucosa involvement | 80 |
| B | Muscular coat penetrated | 60 |
| C | Lymph node involvement | 20 |
| D | Distant metastases | < 1 |

**Table 11.4: Distinctions between Crohn's disease and ulcerative colitis**

| Feature | Crohn's disease | Ulcerative colitis |
|---------|-----------------|--------------------|
| Histology | Transmural inflammation<br>Skip lesions<br>Non-caseating granuloma | Mucosal inflammation<br>Crypt abscesses<br>No granuloma |
| Smoking history | + | − |
| Perianal disease | + | − |
| Small bowel involvement | + | − |
| Large bowel involvement | + | + |
| Oral aphthous ulcers | + | − |
| Malabsorption | + | − |

**Box 11.10: Contributory factors in functional disorders**

Hypermotility
Lowered sensory threshold
Previous gut infection
Altered gut flora
Fibre deficiency
Increased refined carbohydrate in diet
Food additives
Food allergy
Caffeine
Smoking
Alcohol
Anxiety
Depression

**Box 11.11: Symptoms more suggestive of functional disorders**

Flatulence
Borborygmi
Abdominal distension
Bloating
Exacerbated by stress
Pain relief with bowels open
Tenesmus
Urgency of defecation
Proctalgia fugax

- Fatty liver
- Chronic active hepatitis (autoimmune)
- Gallstones
- Hepatic granuloma

### Rheumatological
- Sacroiliitis
- Polyarthritis
- Ankylosing spondylitis

### Eyes
- Conjunctivitis
- Uveitis
- Episcleritis
- Keratitis
- Retinitis
- Retrobulbar neuritis

### Miscellaneous
- Pulmonary fibrosis
- Renal calculi
- Pyelonephritis
- Autoimmune haemolytic anaemia
- Thromboembolism
- Coeliac disease
- Amyloid
- Infertility

# Gastrointestinal haemorrhage

## Causes of haematemesis

### Oesophagus
- Oesophagitis
- Carcinoma
- Ulcer
- Varices
- Mallory–Weiss tear

### Stomach
- Gastric ulcer
- Gastritis
- Carcinoma
- Erosions
- Gastric varices
- Angiodysplasia
- Leiomyoma
- Carcinoid syndrome
- Crohn's disease
- Portal hypertensive gastropathy

### Duodenum
- Duodenal ulcer
- Duodenitis
- Ampullary carcinoma
- Aortoduodenal fistula

### Miscellaneous

- Chronic renal failure
- Thrombocytopenia
- Coagulation disorders
- Anticoagulant therapy
- Telangiectasia
- Vasculitis
- Ehlers–Danlos syndrome
- Mesenteric ischaemia
- Epistaxis
- Pseudoxanthoma elasticum
- Munchausen's syndrome

## Causes of melaena

- Meckel's diverticulum
- Small bowel infarction
- Inflammatory bowel disease
- Right-sided colonic tumours
- *See also: Causes of haematemesis (above)*

## Causes of fresh rectal bleeding

- Large bowel tumour
- Inflammatory bowel disease
- Diverticular disease
- Infective colitis
- Haemorrhoids
- Angiodysplasia
- Ischaemic colitis
- Proctitis

## Management of active upper gastrointestinal bleeding

- Quick initial survey
- Obtain i.v. access (large-bore)
- CVP line may be needed
- If shocked use plasma expanders
- i.v. Normal saline (5% dextrose in hepatic encephalopathy)
- Blood transfusion
- Check clotting and give fresh frozen plasma in severe haemorrhage
- Careful fluid balance
- OGD may be required urgently to allow intervention and aid surgery if subsequently needed
- Begin proton pump inhibitors early
- Keep patient nil by mouth
- Octreotide, vasopressin and Sengstaken tubes are options for bleeding oesophageal varices
- Tranexamic acid may be required
- i.v. Ranitidine is ineffective and extremely expensive
- Surgery may be indicated in non-variceal bleeding, continuing haemorrhage, advanced age or rebleeding

# Miscellaneous gastrointestinal disorders

## Causes of calcification on abdominal x-ray

- Phleboliths
- Calcified lymph nodes
- Calculi
- Calcified organs
- Calcified aorta
- Calcified tumours
- Faecolith
- Fetus
- Cystercicosis
- Calcified hydatid cyst

# Causes of protein-losing enteropathy

## Stomach
- Ménétrièr's disease
- Multiple gastric ulcers
- Gastric tumours

## Small bowel
- Coeliac disease
- Crohn's disease
- Tropical sprue
- Lymphoma
- Lymphangiectasia
- Whipple's disease

## Large bowel
- Crohn's disease
- Ulcerative colitis
- Colonic tumours
- Villous adenoma

## Miscellaneous
- Constrictive pericarditis
- Cardiac failure
- Agammaglobulinaemia
- Erythroderma
- Acrodermatitis

# Gastrointestinal manifestations in HIV

## Normal infections
### Viral
Human papilloma virus
Herpes simplex virus
CMV
EBV
Hepatitis A
Hepatitis B

### Bacterial
*Neisseria gonorrhoeae*
*Chlamydia trachomatis*
*Shigella*
*Campylobacter*

*Salmonella*
Syphilis

### Protozoa
Giardia
*Amoeba*

### Arthropods
Scabies
*Phthirus pubis*

### Helminths
*Enterobius vermicularis*

## Opportunistic infections
- Candida
- Cryptosporidia
- Toxoplasmosis
- *Mycobacterium avium intracellulare*
- *Isospora*
- Microsporidia

## Miscellaneous
- Kaposi's sarcoma
- Lymphoma
- Partial villous atrophy
- Sclerosing cholangitis
- Leukoplakia

# Carcinoid tumours

- Carcinoid tumours are most commonly situated in the gut
- They are derived from neuroendocrine cells (argentaffin cells of the APUD system)
- They are generally of low-grade malignancy
- 90% are found in the terminal ileum and appendix
- Terminal ileal tumours are the most likely to metastasise
- They secrete 5H-tryptamine
- Appendix tumours are usually asymptomatic
- Gastric tumours secrete predominantly

**Box 11.12: Features of carcinoid syndrome**

Secretory diarrhoea
Flushing
Bronchospasm
Pellagra
Hepatomegaly
Pulmonary stenosis
Pulmonary regurgitation
Tricuspid stenosis
Tricuspid regurgitation

histamine
- Colonic tumours are not usually associated with hormone secretion

## Carcinoid syndrome
- Occurs only when the liver is bypassed and cannot metabolise tumour products
- This usually arises due to the presence of liver metastases draining into the hepatic vein
- It may occur in pulmonary, testicular and ovarian tumours draining into the systemic circulation
- Diagnosis usually achieved by demonstrating raised urinary 5H1AA levels

## Treatment of carcinoid syndrome
- Removal of the tumour
- Cyproheptadine
- Methysergide
- $H_1$ and $H_2$ blockers (for gastric carcinoids)
- Imodium and codeine phosphate
- Somatostatin
- Octreotide (particularly useful for flushing and diarrhoea)
- Niacin (for pellagra)

# Pancreatic disease
## Anatomy

- Retroperitoneally situated
- Drains into the second part of the duodenum via the ampulla of Vater
- Exocrine function: production of secretin, trypsin, chymotrypsin
- Endocrine function: islets of Langerhans (1% of volume)
- *B cells*: produce insulin
- *α cells*: produce glucagon
- *D cells*: produce somatostatin
- *PP cells*: produce pancreatic polypeptide
- In pancreatic disease, exocrine function is lost first

# Physiology

## Pancreatic secretions
- Bicarbonate
- VIP
- Pancreatic polypeptide
- Somatostatin
- Maltase
- Amylase
- Lipase
- Trypsinogen
- Chymotrypsinogen
- Aminopeptidases
- Carboxypeptidases

## Control of pancreatic secretions
### Increased
- Gastrin
- Vagal stimulation
- Secretin
- CCK-PZ

Tryptophan ⟶ 5-hydroxytryptophan ⟶ 5-hydroxytryptamine
                                                              ↓
5-hydroxyindole acetic acid (5-HIAA) ⟵ 5-hydroxyindole acetaldehyde

**Fig. 11.3: Serotonin metabolism**

- VIP

**Reduced**
- Pancreatic polypeptide
- Somatostatin

# Tests of exocrine pancreatic function

## Secretin–cholecystokinin (CCK) test
- Fast patient overnight
- Intubate patient with a double-lumen tube with one tube in the stomach and one in the duodenum
- Aspirate gastric and duodenal juice throughout the test but discard all gastric juices
- At the start of the test collect and discard resting duodenal juice
- Give i.v. secretin and collect the duodenal juice every 10 minutes for 30 minutes
- Then give intravenous CCK and collect duodenal juice every 10 minutes for 30 minutes
- Normal results:
  Total volume of aspirate in 60 minutes > 150 ml
  Peak bicarbonate concentration > 60 mmol/l
  Peak tryptic activity > 30 IU/ml
  Total tryptic activity after CCK > 2200 IU

## Lundh test
- Fast patient overnight
- Intubate patient with a single-lumen tube placed in the duodenum
- Aspirate resting duodenal juice and discard
- Give test meal containing corn oil, skimmed milk powder and dextrose
- Aspirate duodenal juice every 30 minutes for 2 hours
- Normal results: normal tryptic activity > 25 IU/ml in at least one sample

## Fluorescein dilurate test
- On day 1 give 0.5 mmol fluorescein dilurate orally
- Ensure adequate fluid intake
- Collect urine for 10 hours
- Measure amount of fluorescein excreted
- On day 2 repeat the test
- False positive results are obtained if bile salt secretion is defective

$$\text{TK index} = \frac{\text{fluorescein excreted on day 1}}{\text{fluorescein excreted on day 2}} \times 100$$

Normal pancreatic function:
  TK index > 30%
In pancreatic insufficiency:
  TK index < 20%

## $^{14}C$ p-aminobenzoic acid (PABA) excretion test
- Fast patient overnight
- Give 0.5 g BT-PABA, $^{14}C$ PABA and 24 g of casein and 500 ml water orally
- Collect urine for 6 hours
- Analyse urine for PABA and $^{14}C$ content
- This test is not suitable for use in pregnancy or renal failure
- Paracetamol and sulphonamides also interfere with the results

$$\text{PABA }^{14}\text{C index} = \frac{\text{PABA excreted / PABA ingested}}{^{14}\text{C excreted / }^{14}\text{C ingested}} \times 100$$

Normal pancreatic function:
  PABA index > 0.76
In pancreatic insufficiency:
  PABA index < 0.76

## Serum amylase
- Useful in acute pancreatitis but of no use in chronic pancreatitis

# Exocrine pancreatic disease

## *Aetiology of acute pancreatitis*

### *Infection*
- Mumps
- Coxsackie B
- EBV
- *Ascaris*
- *Clonorchis sinensis*
- *Mycoplasma pneumoniae*

### *Drugs*
- Alcohol abuse
- Steroids
- Opiates
- Azathioprine
- Sulphonamides
- Combined oral contraceptive pill
- Thiazides
- Frusemide
- Tetracycline

### *Metabolic*
- Hyperlipidaemia
- Hyperparathyroidism
- Hypercalcaemia
- Hypothermia

### *Miscellaneous*
- Common bile duct stones
- Pregnancy
- Post ERCP
- Trauma
- Carcinoma of the pancreas
- Idiopathic
- Laparotomy
- Translumbar aortography
- Polya gastrectomy

## *Complications of acute pancreatitis*

### *Early*
- Cardiac failure
- Renal failure
- ARDS
- Hyperglycaemia

**Box 11.13: Causes of pancreatic exocrine insufficiency**

Acute pancreatitis
Chronic pancreatitis
Cystic fibrosis
Schwachman's syndrome
Carcinoma of the pancreas

- Anaemia
- Biliary obstruction
- DIC
- Paralytic ileus
- Hypocalcaemia
- Hypoalbuminaemia
- Metabolic acidosis
- Hypoxia
- Cullen's sign (umbilical bruising)
- Grey–Turner's sign (flank bruising)
- Fat necrosis

### *Late*
- Pseudocyst
- Abscess
- Pancreatic duct stricture
- Ascites
- Pleural effusion
- Diabetes mellitus

## *Aetiology of chronic pancreatitis*
- Alcohol
- Gallstones

**Box 11.14: Indicators of severity of acute pancreatitis**

White blood count $> 15 \times 10^9$/l
Blood sugar $> 10$ mmol/l
Serum urea $> 16$ mmol/l
$Po_2 < 8$ kPa
Serum calcium $< 2$ mmol/l
Serum albumin $< 32$ g/l
Serum LDH $> 60$ U/l
Serum AST $> 55$ U/l
Age $> 55$ years

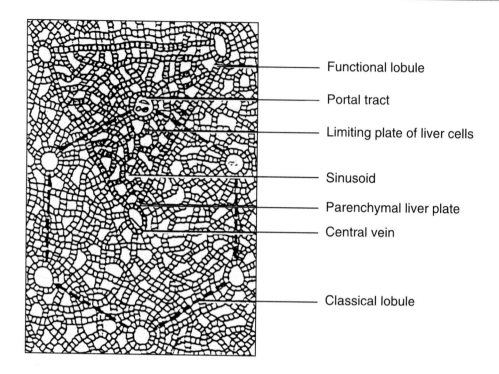

- Functional lobule
- Portal tract
- Limiting plate of liver cells
- Sinusoid
- Parenchymal liver plate
- Central vein
- Classical lobule

**Fig. 11.4: Normal liver histology.**

- Hereditary
- Pancreas divisum
- Malnutrition
- Hyperlipidaemia
- Hypercalcaemia
- Idiopathic
- Primary biliary cirrhosis
- Sclerosing cholangitis

# Liver disease

## Anatomy

- There are two lobes, right and left
- Total liver blood supply is 1300 ml/min
- Blood supply comes from: hepatic artery (provides 25% of blood flow and 50% of oxygen)
  Portal vein (provides 75% of blood

---

**Box 11.15: Composition of bile**

Bile acids
Phospholipid
Cholesterol
Bile pigments (bilirubin, biliverdin)
Protein

---

**Box 11.16: Function of bile acids**

To solubilise cholesterol into micelles
Aid emulsification of fats
Aid absorption of fat-soluble vitamins
Stimulate pancreatic secretion via
  CCK-PZ

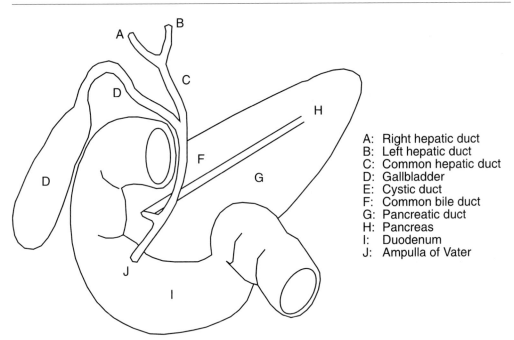

A: Right hepatic duct
B: Left hepatic duct
C: Common hepatic duct
D: Gallbladder
E: Cystic duct
F: Common bile duct
G: Pancreatic duct
H: Pancreas
I: Duodenum
J: Ampulla of Vater

**Fig. 11.5: Anatomy of the biliary tree**

flow and 50% of oxygen)
- Venous drainage is via: hepatic vein into inferior vena cava
Oesophageal veins into the azygous vein
Inferior mesenteric veins into the internal iliacs
Anterior abdominal wall veins into the umbilicus

## Microanatomy
- The liver consists of a series of sinusoids running between plates of hepatocytes
- Sinusoids contain Kupffer cells (phagocytic function)
- Liver cells are divided into lobules centred around a central vein (see Fig. 11.4)

## Biliary tree
Anatomy of the biliary is shown in Fig. 11.5.

# Physiology

## Production of bile salts and bicarbonate to aid digestion
- Once formed, bile salts are excreted into the bile canaliculi and eventually into the duodenum
- Bile salts are reabsorbed in the terminal ileum and recirculated to the liver (enterohepatic circulation)
- 250–1100 ml of bile are produced daily

## Causes of impaired enterohepatic circulation
- Bile salts chelating agents (cholestyramine)
- Terminal ileal disease
- Bacterial overgrowth

## Control of biliary secretion
### Increased
- Vagal stimulation
- Gastrin

- Secretin
- CCK

### Reduced
- Sympathetic stimulation
- Pancreatic polypeptide

## Control of protein metabolism
- Regulates amino acid levels by controlling the rate of gluconeogenesis and transamination
- Converts ammonia to urea by the urea cycle
- Main site for synthesis and degradation of plasma proteins and clotting factors (fibrinogen, Factors II, V, VII–XIII)

## Control of carbohydrate metabolism
- The liver is a major site for glycogen storage, glycogenolysis and gluconeogenesis

## Control of lipid metabolism
- The liver is involved in the synthesis of lipoproteins

## Excretion of waste products
- The liver acts as a major excretory pathway for many drugs

# Signs of liver disease

## Causes of hepatomegaly
### Venous hypertension
- *Cardiac failure*
- Constrictive pericarditis
- Tricuspid stenosis
- Budd–Chiari syndrome
- Inferior vena cava thrombosis

### Degenerative
- Early cirrhosis
- Fatty infiltration

- Reye's syndrome

### Myeloproliferative disorders

### Neoplasia
- Primary and secondary deposits
- Leukaemia
- Lymphoma

### Infection
- Viral hepatitis
- Abscess
- Tuberculosis
- Syphilis
- Brucellosis
- Leptospirosis
- Malaria
- Kala-azar
- Hydatid cysts

### Storage disorders
- Amyloid
- Wilson's disease
- Gaucher's disease
- Niemann–Pick disease
- Histiocytosis X
- Glycogen storage diseases
- Haemochromatosis
- Hurler's syndrome

### Miscellaneous
- Sarcoid
- Biliary obstruction
- Rheumatoid arthritis
- Polycystic disease
- Riedel's lobe
- Hyperinflated lungs

## Causes of ascites
- Neoplasm (ovarian, gastrointestinal)
- Portal hypertension
- Hypoalbuminaemia
- Cardiac failure
- Budd–Chiari syndrome
- Constrictive pericarditis
- Peritonitis
- Lymphatic obstruction (chylous

**Table 11.5: Conjugated or unconjugated jaundice**

| Feature | Conjugated | Unconjugated |
|---|---|---|
| Serum bilirubin | Increased | Increased (rarely > 100 µmol/l) |
| Bilirubinuria | + (dark urine) | – |
| Urine urobilinogen | Reduced | Increased |
| Faecal stercobilinogen | Reduced (pale stools) | Increased |

**Table 11.6: Hepatic or obstructive jaundice**

| Feature | Hepatic | Obstructive |
|---|---|---|
| Pruritus | – | + |
| Alkaline phosphatase | Normal/mildly raised | Very raised |
| Transaminases | Very raised | Normal/mildly raised |
| Transaminase:AP ratio | Increased | Reduced |
| Liver ultrasound | No biliary tree dilatation | Biliary tree dilatation |
| Prothrombin time | Normal | Increased |

ascites)
- Pancreatitis
- Haemodialysis
- Peritoneal dialysis
- Hypothyroidism
- Malnutrition
- Post surgery
- SLE
- Peritoneal mesothelioma
- Pseudomyxoma peritonei
- Whipple's disease
- Sarcoid

## Causes of jaundice
### Pre-hepatic (unconjugated)
- Haemolytic anaemia
- Ineffective erythropoeisis
- Gilbert's syndrome
- Crigler–Najjar syndrome

### Hepatic (conjugated)
- Hepatitis
- Intrahepatic obstruction
- Dubin–Johnson syndrome
- Rotor syndrome

### Posthepatic (conjugated)
- Extrahepatic obstruction

# Investigation of liver disease

## Contraindications to liver biopsy
- Clotting defect
- Thrombocytopenia
- Hydatid cyst
- Haemangioma
- Biliary obstruction
- Patient refusal
- Inability to hold breath

## Complications of liver biopsy
- Pain
- Haemorrhage
- Hypotension
- Perforation of colon
- Perforation of kidney
- Pneumothorax
- Biliary peritonitis
- Peritonitis
- Cholangitis
- Septicaemia
- Mortality

# Intrinsic liver disease

## *Immunopathology of hepatitis B infection*

* Hepatitis B virus is composed of three antigens:

  Surface antigen (s): derived from protein of outer coat. Indicator of active infection

  Core antigen (c): derived from protein of core

  E antigen (e): derived from transcription of part of core protein in the endoplasmic reticulum (major indicator of infectivity)
* Each antigen elicits a corresponding antibody response

In acute infection the appearance of the antigens and antibodies follow a characteristic pattern. (Fig. 11.6)

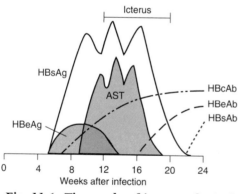
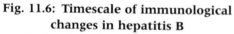

**Fig. 11.6: Timescale of immunological changes in hepatitis B**
*(During phase of HBe antigenaemia HBV particles are present in blood.)*

**Box 11.17: Other viral causes of acute hepatitis**

CMV
Herpes simplex
Herpes zoster
Lassa fever
Marburg virus
Ebola virus
Retrovirus
Coxsackie
Leptospira icterohaemorrhagica

## *Drugs causing hepatitis*
### *Antituberculous drugs*
* PAS
* Isoniazid
* Rifampicin
* Pyrazinamide

### *Antibiotics*
* Sulphonamides
* Co-trimoxazole
* Ketoconazole
* Nitrofurantoin

**Box 11.18: Classification of chronic active hepatitis**

Autoimmune
Chronic viral infection (hepatitis B,C,D)
Drugs (as for cirrhosis)
Wilson's disease
Haemochromatosis
Alcohol

**Table 11.7: Major causes of viral hepatitis**

| Virus | Type | Transmission | Chronicity |
| --- | --- | --- | --- |
| A | RNA | Faecal–oral | No |
| B | DNA | Blood, sex | Yes |
| C | RNA | Blood, sex | Yes |
| D | RNA | Blood, sex | Yes |
| E | RNA | Faecal–oral | No |
| G | RNA | Blood, sex | Yes |

**Table 11.8: Child's classification of severity of cirrhosis**

| Feature | Points scored for increasing abnormalities | | |
|---|---|---|---|
| | 1 | 2 | 3 |
| Encephalopathy | None | Grade 1–2 | Grade 3–4 |
| Ascites | None | Mild | Moderate/severe |
| Serum bilirubin (µmol/l) | < 25 | 25–40 | > 40 |
| Serum albumin (g/l) | > 35 | 28–35 | < 28 |
| Prothrombin time (s) | 1–4 | 4–6 | > 6 |

Total score: 5–6 = grade A; 7–9 = grade B; 10–15 = grade C

*Analgesics*
- Paracetamol
- Aspirin
- NSAIDs

*Psychotropics*
- Monoamine oxidase inhibitors
- Phenothiazines
- Tricyclic antidepressants

*Others*
- Halothane
- Methyldopa
- Thiazides
- Chlorpropramide
- Carbon tetrachloride
- Aflatoxins
- Verapamil
- Diltiazem
- Penicillamine
- Gold
- *Amanita phalloides*
- Phenytoin
- Phenobarbitone
- Sodium valproate
- Carbamazepine

## Causes of cirrhosis
*Infection*
- Hepatitis B
- Hepatitis C
- Hepatitis D
- Congenital syphilis
- Schistosomiasis

*Chronic inflammation*
- Chronic active hepatitis
- Primary biliary cirrhosis
- Sclerosing cholangitis
- Secondary biliary cirrhosis

*Metabolic*
- Galactosaemia
- Fructosaemia
- Cystic fibrosis
- Glycogen storage disease
- $\alpha_1$-Antitrypsin deficiency
- Tyrosinosis
- Abetalipoproteinaemia
- Wilson's disease
- Haemochromatosis

*Vascular*
- Constrictive pericarditis

**Box 11.19: Precipitants of hepatic encephalopathy**

**Infections**
Of any nature
**Dietary indiscretion**
High protein intake
Alcohol excess
**Upper gastrointestinal haemorrhage**
**Electrolyte imbalance**
**Drugs**
Sedatives and diuretics especially implicated
**Development of hepatoma**

- Chronic cardiac failure
- Sickle cell disease
- Hereditary haemorrhagic telangiectasia
- Veno-occlusive disease

### Drugs
- Methotrexate, methyldopa, isoniazid, erythromycin, nitrofurantoin, phenothiazines, azathioprine, combined oral contraceptive pill, thiazides, chlorpropramide, tricyclic antidepressants

### Miscellaneous
- Alcohol abuse
- Idiopathic (cryptogenic)
- Biliary atresia
- Ileoduodenal bypass
- Coeliac disease
- Anorexia nervosa
- Porphyria

## Physiology of hepatic encephalopathy
- Arises from a reduction in the functioning liver cell mass
- This leads to diversion of portal blood past the liver via portosystemic collaterals
- There are two main theories to the development of encephalopathy:
  1. Accumulation of toxins in systemic circulation
     Toxins could include ammonia, amines, indoles, mercaptans
  2. Altered balance of cerebral neurotransmitters
     Increased levels of cerebral aromatic amino acids and reduced levels of branched chain amino acids leads to the formation of false neurotransmitters
     This lead to alterations in the levels of normal cerebral neurotransmitters

**Table 11.9: Grading of hepatic encephalopathy**

| Grade | Features |
|-------|----------|
| 1 | Euphoria |
|   | Occasionally depression |
|   | Fluctuant mild confusion |
|   | Slowness of mentation and affect |
|   | Untidy |
|   | Slurred speech |
|   | Disorder in sleep rhythm |
| 2 | Accentuation of grade 1 |
|   | Drowsy |
|   | Inappropriate behaviour |
| 3 | Sleeps most of the time but rousable |
|   | Incoherent speech |
|   | Marked confusion |
| 4 | Unrousable |

## Management of hepatic encephalopathy
- Identify and treat underlying cause
- Initial low-protein diet
- Neomycin 500 mg–1 g qds
- Lactulose, aiming for 2–3 soft stools per day
- i.v. 5% dextrose infusion
- Careful fluid balance
- CVP monitoring may be required for control of clotting status
- Inotropic support may be needed

## Causes of haemochromatosis
- Idiopathic
- Multiple blood transfusions
- Sideroblastic anaemia
- Thalassaemia
- Sickle cell disease
- Congenital transferrin deficiency
- Chronic liver disease
- Portacaval shunt
- Porphyria cutanea tarda
- Xanthinuria

## Causes of veno-occlusive disease

### Vascular
- Budd–Chiari syndrome
- Hyperviscosity syndromes

### Malignancy
- Renal cell carcinoma
- Hepatoma
- Carcinoma of the stomach
- Carcinoma of the pancreas

### Drugs
- Combined oral contraceptive pill
- Cytotoxic drugs
- Alkaloids

### Infection
- Amoebic cysts
- Schistosomiasis
- Hydatid
- Syphilis

### Miscellaneous
- Graft-versus-host disease
- Mixed connective tissue disease
- Trauma
- Pregnancy
- Inflammatory bowel disease
- Protein-losing enteropathy
- Nephrotic syndrome
- Sarcoid

# Obstructive liver disease

## Causes of obstructive jaundice

### Intrahepatic
- Primary biliary cirrhosis
- Alcohol-induced hepatitis
- *Cirrhosis*
- *Metastases*
- Pregnancy
- Combined oral contraceptive pill
- Methyltesterone
- Total parenteral nutrition
- Lymphoma

- Postoperative
- Caroli's disease (congenital intrahepatic dilatation)
- Viral hepatitis
- Biliary atresia
- Neonatal hepatitis
- Galactosaemia
- $\alpha_1$-Antitrypsin deficiency
- Byler's disease

### Extrahepatic
- Gallstones
- Carcinoma of the pancreas
- Post-traumatic
- Sclerosing cholangitis
- Biliary atresia
- Choledochal cyst
- Acute pancreatitis
- Chronic pancreatitis
- Retroperitoneal fibrosis
- Ascending cholangitis
- Haemobilia
- Carcinoma of the gallbladder
- Cholangiocarcinoma
- Hilar lymphadenopathy
- Carcinoma of the ampulla of Vater

## Gallstones

### Mixed cholesterol stones
- Composed of cholesterol, calcium and bile
- 10% are radio-opaque

---

**Box 11.20: Aetiology of gallstones**

Female gender
Obesity
Advanced age
Advanced parity
Positive family history
Lower social class
Combined oral contraceptive pill
Chronic liver disease
Terminal ileal disease
Chronic haemolytic anaemia
Biliary tract infection

***Pigment stones***
- Contain bilirubin, phosphates and carbonates
- Associated with chronic haemolytic anaemias, *E. coli* infection, *Clostridium* infection and *Bacteroides* infection of the biliary tract
- Radiolucent

# Liver transplantation

## Indications for liver transplantation
- Primary biliary cirrhosis
- Chronic active hepatitis
- Cryptogenic cirrhosis
- Fulminant hepatic failure
- Biliary atresia
- Budd–Chiari syndrome
- Paracetamol
- Primary sclerosing cholangitis
- $\alpha_1$-Antitrypsin deficiency

---

**Box 11.21: Aetiology of malignant liver disease**

**Hepatoma**
Cirrhosis
Hepatitis B
Hepatitis C
Aflatoxin (*Aspergillus flavus*)
Prolonged combined oral contraceptive use
Nitrosamines
Anabolic steroids
Thorotrast (radioactive contrast agent)

**Cholangiocarcinoma**
Gallstones
*Opisthorchis felineus*
*Clonorchis sinensis*
Ulcerative colitis
Primary sclerosing cholangitis
Thorotrast
Congenital hepatic fibrosis
Caroli's disease
Polycystic disease

---

- Wilson's disease
- Galactosaemia
- Hepatoma

# Miscellaneous liver disease

## Causes of hepatic granuloma
### Bacterial infection
- Tuberculosis
- Brucellosis
- Leprosy
- Listeria

### Fungal infection
- Coccidioidomycosis
- Histoplasmosis
- *Nocardia*
- *Aspergillus*
- *Candida*
- Actinomycosis

### Parasitic infection
- Schistosomiasis
- *Ascaris*
- *Toxocara*
- *Amoeba*
- *Strongyloides*
- *Giardia lamblia*

### Viral infection
- CMV
- EBV
- Lymphogranuloma venereum

### Rickettsial infection
- Q fever

### Spirochaete infection
- Syphilis

### Neoplasia
- Hodgkin's lymphoma
- Adenocarcinoma
- Hepatoma

*Connective tissue disease*
- Sarcoid
- Polymyalgia rheumatica
- Whipple's disease
- SLE
- Wegener's granulomatosis
- Polyarteritis nodosa

*Drugs*
- Sulphonamides
- Chlorpropramide
- Phenylbutazone
- Allopurinol
- Hydralazine
- Carbamazepine
- Quinidine
- Aspirin
- Carbimazole
- Halothane
- Quinine

*Miscellaneous*
- Idiopathic
- Chronic granulomatous disease
- Crohn's disease
- i.v. Drug abuse
- Haemodialysis
- Haemophilia
- Ileal bypass surgery
- Berylliosis
- Primary biliary cirrhosis
- Agammaglobulinaemia

*Causes of pyogenic liver abscesses*
- Ascending cholangitis
- Acute cholecystitis
- Amoeba
- Diverticulitis
- Acute pancreatitis
- Appendicitis
- Septicaemia
- Trauma
- Malignancy
- Local extension of subphrenic abscess
- Empyema of gallbladder

# Clinical case scenarios

## Hepatomegaly

There is hepatomegaly as evidenced by a mass in the right hypochondrium which you cannot get above and which moves down with inspiration. It extends $x$ cm below the right costal margin.

Describe whether it is smooth, regular or irregular, tender or pulsatile

- Other features to look for:
    Signs of chronic liver disease
    Signs of congestive cardiac failure
    Elevated JVP with prominent
        v waves and pulsatile liver
        (tricuspid regurgitation)
    Splenomegaly, hyperpigmentation
        (haemochromatosis)
    Erythema nodosum, lupus pernio
        (sarcoid)
    Rheumatoid hands (amyloid)
    Chronic obstructive pulmonary
        disease (apparent hepatomegaly)

## Splenomegaly

There is splenomegaly as evidenced by a mass in the left hypochondrium which you cannot get above and which moves down on inspiration. It extends $x$ cm below the left costal margin.

- Other features to look for:
    Hepatomegaly
    Signs of chronic liver disease
    Lymphadenopathy
        (lymphoproliferative disorders)
    Ruddy complexion (polycythaemia)
    Splinter haemorrhages, cardiac
        murmur (bacterial endocarditis)
    Erythema nodosum, lupus pernio
        (sarcoid)

Rheumatoid hands (Felty's syndrome)
Features of SLE
Thyroid status
Signs of cardiac failure

## Ascites

- The abdomen is distended
- There may be eversion of the umbilicus
- There is dullness to percussion in both flanks, with shifting dullness and a fluid thrill

- Other features to look for: as for hepatomegaly

## Haemochromatosis

- The patient is usually thin
- There is slate-grey hyperpigmentation and decreased body hair
- Gynaecomastia and testicular atrophy
- There will be hepatomegaly and sometimes splenomegaly

- Other features to look for:
    Signs of chronic liver disease
    Signs of diabetes mellitus
    Arthropathy (pseudogout)
    Evidence of cardiomyopathy

## Chronic liver disease

- Prime features:
Jaundice
Hyperpigmentation
Cyanosis
Clubbing
Leukonychia
Palmar erythema
Dupuytren's contracture
Spider naevi

Excoriations
Purpura
Gynaecomastia
Scanty body hair
Gonadal atrophy
Hepatomegaly
Splenomegaly
Peripheral oedema
Ascites
Distended abdominal veins (with flow away from the umbilicus)

- Other features to look for:
    Signs of cardiac failure
    Features of constrictive pericarditis
    Kayser–Fleischer rings, dysarthria (Wilson's disease)
    Features of emphysema ($\alpha_1$-antitrypsin deficiency)
    Abdominal scars (previous surgery for inflammatory bowel disease)
    Xanthelasma in a middle-aged female (primary biliary cirrhosis)
    Tattoos (hepatitis B infection)
    Encephalopathy (flapping tremor, constructional apraxia)

## Primary biliary cirrhosis

- The patient is usually female and middle-aged
- There may be jaundice and hyperpigmentation
- There may be excoriations due to scratching and xanthelasma
- There may be clubbing
- Look for hepatomegaly and splenomegaly

- Other features to look for:
    Signs of associated conditions (Sjögren's syndrome, scleroderma, CREST syndrome, rheumatoid arthritis, dermatomyositis, Hashimoto's thyroiditis)

# Crohn's disease

- There may be a right iliac fossa mass
- Multiple abdominal scars or abdominal wall sinuses
- Perianal disease
- Aphthous ulceration of the mouth
- Ileostomy bag
- Arthropathy
- Erythema nodosum
- Pyoderma gangrenosum
- Iritis
- Ankle oedema (hypoproteinaemia)

# Abdominal mass

- On finding a mass you should define the following:
  Size, shape and consistency
  Whether you can get above or
    below it
  Whether it is bimanually ballottable
  Whether it moves with respiration
  Whether it is tender

## Causes of mass in right iliac fossa
- Carcinoma of the caecum
- Appendix abscess
- Crohn's disease
- Ileocaecal tuberculosis
- Amoebic abscess
- Lymphoma
- Ovarian neoplasm
- Ileal carcinoid

## Causes of mass in left iliac fossa
- Carcinoma of the colon
- Faecal mass
- Diverticular abscess
- Ovarian neoplasm
- Amoebic abscess

## Causes of upper abdominal masses
- Hepatomegaly
- Splenomegaly
- Abdominal aortic aneurysm
- Carcinoma of the stomach
- Carcinoma of the pancreas
- Lymphoma
- Carcinoma of the colon
- Retroperitoneal sarcoma
- Diverticular abscess

# 12 Endocrinology

## Contents

Cells can communicate with each other in four ways:
- Nervous impulses
- Direct contact
- Local chemical release (paracrine activity)
- Hormones (Table 12.1)

## Hormones

- Substances secreted directly into the blood by specialised cells in response to a specific stimulus and in amounts that vary with the strength of the stimulus

### Table 12.1: Types of hormone

| Feature | Peptide hormones | Steroid and thyroid hormones |
|---|---|---|
| Stored | Yes | No |
| Relative concentrations | Low | High |
| Protein-bound | No | Yes |
| Half-life | Short (may be lengthened by addition of sialic acid moieties) | Long |
| Site of target cell receptors | Cell membrane | Cell nucleus |
| Enter target cell | No | Yes |
| Mode of action | Via second messengers , (cAMP phosphatidyl inositol, tyrosine kinase) | Direct effect on metabolism |
| Site of metabolism | All tissues | Liver |
| Method of metabolism | Proteolysis | Conjugation of free hormone (protein-bound hormone protected) |
| Examples | Adrenaline, noradrenaline, glucagon, insulin, ACTH, PTH, ADH, hypothalamic releasing hormones, gastrointestinal hormones | Cortisol, progesterone, oestrogen, testosterone, thyroxine, triiodothyronine |

- Act on specific target cells and regulate pre-existing cellular reactions

# Anterior pituitary gland

## Anatomy

- Comprised of two lobes
- Anterior lobe derived from Rathkes' pouch
- Posterior lobe derived from downgrowth of the floor of the third ventricle (infundibulum)
- Normal adult pituitary weighs 600 mg
- Lies within a depression in the sphenoid bone (sella turcica) (Fig. 12.1)
- Covered by a layer of dura (diaphragma sellae)

- Anterior pituitary consists of three cell types:
  *chromophobes* (do not take up dye) – 50%
  *chromophils* (do take up dye):
    basophils (basic dyes) – 15%
    acidophils (acidic dyes) – 35%

# Causes of hypopituitarism

## *Congenital*
- Pituitary hypoplasia
- Kallman's syndrome (deficient LH, FSH with anosmia)

## *Idiopathic*

## *Malignancy*
- Pituitary adenomas
- Craniopharyngiomas
- Meningiomas
- Secondary deposits

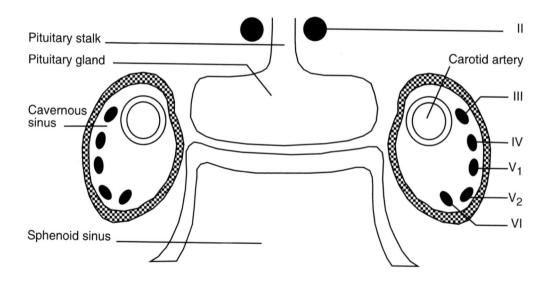

**Fig. 12.1: Coronal view of pituitary gland, showing major anatomical structures**

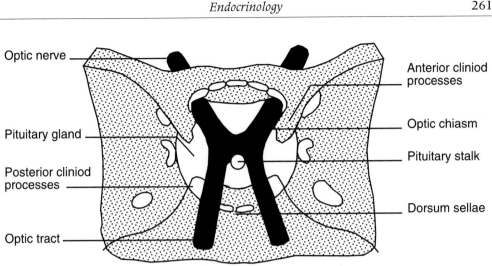

**Fig. 12.2: Superior view of pituitary gland, showing major anatomical structures**

## Infection
- Encephalitis
- Bacterial meningitis
- Syphilis

## Granulomatous infiltration
- Sarcoid
- Histiocytosis X

## Vascular
- Sheehan's syndrome
- Infarction
- Pituitary apoplexy
- Intracranial haemorrhage
- Internal carotid artery aneurysm

## Iatrogenic
- Surgical resection
- Radiotherapy

## Trauma
- Severe head injury

## Miscellaneous
- Anorexia nervosa
- Emotional deprivation
- Malnutrition
- Autoimmune disease

# Pituitary function tests

## Imaging
- *Plain skull X-ray*: may show expansion of pituitary fossa and erosion of dorsum sellae indicative of malignancy, but cannot show whether pituitary is present or absent
- *CT/MRI*: imaging investigations of choice

## Hormonal levels
- *Basal levels*: may give useful clues to diagnosis, but results may be unreliable owing to circadian secretion of hormones and increased secretion due to stress
- *Dynamic levels*: combined pituitary function test (TRH test, GnRH, insulin/glucagon stress test)
  Arginine infusion test (GH)
  Bovril test (GH)
  Exercise test (GH)
  Insulin stress test (GH)
  Glucose tolerance test (GH)
  Synacthen test (ACTH)
  Dexamethasone suppression test (ACTH)

**Table 12.2: Anterior pituitary hormones**

| Hormone | Cell type | Staining reaction | Stimuli | Inhibitors | Main actions |
|---|---|---|---|---|---|
| ACTH | Corticotroph | Basophil | CRH<br>ADH<br>Hypoglycaemia<br>Stress | Cortisol | Increased cortisol production by adrenal cortex<br>Increased adrenal blood flow<br>Increased cholesterol concentration<br>Increased protein synthesis in adrenal cortex |
| MSH | Melanotroph | Basophil | Adrenocortical insufficiency | Melanotroph inhibitory factor<br>Glucocorticoids | Increased skin pigmentation |
| GH | Somatotroph | Acidophil | GHRH, glucagon<br>Bromocriptine<br>Hypoglycaemia<br>Stress, exercise, sleep<br>Raised amino acid levels | Somatostatin<br>Fatty acids<br>Hyperglycaemia<br>Raised cortisol<br>Insulin-like growth factor | Raised blood glucose<br>Increased lipolysis<br>Increased protein synthesis<br>Increased tissue growth |
| TSH | Thyrotroph | Basophil | TRH | Thyroxine<br>Triiodothyronine<br>Somatostatin<br>Dopamine | Increased growth of thyroid<br>Increased iodine uptake by thyroid<br>Increased production of thyroid hormones |
| LH | Luteotroph | Basophil | GnRH, oestradiol<br>Gonadal dysgenesis<br>Clomiphene | Oestradiol<br>Progesterone<br>Testosterone (men) | Controls development of corpus luteum and progesterone secretion (females)<br>Increased testosterone production (males) |
| FSH | Folliculotroph | Basophil | GnRH, TRH (men)<br>Clomiphene<br>Gonadal dysgenesis and spermatogenesis (males) | Inhibin, oestradiol<br>Progesterone<br>Testosterone (men) | Controls development of graafian follicle (females)<br>Increased growth of seminiferous tubules |
| Prolactin | Lactotroph | Acidophil | TRH, oestradiol<br>Exercise, sleep, stress<br>Pregnancy, lactation, Puberty (girls) | Dopamine | Milk synthesis |

TRH test (TSH)
GnRH test (FSH, LH)
Clomiphene test (FSH, LH)

# Management of hypopituitarism

## Emergency treatment of pituitary collapse or coma

- Immediate i.v. hydrocortisone 100–200 mg repeated after 2–4 h
- i.v. fluid replacement

## Subacute treatment

- Thyroid hormones can be started orally but must not be given before steroid replacement has begun (thyroxine increases the clearance of cortisol and exacerbates deficiency)
- Monitor electrolytes, urine output, urine and serum osmolalities carefully (steroid replacement may unmask underlying diabetes insipidus)
- Testosterone should be started early in men to improve muscle strength and wellbeing and hasten recovery

## Long-term treatment

- *Corticosteroids:* usually given as hydrocortisone 20–40 mg/d
  Given in two daily doses, with two-thirds of total daily dose in the morning and one-third in early evening to mimic normal circadian rhythm
- *Thyroxine:* dose monitored using free $T_4$ levels (TSH levels are of no use)
- *Sex hormones:* men – testosterone
  Women with uterus – oestrogen and cyclical progesterone
  Women without uterus – oestrogen only

# Pituitary tumours (Table 12.3)

## Macroadenomas

- Tumours > 10 mm diameter
- All GH-secreting adenomas are macroadenomas
- Some prolactinomas are macroadenomas

## Microadenomas

- Tumours < 10mm diameter

**Table 12.3: Types of pituitary tumour**

| Tumour | Cell type |
|---|---|
| GH-secreting adenoma | Acidophilic (densely granulated) |
| | Chromophobic (sparsely granulated) |
| Prolactinoma | Acidophilic (densely granulated) |
| | Chromophobic (sparsely granulated) |
| ACTH-secreting adenoma | Basophilic (densely granulated) |
| | Chromophobic (sparsely granulated) |
| Undifferentiated adenomas | Chromophobic |
| TSH-secreting adenomas | Chromophobic |
| GnRH-secreting adenomas | Chromophobic |
| Mixed GH-secreting/prolactinoma | Acidophilic (densely granulated) |
| | Chromophobic (sparsely granulated) |
| Craniopharyngioma | Squamous/columnar |
| Ganglioneuromas (third ventricle) | Epithelial |
| Optic chiasm gliomas | Glial |
| Pinealoma | Various |
| Secondary deposits | Various |

- All are microadenomas except GH-secreting tumours and some prolactinomas

## Cell types of pituitary adenomas
- Chromophobic: 70%
- Acidophilic: 15%
- Basophilic: 15%

## Clinical features of pituitary tumours
- Due to hormone oversecretion
- Due to hypopituitarism
- Local effects (Box 12.1)

# Abnormalities of growth hormone status

## Causes of growth hormone deficiency
- Hypopituitarism
- X-linked GH deficiency
- Autosomal dominant GH deficiency
- Laron dwarfism (unresponsive GH receptors, high GH levels)

## Features of growth hormone deficiency
- Short stature
- Delayed growth
- Delayed puberty
- Hypoglycaemia
- Osteoporosis
- Premature cardiovascular disease

## Tests for growth hormone deficiency
### Insulin stress test
- Take blood for basal GH level
- Give 0.1–0.15 U/kg of soluble insulin
- Take blood for GH levels at 30-minute intervals for 2 hours
- Insulin dose should be repeated if hypoglycaemia not precipitated
- Normal response if peak GH > 20 mU/l

---

**Box 12.1: Local effects of pituitary tumours**

Headache
Bitemporal hemianopia
Rhinorrhoea
Meningitis
Palsies of cranial nerves III, IV, V, VI
Cavernous sinus thrombosis
Hydrocephalus
Optic atrophy
Korsakoff's syndrome

---

### Glucagon stress test
- Take blood for basal GH level
- Give glucagon 1 mg i.m.
- Take blood for GH level at 30 minute intervals for 4 hours
- Normal response if peak GH > 15 mU/l (male), > 20 mU/l (female)

### Arginine infusion test
- Take blood for basal GH level
- Give i.v. infusion of 0.5 g/kg arginine (maximum dose 30 g)
- Take blood for GH level at 30-minute intervals for 2 hours
- Normal response if peak GH > 15 mU/l

### Bovril test
- Take blood for basal GH level
- Give Bovril 20 g /1.5m$^2$ body surface area in water
- Take blood for GH level at 30-minute intervals for 2 hours
- Normal response if peak GH > 20 mU/l

### Exercise test
- Take blood for basal GH level
- Ask patient to run up and down stairs as fast as possible for 10 minutes
- Take blood for GH level after 10 minute period of exercise
- Normal response if peak GH > 20 mU/l

## Other causes of short stature
### Constitutional
- Racial
- Familial
- Sporadic

### Nutritional
- Starvation
- Malabsorption
- Protein loss

### Chromosomal defects
- Down's syndrome
- Turner's syndrome

### Skeletal defects
- Rickets
- Achondroplasia
- Hurler's syndrome

### Chronic systemic disease
- Cyanotic congenital heart disease
- Renal failure
- Liver failure
- Pulmonary disease
- Anaemia
- Infections
- Long-term steroid treatment

### Endocrine disease
- Sexual precocity
- Hypopituitarism
- Hypothyroidism
- Congenital adrenal hyperplasia

### Miscellaneous
- Progeria

## Causes of acromegaly
### Pituitary disease
- GH-secreting adenomas
- GH cell hyperplasia
- GH cell carcinoma

### Extra-pituitary disease
- Ectopic GH-secreting adenoma
- Ectopic GH-secreting tumours (lung,
  ovary, breast, pancreas, carcinoids)
- Excess GRF production (hypothalamic
  hamartoma)

## Clinical features of acromegaly
### Cardiorespiratory
- Cardiomyopathy
- Hypertension
- Increased lung volume
- Upper respiratory tract
  obstruction

### Dermatological
- Thickened, coarse skin
- Hyperhidrosis
- Lipomas
- Hirsutism
- Hyperpigmentation
- Raynaud's phenomenon
- Acne

### Musculoskeletal
- Arthropathy
- Proximal myopathy
- Osteoporosis

### Endocrine
- Diabetes mellitus
- Hyperprolactinaemia
- Goitre
- Hyperthyroidism
- Diabetes insipidus

### Neurological
- Nerve entrapment syndromes
- Hypertrophic neuropathy

### Metabolic
- Hypercalcaemia
- Hypercalciuria
- Hyperphosphataemia
- Increased metabolic rate

## Tests for growth hormone excess
### Glucose tolerance test (Fig. 12.3)
- Typically, there is a high basal level of
  GH

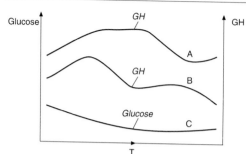

**Fig. 12.3: Typical changes in serum glucose and growth hormone levels during glucose tolerance test**

*A= acromegaly; B and C = normal subjects*

- Following glucose load there is failure of suppression of GH levels
- In some patients there is a paradoxical rise in GH levels following glucose loading

# Hyperprolactinaemia

## Non-physiological causes of hyperprolactinaemia
### Malignancy
- Prolactinoma
- Craniopharyngioma
- Glioma
- Pinealoma

### Pituitary infiltration
- Sarcoid
- Histiocytosis X
- TB meningitis

### Drugs
- Dopamine receptor blockers (neuroleptics, metoclopramide, domperidone)
- Dopamine-depleting agents (reserpine, methyldopa)
- Oestrogen
- TRH
- Opiates
- $H_2$ receptor blockers

**Box 12.2: Features of hyperprolactinaemia**

**Women**
Amenorrhoea
Oligomenorrhoea
Galactorrhoea
Infertility
Hirsutism

**Men**
Impotence
Galactorrhoea
Oligospermia
Prostate hypoplasia
Reduced semen volume
Infertility
Female-pattern body fat distribution

### Miscellaneous
- Pituitary trauma
- Idiopathic
- Hypothyroidism
- Chronic renal failure
- Ectopic secretion (renal cell carcinoma, carcinoma bronchus)
- Grand mal seizure
- Polycystic ovarian syndrome
- Adrenocortical insufficiency
- Cushing's syndrome

# Thyroid gland

## Anatomy

- Derived from floor of the pharynx and the fourth pharyngeal pouch
- Normal adult weight 20 g
- Gland consists of two lobes joined by the isthmus
- The isthmus overlies the 2nd–4th tracheal rings
- Gland composed mainly of follicular cells which contain colloid, rich in thyroglobulin

- Also composed of parafollicular cells (C cells), which secrete calcitonin

# Hormone synthesis

- Synthesis of thyroid hormones dependent on iodine
- Average daily intake of iodine is 100 μg
- Main food sources of iodine are iodised salt, seafish, milk, bread
- Absorbed as iodide in the small intestine
- Iodide is transported into thyroid cells and converted into iodine
- Iodine is incorporated into monoiodotyrosine (MIT) and diiodotyrosine (DIT)
- Two DIT molecules combine to form thyroxine (T$_4$)
- One MIT and one DIT molecule combine to form triiodothyronine (T$_3$)
- Production of thyroid hormones regulated by TSH
- Thyroid hormones metabolised in the liver by conjugation
- Most of the iodine is recirculated and reused

*Thyroxine*: comprises 90% of the active thyroid hormone
Mainly protein-bound:
thyroid-binding globulin (TBG): 75%
thyroid-binding pre-albumin (TBPA): 15%
albumin:10%
Only 0.05% exists in an active, free, unbound form
*Triiodothyronine*: five times as potent as T$_4$
Less strongly protein-bound
0.5% in an active, free, unbound form
T$_3$ is the major active hormone at tissue level
One-third of T$_4$ is converted into T$_3$

---

**Box 12.3: Actions of thyroid hormones**

Increased metabolic rate
Skeletal growth
Sexual maturation
Brain development
Glucose absorption from the gastrointestinal tract
Reduced blood glucose
Conversion of carotene to vitamin A
Reduced serum cholesterol
Upregulation of cardiac β-receptors (potentiation of catecholamines)

---

by deiodination at tissue level
85% of T$_3$ is produced in this fashion

# Hypothyroidism

## *Causes of hypothyroidism*
### *Congenital*
- Thyroid aplasia
- Ectopic thyroid
- Maternal iodine deficiency (endemic cretinism)
- Pituitary insufficiency
- Hypothalamic insufficiency
- Maternal antithyroid drugs
- Maternal Graves' disease
- Defects in thyroid hormone synthesis

### *Acquired: Primary*
- Autoimmune (Hashimoto's thyroiditis)
- Previous treatment of hyperthyroidism
- Iodine deficiency
- Riedel's thyroiditis
- Drugs: phenylbutazone, para-aminosalicylic acid (PAS), lithium, amiodarone

### *Acquired: Secondary*
- Hypopituitarism
- Hypothalamic lesions

## Clinical features of hypothyroidism

### Cardiorespiratory
- Angina
- Bradycardia
- Cardiomyopathy
- Pericardial effusion
- Pleural effusions

### Metabolic
- Hypercholesterolaemia
- Hyponatraemia
- SIADH

### Miscellaneous
- Lethargy
- Weight gain
- Cold intolerance
- Deafness
- Hypothermia
- Malar flush
- Husky voice
- Myalgia
- Arthralgia

### Gastrointestinal
- Constipation
- Ascites

### Neurological
- Hyporeflexia
- Carpal tunnel syndrome
- Cerebellar ataxia
- Myotonia
- Coma

### Haematological
- Macrocytic anaemia
- Microcytic anaemia
- Normocytic anaemia

### Dermatological
- Dry skin
- Alopecia
- Coarse hair
- Puffy face

### Endocrine
- Menorrhagia
- Galactorrhoea
- Goitre

### Psychiatric
- Cognitive impairment
- Depression
- Psychosis

# Hyperthyroidism

## Causes of hyperthyroidism
- Graves' disease
- Multinodular goitre
- Thyroid adenoma
- Thyroiditis
- Ectopic TSH (choriocarcinoma, struma ovarii)
- Metastatic thyroid cancer
- Drugs: thyroxine, amiodarone
- Polyostotic fibrous dysplasia

## Clinical features of hyperthyroidism

### Cardiorespiratory
- Tachycardia
- Palpitations
- Atrial fibrillation
- Collapsing pulse
- High-output cardiac failure
- Angina
- Dyspnoea

### Dermatological
- Palmar erythema
- Spider naevi
- Vitiligo
- Hyperpigmentation
- Onycholysis
- Pretibial myxoedema
- Clubbing
- Hyperhidrosis
- Alopecia

**Box 12.4: Causes of goitre**

Simple goitre
Multinodular goitre
Iodine deficiency
Puberty
Pregnancy
Graves' disease
Hashimoto's thyroiditis
De Quervain's thyroiditis
Thyroid adenoma
Thyroid cyst
Thyroid carcinoma
Acromegaly

*Miscellaneous*
- Weight loss
- Heat intolerance
- Fatigue
- Anxiety
- Gritty eyes
- Lid retraction
- Lid lag
- Exopthalamos
- Proptosis
- Proximal myopathy

*Neurological*
- Tremor

- Visual disturbance
- Ophthalmoplegia
- Papilloedema
- Choreoathetosis

*Gastrointestinal*
- Anorexia
- Nausea
- Vomiting
- Diarrhoea
- Steatorrhoea

*Endocrine*
- Oligomenorrhoea
- Loss of libido
- Gynaecomastia
- Goitre
- Goitre bruit

*Metabolic*
- Hypercalcaemia

# Thyroid emergencies

## *Treatment of myxoedema coma*
- Requires urgent administration of thyroxine 400–500 µg i.v. or orally
- After this, no further thyroid hormone

**Table 12.4: Thyroid carcinoma**

| Types of thyroid carcinoma | Features |
|---|---|
| Papillary | Represents 60–80% of thyroid carcinomas |
| | Typically slow growing |
| | Prognosis good |
| | Responds to thyroxine |
| Follicular | Accounts for 20–25% of thyroid carcinomas |
| | Presents in the fifth decade |
| | Usually well differentiated with good prognosis |
| | Responds to thyroxine |
| Medullary | Accounts for 3–5% of thyroid carcinomas |
| | Arises from parafollicular or C cells |
| | Secretes calcitonin |
| | Prognosis poor |
| Anaplastic | Usually affects the elderly |
| | Carries the worst prognosis |

| Box 12.5: Abnormalities of TBG | |
| --- | --- |
| **Increased** | **Reduced** |
| Hereditary | Hereditary |
| Pregnancy | Androgens |
| Oestrogen | Corticosteroids |
| Phenothiazines | Cushing's syndrome |
| Clofibrate | Active acromegaly |
| Viral hepatitis | Nephrotic syndrome |
| Acute intermittent | Malnutrition |
| porphyria | Malabsorption |
| Hypothyroidism | Major illness |
| | Hyperthyroidism |

# Tests of thyroid function

## Thyroid binding globulin (TBG) levels

- Raised TBG leads to raised total $T_4$ levels but normal free $T_4$ levels
- Reduced TBG leads to reduced total $T_4$ levels but normal free $T_4$ levels

## Autoantibodies

- *TSH receptor antibody* (long-acting thyroid stimulator): Graves' disease
- *Microsomal antibody*: Hashimoto's thyroiditis

## TRH test

- Take blood sample for basal TSH level
- Give TRH 200 µg i.v.
- Measure TSH levels at 20 and 60 minutes

  *Normal result*
  TSH increment of > 3 mU/l in older people and > 5 mU/l in young adults

  *Hyperthyroidism*
  Low basal TSH
  Little or no increase in TSH levels (< 1 mU/l)

  *Hypothyroidism*
  High basal TSH
  Exaggerated TSH increase

  *Hypopituitarism*
  TSH increment usually normal or low normal

  *Hypothalamic disorders*
  Delayed TSH increment

replacement is required for a week
- Supportive treatment should be given to maintain respiration and correct hypothermia
- Despite best treatment it carries a mortality of 50%

## Treatment of thyroid storm

- Requires urgent treatment with antithyroid drugs, usually propylthiouracil 600–1200 µg or carbimazole 60–120 mg orally
- β-Blockers should also be given (propranolol 1–5 mg i.v. or 20–80 mg 6-hourly orally)
- Other supportive treatment should also be given, such as fluid replacement, treatment of cardiac failure and infection

**Table 12.5: Typical radioimmunoassay findings in thyroid disease**

| | Hyper-thyroidism | Hypo-thyroidism | Hypo-pituitarism | Hypothalamic dysfunction | Sick thyroid |
| --- | --- | --- | --- | --- | --- |
| $T_4$ | Raised | Reduced | Reduced | Reduced | Reduced |
| $T_3$ | Raised | Reduced | Reduced | Reduced | Reduced |
| TSH | Reduced | Raised | Reduced | Reduced | Normal |

# Adrenal glands

## Anatomy

- Situated at the upper poles of both kidneys
- Each gland weighs 4–5 g
- Each gland consists of adrenal cortex and adrenal medulla

- *Adrenal cortex*: comprised of outer capsule surrounding three hormone-producing layers:
  *zona glomerulosa*: synthesises mineralocorticoids
  *zona fasciculata*: synthesises cortisol
  *zona reticularis*: synthesises androgens, oestrogen, progesterone
- *Adrenal medulla*: synthesises adrenaline and noradrenaline in chromaffin cells

## Physiology

### Glucocorticoids
- Predominantly cortisol
- Small amounts of corticosterone:
  75% bound to cortisol-binding globulin (transcortin)
  15% bound to albumin
  10% free and active
- Production regulated by ACTH

### Mineralocorticoids
- Principally aldosterone
- Renin secreted by the juxtaglomerular apparatus acts on angiotensinogen in the bloodstream, leading to the production of angiotensin 1.
  This is then converted to angiotensin 2 in the lungs by the angiotensin-converting enzyme.
  Angiotensin 2 then acts through cell surface receptors in the adrenal cortex to stimulate aldosterone production.

**Box 12.6: Alterations in renin release**

| Increased | Decreased |
|---|---|
| Hypovolaemia | Angiotensin 2 |
| Sodium depletion | ADH |
| Catecholamines | Hypernatraemia |
| Oral contraceptives | Hyperkalaemia |
| Hepatic cirrhosis | Indomethacin |
| Congestive | β-Blockers |
| cardiac failure | ACE inhibitors |
| Nephrotic | |
| syndrome | |
| Upright posture | |

### Catecholamines
- Adrenaline 80%, noradrenaline 20%
- Bound to ATP and protein
- Stored as membrane–bound granules (chromaffin granules)
- Half-life 1–3 min
- Release stimulated by stress, hypoglycaemia
- Metabolised by monoamine oxidase inhibitor (MAOI), catechol-*o*-methyl transferase (COMT)

## Causes of hyperaldosteronism

### Primary
- Conn's syndrome

### Secondary
- Upright posture
- Ambulation
- Hyperkalaemia
- Hyponatraemia
- Hypovolaemia
- Surgery
- Anxiety
- Cardiac failure
- Cirrhosis
- Nephrotic syndrome
- Renal artery stenosis

**Box 12.7: Actions of glucocorticoids**

Glycogenolysis
Gluconeogenesis
Increased protein catabolism
Lipolysis
Increased free fatty acid mobilisation
Increased ketone production
Hyperglycaemia
Anti-inflammatory properties
Increased resistance to stress
Mineralocorticoid activity
Reduced lymphocytes and eosinophils
Increased neutrophils, platelets and red
blood cells
Hypercalcuria
Increased secretion of gastric acid
Increased secretion of pepsin

- Bartter's syndrome
- Renin-secreting tumours
- Salt-losing nephropathy

# Adrenocortical insufficiency

## Primary causes of adrenocortical insufficiency (increased ACTH)
### Infections
- Tuberculosis
- Histoplasmosis
- HIV
- Meningococcal septicaemia (Waterhouse–Friedrichsen syndrome)

### Congenital
- 21-hydroxylase deficiency
- Congenital adrenal hypoplasia
- Adrenoleukodystrophy

### Vascular
- Adrenal haemorrhage
- Adrenal infarction

**Box 12.8: Actions of catecholamines**

Increased glycogenolysis
Increased gluconeogenesis
Increased lipolysis
Hyperglycaemia
Increased ketone production

### Malignancy
- Secondary deposits

### Miscellaneous
- Autoimmunity
- Adrenalectomy
- Amyloid
- Haemochromatosis

### Drugs
- Metyrapone
- Cytotoxics
- Etomidate
- Ketoconazole
- Rifampicin
- Carbamazepine

## Secondary causes of adrenocortical insufficiency (reduced ACTH)
- Hypopituitarism
- Glucocorticoid therapy withdrawal
- Post treatment of Cushing's syndrome

## Clinical features of Addison's disease
### Gastrointestinal
- Nausea
- Vomiting
- Abdominal pain
- Acute abdomen

### Cardiovascular
- Postural hypotension
- Tachycardia

### Metabolic
- Hypovolaemia
- Hypoglycaemia

- Raised serum urea
- Hyperkalaemia
- Hyponatraemia
- Hypercalcaemia
- Anaemia
- Lymphocytosis
- Eosinophilia

*Miscellaneous*
- Malaise
- Lassitude
- Somnolence
- Depression
- Dizziness
- Nocturia
- Muscle cramps
- Anorexia
- Weight loss
- Fever
- Hyperpigmentation

## Emergency treatment of Addisonian crisis
- Admit to hospital
- Fluid replacement
- Correction of electrolyte abnormalities
- i.v. Hydrocortisone 200 mg stat followed by 100mg i.v. 6-hourly
- Mineralocorticoid replacement is not required urgently
- Treatment of any precipitating illness

# Cushing's syndrome

## Causes of Cushing's syndrome
### ACTH-driven
- Pituitary dependent:
  Pituitary adenoma (Cushing's disease)
  Pituitary carcinoma
  Hypothalamic tumour (corticotrophin-releasing hormone-secreting)
- Ectopic ACTH:
  Small-cell carcinoma of the bronchus
  Bronchial carcinoid
  Thymus carcinoid
  Pancreatic carcinoid

Medullary carcinoma of the thyroid
Carcinoma of the pancreas
Phaeochromocytoma
Thymoma

### Non-ACTH-driven
Glucocorticoid therapy
Adrenal adenoma
Adrenal carcinoma
Adrenal hyperplasia

### Miscellaneous
Alcohol-induced pseudo-Cushing's

## Clinical features of Cushing's syndrome
### Metabolic
- Hyperglycaemia
- Hypernatraemia
- Hypokalaemia (suggests ectopic ACTH)
- Reduced luteinising hormone (LH)
- Reduced testosterone

### Dermatological
- Hirsutism
- Striae
- Thin skin
- Purpura
- Hyperpigmentation (suggests ectopic ACTH)
- Acne
- Poor wound healing

### Endocrine
- Reduced libido
- Amenorrhoea
- Oligomenorrhoea

### Neuropsychiatric
- Proximal muscle weakness
- Depression
- Psychosis
- Mania

### Miscellaneous
- Weight gain
- Weight loss (malignancy)

- Hypertension
- Centripetal obesity
- Osteoporosis
- Oedema

# Phaeochromocytoma

- Tumour of the adrenal medullary tissue (chromaffin tissue)
- 10% bilateral
- 10% extra-adrenal
- 10% malignant
- 10% multiple
- Most secrete noradrenaline
- Associated with neurofibromatosis, von Hippel–Lindau syndrome and multiple endocrine neoplasia type 2

## Clinical features
- Sustained hypertension and catecholamines crises which consist of attacks of palpitation, headache, sweating, hypertension, flushing, anxiety and postural hypotension

## Treatment
- Combined α and β blockade

# Tests of adrenal function

## Basal levels
### Cortisol assays
- Random serum cortisol can be unreliable owing to circadian rhythm of secretion and increased secretion in response to stress
- In Cushing's syndrome normal diurnal variation is lost
- Morning serum cortisol < 100 nmol/l supports the diagnosis of hypoadrenalism
- Morning serum cortisol > 400 nmol/l excludes hypoadrenalism
- 24-hour urinary cortisol correlates well with mean 24-hour serum cortisol level
- Normal 24-hour urinary cortisol < 300 nmols/24 hours
- More useful in diagnosing Cushing's syndrome

### Mineralocorticoid assays
- Renin and aldosterone levels can be measured by radioimmunoassay from urine or serum
- Can be affected by diuretics and must be interpreted in conjunction with electrolyte levels

### Adrenal androgen levels
- Serum testosterone can be a useful measurement to exclude virilising adrenal tumours
- Serum androstenedione and dehydroepiandrosterone (DHEA) can also be measured

## Suppression tests
- Used to investigate for Cushing's syndrome and to identify the cause of Cushing's syndrome

### Overnight dexamethasone suppression tests
- 1 mg dexamethasone orally at midnight
- Take blood for serum cortisol at 8 am
- Normal 8 am cortisol < 50 nmol/l
- In Cushing's syndrome serum cortisol level is not suppressed
- False positive overnight dexamethasone suppression tests found if: liver enzyme induction Depression Obesity Pregnancy

### Low-dose dexamethasone suppression test
- Give 0.5 mg dexamethasone 6-hourly for 48 hours
- In Cushing's syndrome serum cortisol not suppressed

- In normal individuals serum cortisol < 100nmol / l
- Used to make the diagnosis of Cushing's syndrome

### High-dose dexamethasone suppression test

- Give 2 mg dexamethasone 6-hourly for 48 hours
- Used to differentiate causes of Cushing's syndrome
- In Cushing's syndrome there is normal cortisol suppression but in adrenal tumours and ectopic ACTH production there is no cortisol suppression

## Stimulation tests

These are used to diagnose hypoadrenalism.

### Short synacthen test

- Take 9 am blood sample for basal cortisol
- Give synacthen 200 µg intramuscularly
- Take blood for cortisol at 30 and 60 minutes
- Normal result: base line > 190 nmol/l Increment of 200 nmol/l following synacthen Peak cortisol > 550 nmol/l

### Long synacthen test

- On day 1 take 9 am blood sample for serum cortisol
- Inject 1 mg of synacthen i.m.
- On days 2 and 3 repeat dose of synacthen
- On day 4 take 9 am blood sample for serum cortisol
- In primary adrenal insufficiency day-4 cortisol < 200 nmol/l
- In secondary adrenal insufficiency day-4 cortisol > 200 nmol above baseline

### CRH Test

- Useful in distinguishing between

Cushing's disease and ectopic ACTH
- In Cushing's disease CRH administration leads to a rise in ACTH levels
- In ectopic ACTH production there is no increase in ACTH levels following CRH

## Tests of adrenal medulla

### Urinary vanillylmandelic acid (VMA)/metanephrines

- Used for the diagnosis of phaeochromocytoma
- Urinary metanephrines are more reliable
- Urinary VMA can be affected by food (tea, coffee, chocolate, bananas, vanilla) and some drugs

### Meta-iodobenzyl guanidine (MIBG) scan

- $^{131}$I-radiolabelled MIBG (a catecholamine precursor) can be used to localise phaeochromocytomas

# Disorders of sex hormones

## Physiology

### Normal development

- Development of testes controlled by testis-determining gene (SRY on Y chromosome)
- Sertoli cells in testes produce antimüllerian hormone
- Antimüllerian hormone causes müllerian ducts to disappear
- Persistence of müllerian ducts leads to the development of female genital tract
- In contrast, Wolffian ducts persist in males and disappear in females

## Early life

### Males

- Testicular development is stimulated by testosterone produced by Leydig cells
- Late in utero the pituitary begins to secrete LH
- In the first 6 months of life LH levels rise, leading to the rise in serum testosterone levels
- After this period all hormones fall to low levels

### Females

- The ovaries play no role in development of the female genitalia
- There is a similar transient increase in LH after birth, as in males

## Puberty

### Males

- Puberty begins with pulsatile nocturnal LH secretion which leads to pulsatile nocturnal testosterone secretion
- Later the secretion of testosterone becomes continuous
- Follicle-stimulating hormone (FSH) levels also rise and, with testosterone, stimulate spermatogenesis
- During puberty, testis volume increases from 1 ml to 15–25 ml
- LH acts on Leydig cells to promote spermatogenesis
- The rise in serum testosterone levels leads to development of the secondary sexual characteristics
- Plasma sex hormone-binding globulin (SHBG) levels fall by 50%

### Females

- Puberty starts earlier than in males (on average by 2 years)
- The full complement of ovarian follicles is present at birth and the numbers decline thereafter until the menopause

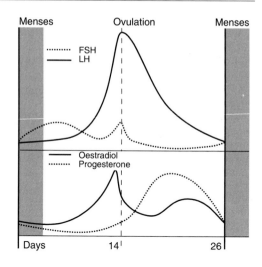

**Fig. 12.4: Menstrual cycle hormonal changes**

- Rises in FSH levels lead to follicular maturation and oestrogen production
- Breast development is stimulated by a rise in oestradiol levels, which affect the duct epithelium
- Progesterone causes increases in breast volume

# Causes of male hypogonadism (androgen deficiency)

## Low LH and FSH

- Simple delayed puberty
- Hypopituitarism
- Cyproterone acetate
- Malnutrition
- Anorexia nervosa
- Isolated GnRH deficiency
- Kallman's syndrome

## High LH and FSH

- Klinefelter's syndrome
- Trauma
- Testicular degeneration
- Mumps

- Radiation
- Cyclophosphamide
- Dystrophia myotonica

### Variable LH and FSH
- Prader–Willi syndrome
- Hyperprolactinaemia
- Noonan's syndrome
- Hepatic cirrhosis
- Cushing's syndrome
- Spironolactone
- Alcohol
- Russell–Silver syndrome
- Werner's syndrome

# Causes of impotence

### Psychogenic
- Depression
- Stress

### Vascular
- Atherosclerosis
- Hypertension

### Neurological
- Autonomic neuropathy
- Spinal cord damage

### Genitourinary
- Hypospadias
- Peyronie's disease
- Phimosis
- Prostatic surgery
- Rectal surgery
- Pelvic fracture

### Drugs
- Antihypertensives
- Antidepressants
- Sedatives
- Alcohol
- Antiandrogens
- Cocaine
- Amphetamines

### Endocrine
- Diabetes mellitus
- Hyperprolactinaemia
- Hypogonadism
- Oestrogen-secreting tumours
- Hyperthyroidism
- Hypothyroidism
- Cushing's syndrome

### Miscellaneous
- Cardiac failure
- Hepatic failure
- Renal failure
- Chronic lung disease
- Advanced age

# Causes of gynaecomastia

### Physiological
- Neonatal
- Pubertal
- Advanced age
- Post malnutrition

### Pathological
- Idiopathic
- Hypogonadism
- Testicular feminisation
- Hepatic cirrhosis
- Hyperthyroidism
- HcG secreting tumours
- Leydig cell tumour
- Adrenal tumours
- Breast tumour

### Drugs
- Spironolactone
- Digoxin
- Cannabis
- Cyproterone acetate
- Oestrogen
- Alcohol
- Ketoconazole
- Cimetidine
- Cytotoxics

# Causes of amenorrhoea

## Structural abnormalities
- Malformed uterus/vagina
- Imperforate hymen
- Müllerian agenesis
- Loss of endometrium

## Endocrine disease
- Hypopituitarism
- Hyperprolactinaemia
- Congenital adrenal hyperplasia
- Hypothyroidism
- Hyperthyroidism
- Cushing's syndrome

## Failure of normal ovarian development
- Turner's syndrome
- Familial XX gonadal dysgenesis
- Ovarian enzyme deficiencies

## Premature ovarian failure
- Idiopathic
- Autoimmune
- Mumps
- Radiotherapy
- Cytotoxic drugs
- Surgical

## Ovarian dysfunction
- Polycystic ovary syndrome
- Resistant ovary syndrome

## Miscellaneous
- Pregnancy
- Post menopause
- Severe systemic illness

# Diabetes mellitus

## Physiology

### Insulin
- Insulin is synthesised and secreted by

---

**Box 12.9: Actions of insulin**

Increased glycogen formation
Reduced gluconeogenesis
Increased glucose uptake
Reduced blood glucose level
Reduced lipolysis
Reduced ketogenesis
Increased triglyceride formation
Increased protein synthesis
Increased fatty acid synthesis
Increased lipid storage

---

β cells of the pancreas gland (islets of Langerhans)
- Pre-proinsulin is cleaved to produce proinsulin, which is then cleaved to produce equal amounts of insulin and C peptide
- Insulin consists of A and B chains linked by two disulphide bonds
- C peptide is biologically inert: it is cleared more slowly than insulin and is therefore a better marker of insulin secretion
- Basal insulin secretion occurs in regular l0–l5-minute pulses

### Control of insulin secretion
*Increased*
- Carbohydrate meal
- Fatty acids
- Ketone bodies
- Vagal nerve stimulation
- Amino acids
- Gastrin
- Cholecystokinin
- Pancreozymin
- Secretin
- Glucagon
- GIP
- Sulphonylureas
- β-agonists
- Prostaglandins

*Reduced*
- Sympathetic nerve stimulation
- α-agonists
- β-blockers
- Dopamine
- Serotonin
- Somatostatin
- Cortisol
- Adrenaline
- Glucagon
- Growth hormone
- Oestrogen
- Thyroxine

## Control of glucagon secretion
### Increased
- Aminoacids
- Insulin
- β-adrenergic stimulation
- Fasting
- Exercise
- Hypoglycaemia
- Gastrin
- Cholecystokinin
- Cortisol

### Reduced
- Glucose
- Somatostatin
- Free fatty acids
- Ketones
- Insulin

---

**Box 12.10: Actions of glucagon**

Glycogenolysis
Gluconeogenesis
Increased lipolysis
Increased ketone formation
Increased secretion of growth hormone, insulin and somatostatin
Reduced intestinal motility
Reduced gastric acid secretion
Increased amino acid catabolism
Reduced fatty acid synthesis

---

# Diagnosis of diabetes mellitus

## Fasting blood glucose
- Normal < 6.1 mmol/l
- Impaired fasting glucose ≥ 6.1 – < 7 mmol/l
- Diabetes mellitus ≥ 7 mmol/l

## Glucose tolerance test
- Fast patient overnight
- Take morning blood sample for basal glucose level
- Give 75 g of glucose in water orally
- Take blood samples for glucose every 30 minutes for 2 hours
- Patient should be resting throughout and should not be allowed to eat during the test. Smoking is also not

**Table 12.6: Differences between insulin-dependent diabetes mellitus (IDDM) and non-insulin-dependent diabetes mellitus (NIDDM)**

| Feature | IDDM | NIDDM |
|---|---|---|
| Typical age of onset | Childhood, young adult | Middle/Older age |
| Onset | Acute | Gradual |
| Body mass index | Lean | Obese |
| Weight loss | Common | Uncommon |
| Ketone production | Common | Uncommon |
| Serum insulin | Low | Normal/high |
| Insulin resistance | No | Yes |
| Family history | Uncommon | Common |
| HLA association | DR3, DR4 | None |

permitted
- Normal 2-hour blood glucose < 7.8 mmol/l
- Impaired glucose tolerance ≥ 7.8 – < 11.1 mmol/l
- Diabetes mellitus ≥ 11.1 mmol/l

### Glycosylated haemoglobin
- Normal HbA1c < 7%

# Types of diabetes mellitus

Type 1: immune-mediated idiopathic forms of β-cell dysfunction, leading to absolute insulin deficiency
Type 2: diabetes of adult onset originating from insulin resistance or relative insulin deficiency
Type 3: diabetes due to diseases of the exocrine pancreas or genetic defects of β-cell function and insulin action
Type 4: gestational diabetes

# Drug treatment of diabetes mellitus

## Sulphonylureas
First generation: chlorpropamide, tolbutamide
Second generation: glibenclamide, gliclazide, glipizide

- Sulphonylureas act primarily by enhancing basal and prandial insulin secretion
- They are ineffective in insulin-deficient patients
- Most are metabolised through the kidneys (glipizide is metabolised by the liver)

### Complications
- Hypoglycaemia
- Weight gain
- Reduced insulin sensitivity

---

**Box 12.11: Chronic complications of diabetes mellitus**

**Microvascular disease**
Retinopathy
Nephropathy
Sensory neuropathy
Autonomic neuropathy

**Macrovascular complications**
Ischaemic heart disease
Hypertension
Stroke
Peripheral vascular disease

**Miscellaneous**
Cataracts
Maculopathy
Necrobiosis lipoidica
Granuloma annulare
Hyperlipidaemia

---

- Allergic skin reactions
- Alcohol induced facial flushing
- SIADH
- Blood dyscrasias

### Biguanides
- Metformin acts by stimulating glucose uptake into peripheral tissues and by inhibiting gluconeogenesis in the liver
- It has no effect on insulin secretion and therefore does not cause hypoglycaemia
- Metformin is particularly indicated in obese patients
- Contraindicated in renal failure, hepatic failure, cardiac or respiratory failure

### Complications
- Lactic acidosis
- Nausea
- Vomiting
- Diarrhoea
- Dyspepsia
- Anorexia
- Megaloblastic anaemia

**Table 12.7: Types of insulin**

| Type | Examples | Onset of action (hours) | Peak of action (hours) | Duration of action(hours) |
|---|---|---|---|---|
| Short-acting (soluble insulins) | Actrapid Velosulin Humulin S | 0.5–1 | 2–4 | 5–8 |
| Intermediate (isophanes) | Isophane Neuphane Protophane Humulin I Humulin M1-5 Mixtard Insulatard | 2–4 | 6–10 | 12–24 |
| Long-acting (insulin–zinc suspensions) | Humulin lente Humulin Zn Ultratard Monotard | 3–4 | 12–18 | 24 |

## Acarbose

- Acarbose is an $\alpha$-glucosidase inhibitor
- It acts at the intestinal brush border by preventing the breakdown of polysaccharides
- Its main effect is therefore to reduce postprandial hyperglycaemia
- Its main side effects are gastrointestinal upset, with borborygmi, flatus and diarrhoea

**Box 12.12: Complications of insulin use**

Hypoglycaemia
Lipoatrophy
Lipohypertrophy
Anaphylaxis
Psychological problems
Transient worsening of retinopathy from tight glycaemic control

# Diabetic emergencies

## Causes of diabetic coma

- Diabetic ketoacidosis
- Hyperosmolar non-ketotic coma
- Hypoglycaemia
- Lactic acidosis
- Stroke
- Postictal
- Drug overdose
- Alcohol

## Diabetic ketoacidosis

### Correct fluid and electrolyte depletion

- Start with normal saline as per the following regimen:
  1 litre in 1 hour
  then 1 litre in 2 hours
  then 1 litre in 4 hours
  then continue with 1 litre 6-hourly
- Strictly monitor fluid balance
- CVP readings may be required
- Ensure that first 2 litres contain potassium supplements but monitor potassium frequently to watch for hyperkalaemia
- When blood glucose has fallen to

< 15 mmol/l, continue fluid replacement with 5% dextrose

### Insulin replacement
- Best given as a continuous i.v. infusion made up of 50 units of soluble insulin in 50 ml normal saline
- Infusion should be guided by hourly sliding scale
- Continue with intravenous fluids and i.v. insulin until patient is eating and drinking normally

### Other measures
- Identify and treat underlying cause of ketoacidosis
- Prophylactic subcutaneous heparin
- Treatment of shock with plasma expanders and inotropes
- Acidosis usually corrects itself following the above treatment but sometimes bicarbonate infusions are required
- The patient should also be monitored for signs of cerebral oedema and adult respiratory distress syndrome (ARDS)
- Nasogastric tube should be inserted if the patient is vomiting or shows signs of gastric dilatation

### Hyperosmolar non-ketotic coma
- In this condition hyperglycaemia is generally greater than in ketoacidosis but there is no hyperketonaemia or ketonuria
- Treatment is similar to diabetic ketoacidosis but, although dehydration is more severe, fluid replacement is more cautious because of the greater risk of cerebral oedema
- Fluid replacement should be with half-strength normal saline (because of hypernatraemia)
- Give the first litre in 2 hours, second litre in 4 hours, then continue with 1 litre every 6 hours

- Again, careful monitoring of fluid balance is required and CVP readings may be needed
- Hypokalaemia more marked than in diabetic ketoacidosis
- Prophylactic heparin should be given as hyperviscosity is more marked
- Again, treatment of underlying illnesses should be vigorous
- Insulin should be given as an intravenous sliding scale as in diabetic ketoacidosis (insulin requirements usually less than in ketoacidosis)

### Lactic acidosis
- In this condition blood glucose levels are usually lower than in the previous two emergencies and therefore little insulin is required
- Bicarbonate infusions often exacerbate acidosis
- Often only supportive treatment can be offered

# Hypoglycaemia

Hypoglycaemia is defined as a blood glucose level < 2.2 mmol/l.

## Causes of hypoglycaemia

### Malignancy
- Insulinoma
- Nesidioblastoma
- Mesenchymal tumours
- Hepatomas

### Drugs and toxins
- Insulin
- Oral hypoglycaemics
- Pentamidine
- Ethanol
- Salicylate overdose
- Ackee poisoning

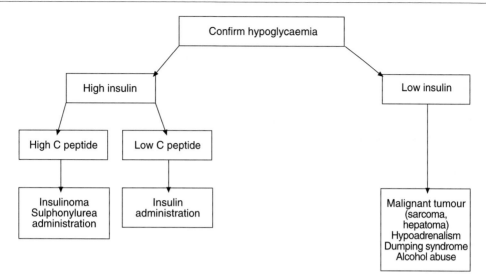

**Fig. 12.5: Investigation of hypoglycaemia**

## Endocrine
- Addison's disease
- Congenital adrenal hyperplasia
- Hypopituitarism

## Hepatic disease
- Acute hepatic failure
- Glycogen storage disease (I and II)

## Miscellaneous
- Starvation
- Prolonged exercise
- Post gastric surgery
- Hereditary fructose intolerance
- Falciparum malaria
- Neonatal
- Autoimmune
- Idiopathic
- Factitious

## Type 1
- Parathyroid
- Pancreas
- Anterior pituitary
- Bronchus
- Bowel

## Type 2a
- Thyroid (C cell)
- Adrenal medulla
- Parathyroid

## Type 2b
- Thyroid (C cell)
- Adrenal medulla
- Mucosal neuromas
- Marfanoid appearance

# Multiple endocrine neoplasia

All types are inherited in an autosomal dominant fashion.

# Clinical case scenarios

## Addisons disease

- There is generalised pigmentation, most marked in skin creases and scar tissue

- Other features to look for:
  Signs of hypopituitarism
  Vitiligo
  Signs of hypothyroidism
  Abdominal scar (bilateral
    adrenalectomy)
  Signs of tuberculosis
  Signs of diabetes mellitus
  Bitemporal hemianopia (pituitary
    tumour)

# Cushing's syndrome

The patient has centripetal obesity with a moon face, truncal obesity and buffalo hump. The skin is thin. There are striae with areas of purpura.

- Other features to look for:
  Gynaecomastia
  Hirsutism
  Proximal myopathy
  Peripheral oedema
  Hyperpigmentation
  Bitemporal hemianopia
  Third-nerve palsy
  Signs of steroid-treated conditions
    (rheumatoid arthritis, fibrosing
    alveolitis, chronic active hepatitis)
  Signs of bronchial carcinoma
    (ectopic ACTH)

# Hypopituitarism

The patient's skin is soft, wrinkled and pale. The secondary sexual characteristics are underdeveloped. The patient may show signs of hypothyroidism and addisons disease

# Gynaecomastia

The presence of increased glandular breast tissue will be obviously apparent.

- Look for signs of underlying cause:
  Signs of hepatic cirrhosis
  Signs of carcinoma of the lung
  Signs of heart failure
    (spironolactone treatment)
  Age of patient (pubertal, advanced
    age)
  Signs of hypogonadism
    (Klinefelter's syndrome)
  Sense of smell (Kallman's
    syndrome)
  Bitemporal hemianopia (pituitary
    adenoma)
  Signs of Addison's disease
  Thyroid status
  Atrial fibrillation (digoxin
    treatment)

# Diabetic foot

- There is usually an ulcer on the sole of the foot over pressure points
- Some of the toes may have been amputated
- The patient may be rather flat-footed
- There may be signs of peripheral neuropathy in a stocking distribution
- Peripheral pulses may be absent and there may be digital gangrene

# Acromegaly

- The patient has prominent supra-orbital ridges and a large lower jaw
- The features are coarse and exaggerated
- There is poor occlusion of the teeth
- The nose, tongue and ears are enlarged
- The patient may be kyphotic
- The hands are large and spade shaped
- The skin is thickened

- Other features to look for:
  Hyperhidrosis

Hirsutism
Wasting of thenar eminence (carpal tunnel syndrome)
Bitemporal visual field defect
Bowed legs
Goitre
Gynaecomastia
Hypogonadism
Greasy skin, acne
Proximal myopathy
Cardiomyopathy
Third cranial nerve palsy
Hypopituitarism

# Exophthalmos

Exophthalmos is defined as protrusion of the eye, revealing the sclera above the lower eyelid in the position of forward gaze. This may be associated with chemosis, corneal ulceration and ophthalmoplegia. Convergence may be impaired

### Causes of exophthalmos
- <u>Graves' disease</u>
- Cavernous sinus thrombosis
- Caroticocavernous fistula (pulsating exophthalmos)
- Retro-orbital tumour (unilateral exophthalmos)
- Orbital cellulitis (unilateral exophthalmos)

- Other features to look for:
    Thyroid status

# Graves' disease

- The patient is usually thin
- Thyroid eye signs are present which include exophthalmos, proptosis, lid lag
- There may be a goitre with a bruit
- The patient may show signs of hyperthyroidism, or may be euthyroid or hypothyroid in treated cases

- Other features to look for:
    Thyroidectomy scar

# Goitre

- The goitre may be obviously visible in the anterior neck
- Note its size and regularity, the presence of a bruit and patient's thyroid status
- Other features to look for: tenderness (De Quervain's thyroiditis)
    Features of acromegaly

# Hypothyroidism

- The patient is overweight with myxoedematous facies (thickened and coarse facial features, periorbital puffiness and pallor)
- The skin is rough, dry, cold and inelastic
- There may be generalised non-pitting swelling of subcutaneous tissues
- The patient's voice is hoarse and croaky
- The patient may be hard of hearing and their movements slow
- There may be alopecia and dry and brittle nails
- Some patients may lose the outer third of their eyebrows

- Other features to look for:
    Presence of eye signs indicating previously treated Grave's disease
    Thyroidectomy scar
    Evidence of hypopituitarism

# Landmark endocrinology studies

## Diabetes Mellitus Insulin Glucose Infusion in Acute Myocardial Infarction (DIGAMI) Study Group

Prospective randomised study of intensive insulin treatment on long term survival after acute myocardial infarction in patients with diabetes mellitus

*Br Med J* 1997; 314: 1512–15

*This Swedish study showed that immediate treatement with insulin-glucose infusion followed by long-term intensive subcutaneous insulin treatment in diabetic patients with acute myocardial infarction improves long-term survival. Mortality was reduced by 11%, equating to one life saved per nine patients treated. The benefits were most apparent in patients not previously treated with insulin and who were at low cardiovascular risk.*

## UK Prospective Diabetes Study Group 1998

Multiple references

*This major British study of Type II diabetic patients has resulted in many publications. The major results showed that tight glycaemic control, cholesterol reduction and blood pressure lowering to around 140/85 mmHg in these patients reduces the risk of micro- and macrovascular complications and improves longterm survival.*

# 13 Rheumatology

## Contents

## Anatomy

### Joint capsule

- Composed of collagen fibres and ligaments
- Continuous with periosteum of the bone
- Contains proprioceptive nerve endings which are sensitive to tension

### Synovial tissue

- Specialised lining of connective tissue composed of two cell types:
  *Type A*: macrophage-like with a phagocytic function
  *Type B*: secretory fibroblast-like. Main function to provide synovial fluid

### Synovial fluid

- Dialysate of plasma and hyaluronic acid
- Most abundant protein is albumin
- Hyaluronic acid conveys viscosity to synovial fluid and is reduced in inflammatory synovitis
- Main function is lubrication and nutrition of cartilage

| Box 13.1: Terminology | |
|---|---|
| *Arthralgia* | Pain arising from a joint |
| *Arthritis* | Joint destruction |
| *Bursitis* | Inflammation of a bursa |
| *Monoarthropathy* | Affects one joint |
| *Oligoarthropathy* | Affects two to four joints |
| *Polyarthropathy* | Affects more than four joints |
| *Synovitis* | Inflammation of a synovial joint |
| *Tendinitis* | Inflammation of a tendon |
| *Tenosynovitis* | Inflammation of a tendon sheath |
| *Seropositive arthropathy* | Positive rheumatoid factor |
| *Seronegative arthropathy* | Negative rheumatoid factor |

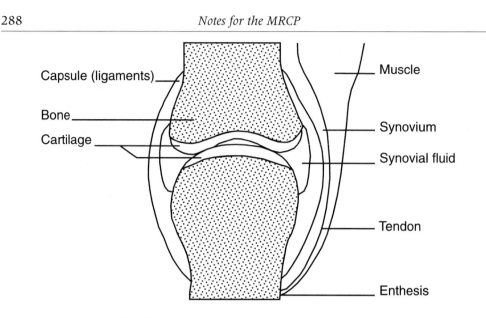

**Fig. 13.1: Longitudinal section through knee joint showing major anatomical structures**

# Articular cartilage

- Composed of cells (chondrocytes), matrix (proteoglycans), fibres (collagen)

# Joint abnormalities

## Causes of polyarthritis

- Osteoarthritis
- Rheumatoid arthritis
- Viral infections
- Henoch–Schönlein purpura
- Palindromic rheumatism
- Juvenile chronic arthritis
- Rheumatic fever
- SLE
- Reiter's disease
- Psoriatic arthritis
- Gonococcal arthritis
- Gout
- Pyrophosphate arthropathy
- Serum sickness
- Sarcoid
- Familial Mediterranean fever
- Type 2 hyperlipidaemia
- Leukaemia

## Causes of hypermobile joints

- Idiopathic

> **Box 13.2: Definition of hypermobile joints**
>
> Extend little finger more than 90° (*1 point for each finger*)
>
> Bring thumb back parallel to or touching forearm (*1 point for each thumb*)
>
> Extend elbows more than 10° (*1 point for each elbow*)
>
> Extend knee more than 10° (*1 point for each knee*)
>
> Touch the floor with palms of hands keeping legs straight (*1 point*)
>
> *Total = 9*
> Score > 6 indicates hypermobility

- Ehlers–Danlos syndrome
- Marfan's syndrome
- Osteogenesis imperfecta
- Homocystinuria
- Hyperlysinaemia

# Rheumatoid arthritis

## Pathology

- Increase in synovial membrane type A cells

- Synovium becomes oedematous, thickened and vascular
- Fibrin is deposited in the synovium
- Inflammatory infiltrate (macrophages, T and B lymphocytes, mast cells)
- Increase in neutrophils in the synovial fluid
- Chronic inflammatory process leads to articular and bone destruction
- Progressive destruction leads to deformity and subluxation
- T lymphocytes produce cytokines
- Synovial membrane produces immunoglobulins (rheumatoid factor)

---

**Box 13.3: Extra-articular manifestations of rheumatoid arthritis**

**Periarticular**
Rheumatoid nodules
Synovitis
Bursitis

**Muscular**
Myositis
Myopathy

**Respiratory**
Pleural effusion
Pleurisy
Empyema
Pulmonary nodules
Fibrosing alveolitis
Obliterative bronchiolitis
Caplans syndrome
Pulmonary hypertension

**Eye**
Keratoconjunctivitis sicca
Scleritis
Episcleritis
Uveitis
Scleromalacia perforans

**Gastroenterological**
Amyloid

**Neurological**
Entrapment neuropathies
Peripheral neuropathy
Cervical myelopathy
Mononeuritis multiplex

**Cardiovascular**
Pericarditis
Pericardial effusion
Myocarditis
Coronary arteritis
Valvular disease
Endocarditis

**Miscellaneous**
Anaemia
Vasculitis
Osteoporosis
Depression
Weight loss
Pyoderma gangrenosum
Renal failure
Oedema
Splenomegaly (Feltys syndrome)
Leg ulcers

# Major disease-modifying drugs used in rheumatoid arthritis

## Sulphasalazine
- Acid azo compound of sulphapyridine and 5-aminosalicylic acid
- Active moiety is sulphapyridine
- Major side effects are nausea, dyspepsia, hepatotoxicity, blood dyscrasias, oligospermia

## Gold
- Common side effects include rash, stomatitis, thrombocytopenia, leukopenia, bone marrow aplasia, glomerulonephritis, pneumonitis
- Regular FBC and urinary protein analysis required

## Penicillamine
- Sulphur-containing amino acid
- Similar side effects to gold, plus myasthenia gravis and lupus syndrome

## Antimalarials
- Chloroquine and hydroxychloroquine
- Major side effects are ophthalmic complications

# Other disease-modifying drugs used in rheumatoid arthritis

- Methotrexate
- Corticosteroids
- Azathioprine
- Cyclophosphamide
- Cyclosporin

# Patterns of rheumatoid arthritis

- Gradual-onset symmetrical arthropathy affecting PIP joints and MCP joints
- Acute-onset polyarthritis
- Gradual monoarticular presentation
- Acute-onset monoarthritis
- Palindromic rheumatism (episodic arthritis)

# Osteoarthritis

## Pathology

- Reduced joint space
- Loss of cartilage
- Sclerosis of subchondral bone
- Osteophyte formation
- Increased proteoglycan turnover
- Increased type 2 collagen
- Chondrocyte loss
- Hydroxyapatite and calcium pyrophosphate deposits

## Causes of secondary osteoarthritis

- Previous inflammatory arthritis
- Occupational strain
- Obesity
- Intra-articular fracture
- Previous septic arthritis
- Avascular necrosis
- Joint dysplasia
- Congenital dislocation of the hip
- Perthes' disease
- Acromegaly
- Alkaptonuria
- Haemochromatosis
- Kashin–Beck disease

# Seronegative arthropathy

## Patterns of psoriatic arthritis

- Asymmetrical or oligoarthritis
- Symmetrical polyarthritis (resembling rheumatoid arthritis)
- Arthritis mutilans
- Spondylitis
- Nail disease

## Causes of Reiter's syndrome

### Genitourinary infection
- *Chlamydia trachomatis*
- *Ureaplasma urealyticum*
- *Neisseria gonorrhoeae*
- *Escherichia coli*

### Gastrointestinal infection
- *Shigella*
- *Salmonella*
- *Yersinia*
- *Campylobacter jejuni*
- *Clostridium dificile*
- *Giardia lamblia*

---

**Box 13.4: Types of seronegative arthropathy**

Ankylosing spondylitis
Psoriatic arthritis
Reiter's syndrome
Gout
Pseudogout
Behçet's syndrome
Whipple's disease
Ulcerative colitis
Crohn's disease

---

### Other infections
- Lyme disease
- *Chlamydia pneumoniae*
- HIV

## Causes of pseudogout (pyrophosphate arthropathy)

- Idiopathic
- Hyperparathyroidism
- Diabetes mellitus
- Osteoarthritis
- Hypothyroidism
- Haemochromatosis
- Wilson's disease
- Hyperuricaemia
- Hypophosphatasia
- Hypomagnesaemia
- Hypertension
- Hypermobility
- Trauma
- Alkaptonuria

# Infective arthritis

## Causes of infective arthritis

### Bacterial
- *Staphylococcus aureus*
- *Streptococcus pyogenes*
- *Streptococcus pneumoniae*
- *Neisseria gonorrhoea*
- *Neisseria meningitidis*
- *Salmonella typhimurium*
- Tuberculosis
- Syphilis
- Lyme disease

### Fungal
- Actinomycosis
- Blastomycosis

**Box 13.5: Rheumatological features of HIV infection**

Septic arthritis
Reiter's syndrome
Acute oligoarthropathy
Polymyositis
Vasculitis
Lupus-like illness
Sjögren's syndrome
Psoriatic arthritis

- Coccidiodomycosis
- Histoplasmosis
- Sporotrichosis

## Viral
- Rubella
- Hepatitis A
- Hepatitis B
- Mumps
- Chickenpox
- Adenovirus
- EBV
- Arbovirus
- Parvovirus
- HIV (Box 13.5)

# Connective tissue diseases

## Clinical features of SLE

### Musculoskeletal
- Arthralgia
- Myalgia
- Proximal myopathy
- Aseptic necrosis
- Deforming arthritis

### Skin
- Butterfly rash
- Alopecia
- Photosensitivity

- Livedo reticularis
- Telangiectasia
- Vasculitis
- Chilblains
- Erythema nodosum
- Raynaud's syndrome

### Neuropsychiatric
- Seizures
- Cranial nerve palsies
- Chorea
- Psychosis
- Cerebellar ataxia
- Transverse myelitis
- SIADH
- Aseptic meningitis
- Peripheral neuropathy

### Haematological
- Lymphocytopenia
- Neutropenia
- Haemolytic anaemia
- Thrombocytopenia
- Anaemia of chronic disease
- Antiphospholipid syndrome

### Cardiovascular
- Pericarditis
- Myocarditis
- Hypertension
- Libman–Sachs endocarditis
- Valvular disease
- Coronary ischaemia

### Pulmonary
- Pleurisy
- Pneumonitis
- Fibrosis

### Renal
- Glomerulonephritis
- Nephrotic syndrome

### Gastrointestinal
- Serositis
- Hepatosplenomegaly
- Pancreatitis

**Table 13.1: Distinctions between drug induced lupus and SLE**

| Feature | Drug-induced | Idiopathic |
|---|---|---|
| Peak age at onset | 50–60 years | 20–30 years |
| Race | White >black | Black >white |
| Female: Male | 5:4 | 9:1 |
| Joint symptoms | Very common | Very common |
| Cutaneous | Uncommon | Very common |
| Pulmonary | Very common | Common |
| Renal | Rare | Common |
| CNS | Rare | Common |
| ANF | + | + |
| DNA antibody | – | + |
| Antihistone antibody | + | + |
| Serum complement | Normal | Low |

# Causes of drug-induced lupus syndrome

## Antibiotics
- Isoniazid
- Sulphonamides
- Tetracycline
- Penicillin
- Streptomycin
- Dapsone
- Griseofulvin

## Anticonvulsants
- Phenytoin
- Carbamazepine
- Primidone
- Ethosuximide

## Miscellaneous
- Hydralazine
- Procainamide
- Chlorpromazine
- Combined oral contraceptive pill
- Nitrazepam
- Methyldopa
- Gold
- Phenylbutazone
- Penicillamine
- L-Dopa
- Propylthiouracil
- Quinidine
- Allopurinol

# Clinical features of scleroderma

## Skin
- Oedema
- Thickening
- Tightening
- Atrophy
- Alopecia
- Hyperpigmentation
- Vitiligo
- Telangiectasia
- Subcutaneous calcification
- Raynaud's phenomenon
- Vasculitis (Box 13.6)

## Gastrointestinal
- Oesophageal stricture
- Oesophageal dilatation
- Malabsorption

## Musculoskeletal
- Flexion contractures
- Arthralgia
- Arthritis
- Myopathy

**Box 13.6: Classification of vasculitis**

**Large artery**
Giant-cell arteritis
Takayasu's arteritis
Syphilis

**Medium artery**
Polyarteritis nodosa
Kawasaki's disease

**Medium and small arteries**
Wegener's granulomatosis
Churg–Strauss syndrome
Connective tissue disease

**Small artery**
Henoch–Schönlein purpura
Drugs
Sepsis
Essential mixed cryoglobulinaemia

## Miscellaneous
- Conduction defects
- Pericarditis
- Cardiomyopathy
- Chronic renal failure
- Hypertension
- Pleurisy
- Pulmonary hypertension

# Miscellaneous conditions

## Causes of Sjögren's syndrome

- Connective tissue disease
- Hashimoto's thyroiditis
- Peripheral neuropathy
- Renal tubular acidosis
- Primary biliary cirrhosis
- Pulmonary fibrosis
- Cryoglobulinaemia

- Waldenström's macroglobulinaemia
- Lymphoma
- Pancreatitis
- HIV
- Pernicious anaemia
- Glomerulonephritis
- Raynaud's phenomenon
- Gold

## Causes of reflex sympathetic dystrophy (shoulder–hand syndrome or Sudek's atrophy)

- Stroke
- Acute myocardial infarction
- Trauma
- Cervical spine lesion
- Space-occupying lesion
- Electroconvulsive therapy (ECT)
- Herpes zoster virus
- Phenobarbitone
- Isoniazid

## Causes of carpal tunnel syndrome

- Idiopathic
- Post menopause
- Rheumatoid arthritis
- Pregnancy
- Hypothyroidism
- Acromegaly
- Scaphoid fracture
- Amyloid
- Chronic renal failure
- SLE
- Scleroderma

# Causes of aseptic necrosis

- Trauma
- Osteomyelitis
- Septic arthritis
- Sickle cell disease
- Corticosteroids
- Caisson disease
- Gaucher's disease
- Irradiation
- Perthes' disease

# Causes of back pain

## Mechanical
- Prolapsed disc
- Soft tissue injury
- Osteoarthritis
- Spinal stenosis
- Spondylolisthesis
- Scheurmann's osteochondritis
- Fracture

## Inflammatory
- Seronegative arthropathy
- Rheumatoid arthritis
- Infection

## Referred pain
- Pelvic carcinoma
- Dysmenorrhoea
- Renal colic
- Biliary colic
- Abdominal aortic aneurysm
- Duodenal ulcer
- Pancreatitis
- Carcinoma of the pancreas

## Malignancy
- Bone
- Spine (primary or secondary)

## Metabolic
- Osteoporosis
- Osteomalacia
- Alkaptonuria
- Paget's disease
- Chondrocalcinosis

## Depression

# Causes of Raynaud's phenomenon

## Connective tissue disease
- Systemic sclerosis
- SLE
- Rheumatoid arthritis
- Sjögren's syndrome

## Vasoconstriction
- Raynaud's disease
- Vibrating machinery
- β-blockers
- Vinyl chloride
- Ergot
- Heavy metals
- Tobacco

## Arterial occlusion
- Thoracic outlet obstruction
- Embolism
- Thrombosis
- Stenosis
- Atherosclerosis
- Buerger's disease
- Trauma (Volkmann's ischaemia)
- Hyperviscosity

## Miscellaneous
- Paralysis (disuse atrophy)
- Frostbite
- Cachexia
- Typhoid
- Amyloid
- Hypothyroidism
- Paroxysmal cold haemoglobinuria
- Cervical rib
- Syringomyelia
- Tabes dorsalis

# Clinical case scenarios

## Ankylosing spondylitis

- The patient is male
- There is loss of the lumbar lordosis and kyphosis, leading to a protuberant abdomen
- The spine is rigid with little movement
- When the patient attempts to turn his head to look to the side the whole body turns as a block
- The patient is unable to touch his toes
- The above features may not be obvious if the patient is resting in bed

- Other features to look for:
    Reduced chest expansion
    Apical pulmonary fibrosis
    Iritis
    Aortic regurgitation

## Osteoarthritis

- There are Heberden's nodes over the distal interphalangeal joints and there may be similar nodes over the proximal interphalangeal joints (Bouchard's nodes)
- The thumb is a commonly affected site where subluxation of the base of the first metacarpal may lead to a thumb-in-palm deformity
- There is restricted movement and crepitus of affected joints
- Other commonly affected sites include hips, knees and neck

- Other features to look for:
    Nerve entrapment syndromes (ulnar and carpal tunnel syndrome)
    Features of causes of secondary osteoarthritis

## Rheumatoid arthritis

- There is a symmetrical deforming arthropathy involving proximal interphalangeal and metacarpophalangeal joints
- There is generalised wasting of the small muscles of the hand
- The functional use of the hand is poor owing to muscle weakness, pain and deformity (ask the patient to pick up cup, use cutlery or undo buttons, depending on what is around the bedside)
- There may be nodules over the extensor tendons and at the elbows
- A variety of deformities may be present: swan neck deformity
  Boutonnière deformity
  Ulnar deviation
  Z thumb

- Other features to look for:
    Psoriatic plaques (differential diagnosis)
    Palmar erythema, nailfold infarcts (vasculitis)
    Cushingoid facies (steroid treatment)
    Triggering of fingers (flexor tendon nodules)
    Other joint involvement
    Carpal tunnel syndrome
    Eye signs
    Splenomegaly (Felty's syndrome)
    Leg ulcers
    Hyposplenism (amyloid)
    Pulmonary fibrosis
    Pyoderma gangrenosum
    Pleural effusion

## Swollen knee

- The swelling will be obvious
- Comment on the loss of lateral dimpling

- Patella tap sign is performed by massaging fluid from the suprapatellar pouch into the knee joint using the left hand; with the index finger of the right hand depress the patella sharply If the patella rebounds it indicates that fluid is present within the knee joint It may be negative if only a small amount of fluid is present
- Check for extension of fluid into the popliteal fossa (Baker's cyst)
- Look at both calves (calf may be swollen owing to a ruptured Baker's cyst)
- Joint function is impaired because of limited movement
- Check temperature of the joint: if warm, suspect septic arthritis

- Other features to look for:
  Hands (rheumatoid arthritis, osteoarthritis)
  Gouty tophi
  Psoriasis
  Acromegaly
  Thyroid status
  Hepatomegaly (pseudogout)
  Argyll Robertson pupils (tabes dorsalis)

# 14 Dermatology

## Contents

## Normal anatomy

- Skin surface area is about 2 m$^2$ in adults
- Skin weight is about 4 kg (6% of adult body weight)

### Epidermis

- This is the outer layer of the skin
- It is derived from the ectoderm
- The main cell type of epidermis is the keratinocyte (90%)

  *Keratinocytes*: arise from the basal layer which lies above the epidermo-dermal junction
  As they mature they move outwards

---

**Box 14.1: Functions of the skin**

Maintains thermoregulation
Protects against mechanical injury
Prevents entry of noxious chemicals and microorganisms
Screens and reduces penetration of ultraviolet radiation (melanocytes)
Prevents loss of body contents
Provides a frictional surface for grip
Discourages microbial growth
Serves as the outpost of the immune system (Langerhan's cells)
Restricts electrical conductivity
Serves as the outpost of the sensory nervous system
Signals emotions via the autonomic nervous system
Synthesises vitamin D (keratinocytes)

Epidermis

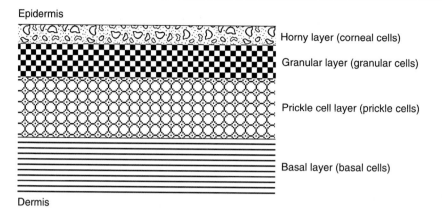

Horny layer (corneal cells)

Granular layer (granular cells)

Prickle cell layer (prickle cells)

Basal layer (basal cells)

Dermis

**Fig. 14.1: Layer construction of the skin**

As the cells mature they produce large
    amounts of keratin
    Also synthesise vitamin D
*Melanocytes*: derived from the ectoderm
    Lie in the basal layer of the epidermis
*Langerhans' cells*: dendritic cells in the
    basal layer of the epidermis
    Express HLA-DR antigens and
    receptors for complement fraction
    C3 and the Fc fragment of IgG on
    the cell surface
    Act as antigen-presenting cells
*Merkel cells*: found in the basal layer of
    the epidermis
    Closely related to sensory nerve ends
    May be involved in sensory touch
    reception

## Dermis

* The dermis consists of a matrix of
  fibrous collagen and elastin and has a
  rich vascular supply
* It is also full of terminal lymphatic
  vessels and cutaneous nerve endings
* Within the dermis can be found
  fibroblasts, mast cells and the skin
  appendages
  *Fibroblasts*: involved in the production
      of collagen and elastin
  *Mast cells*: involved in acute

inflammatory responses (type 1
    hypersensitivity reactions)
*Skin appendages*: derived from the
    epidermis and found in the dermis
    Hair follicles, sebaceous glands,
    eccrine and apocrine sweat glands
    are all ectodermal in origin
*Eccrine sweat glands*: found in the
    axillae and on the palms and soles
*Apocrine sweat glands*: found mainly in the
    genital and anal regions and axillae
*Sebaceous glands*: found in hair-bearing
    areas
*Hair follicles*: found all over the body
    except on the palmar and plantar
    skin, the glans penis and vulval
    introitus
    Each follicle undergoes alternating
    phases of growth (anagen) and rest
    (telogen)
    The rate of hair growth is about
    0.45 mm/day on the scalp

# Skin Examination

## Causes of purpura

### *Haematological*
* Thrombocytopenia
* Haemophilia A and B

- Von Willebrand's disease
- Haemolytic–uraemic syndrome
- Paraproteinaemia

## Infection
- Scarlet fever
- Rubella
- Typhoid
- Infective endocarditis

## Drugs
- Chloramphenicol
- Thiazides
- Steroids
- Warfarin
- Aspirin

## Miscellaneous
- Advanced age
- Henoch–Schönlein purpura
- Hereditary haemorrhagic telangiectasia
- Venous stasis
- Scurvy
- Amyloidosis
- Renal failure
- Fat embolism
- Cyanotic congenital heart disease

# Causes of Koebner's phenomenon

- Psoriasis
- Lichen planus
- Contact dermatitis

---

**Box 14.2: Terminology**

| | |
|---|---|
| *Erythema* | Redness due to vascular dilatation. Blanches on pressure |
| *Telangiectasia* | Caused by dilated blood vessels in the skin. Individual blood vessels are visible |
| *Weal* | Transient pink elevation of the skin due to dermal oedema |
| *Purpura* | Caused by extravasation of red blood cells. Usually dark red and non-blanching |
| *Petechiae* | Small purpuric lesions |
| *Ecchymoses* | Large purpuric lesions |
| *Macule* | Flat circumscribed, palpable and coloured area |
| *Papule* | Small solid elevation of the skin less than 0.5 cm in diameter |
| *Nodule* | Large solid elevation of the skin greater than 0.5 cm in diameter |
| *Plaque* | Flattened lesion with large surface area (over 2 cm) in diameter |
| *Vesicle* | Fluid-containing blister less than 0.5 cm in diameter |
| *Bulla* | Large fluid-containing blister greater than 0.5 cm in diameter |
| *Pustule* | Visible collection of pus in the skin (not necessarily infective) |
| *Atrophy* | Thinning of the skin with loss of normal skin markings and increased transparency |
| *Sclerosis* | Hardening of the skin due to dermal changes |
| *Lichenification* | Chronic thickening of epidermis with exaggeration of normal skin markings |
| *Erosions* | Caused by partial loss of epidermis, dermis unharmed |
| *Ulcers* | Due to loss of the entire epidermis and dermis |
| *Excoriations* | Scratch marks |
| *Koebner's phenomenon* | Development of new lesions along a scratch line |
| *Nicolsky's sign* | Development of blisters on skin pressure |

- Keloid scars
- Sarcoid
- Viral warts
- Vitiligo

# Bullous diseases

## Causes of blistering

### *Common*
- Friction
- Insect bites and stings
- Burns
- Contact dermatitis
- Impetigo
- Erysipelas
- Herpes simplex infection
- Herpes zoster infection
- Frostbite

### *Uncommon*
- Pemphigus vulgaris
- Bullous pemphigoid
- Pemphigus foliaceus
- Pemphigoid gestationis
- Pemphigus vegetans
- Cicatricial pemphigoid
- Dermatitis herpetiformis
- Linear IgA disease
- Epidermolysis bullosa
- Urticaria pigmentosa
- Incontinentia pigmenti
- Ichthyosiform erythroderma
- Erythema multiforme
- SLE
- Diabetes mellitus
- Lichen planus
- Porphyria cutanea tarda
- Drugs: Sulphonamides
  Penicillamine
  Captopril
  Rifampicin
  Tetracyclines

**Table 14.1:  Distinctions between pemphigus and pemphigoid**

| Feature | Pemphigus vulgaris | Bullous pemphigoid |
|---|---|---|
| Age of patient | Middle-aged | Elderly |
| Typical site of blisters | Axillae and trunk | Limbs |
| Mucosal involvement | Yes | No |
| Stability of blisters | Thin-walled, frequently rupture | Thick-walled, tense, rarely rupture |
| Nicolsky's sign | Yes | No |
| Histological site of blister | Intraepidermal | Subepidermal |
| Immunopathology | Intraepidermal IgG | Linear IgG at epidermodermal junction |
| Acantholysis | Yes | No |

**Table 14.2:  Distinctions between irritant and allergic contact dermatitis**

| Factor | Irritant | Allergic contact |
|---|---|---|
| Site | Usually hands | Hands, face and elsewhere |
| Spread | Localised | Disseminates |
| Eyelid involvement | No | Often |
| Occupations | Engineering, mining, kitchen work | Metal work, rubber work, adhesive work, dye work |
| Patch testing valuable | No | Yes |

---

**Box 14.3: Common causes of exogenous dermatitis**

| Agent | Common sources |
|---|---|
| Nickel | Jewellery, watchbands, silver coins |
| Lanolin | Cosmetics and medicaments |
| Perfumes | Cosmetics and medicaments |
| Cobalt | Jewellery, cement, dental plates, pottery pigments, dryers in paints, printing inks |
| Chromate | Cement, antirust coatings, galvanised metal surfaces, primer paints, anticorrosives, welding materials, leather |
| Rubber | Clothing, tyres, shoes, condoms |
| Epoxy resins | Glues |
| Organic dyes | Hair dyes, photographic colour developers |
| Preservatives | Cosmetics and medicaments |
| Colophony | Sticking plasters, inks, newsprint |
| Drugs | Sulphonamides, tetracycline, fusidic acid, gentamicin, sulphonylureas, phenylbutazone, methyldopa, gold |

---

Naproxen
Pyridoxine
Barbiturate overdose
Photosensitivity (nalidixic acid, high-dose frusemide)

# Dermatitis

## Classification of dermatitis

### *Endogenous*
- Atopic dermatitis (allergic)
- Gravitational dermatitis (chronic venous insufficiency)
- Pompholyx (idiopathic)
- Asteatotic dermatitis (elderly, hypothyroidism, diuretics)
- Seborrhoeic dermatitis
- Discoid dermatitis (idiopathic)

### *Exogenous (Box 14.3)*
- Irritant contact dermatitis
- Allergic contact dermatitis

# Psoriasis

## Provocative factors in psoriasis

- Trauma
- Sepsis
- Hormonal changes
- Drugs: Lithium, Chloroquine
- Psychological stress
- Sunlight
- Hypocalcaemia

# Pruritus

## Systemic causes of pruritus

- Obstructive biliary disease
- Carcinoma of the bronchus, stomach, colon, breast
- Chronic renal failure
- Psychogenic
- Hyperthyroidism

**Table 14.3: Clinical manifestations of psoriasis**

| Pattern | Features |
|---|---|
| Discoid psoriasis | Well-defined plaques primarily affecting extensor surfaces of limbs, lower back, knees and elbows |
| Napkin psoriasis | Eruptions spreading from the napkin area in infants |
| Guttate psoriasis | Numerous small papules and plaques, commonly following respiratory infections in children; uniformly distributed on trunk and limbs |
| Pustular psoriasis | Pustular development primarily affecting palms of hands and soles of feet |
| Flexural psoriasis | Predominantly affects flexural areas (axillae, anogenital and submammary folds) |
| Scalp psoriasis | Predominantly affects the scalp |
| Nail involvement | Characteristically produces small thimble-like pits with subungual keratoses and onycholysis |
| Psoriatic arthropathy | Affects 5% of people with psoriasis |
| | Typically produces asymmetrical distal arthropathy affecting terminal interphalangeal joints of fingers and toes |
| | May also cause single-joint arthropathy and sacroiliitis |
| | May resemble rheumatoid arthritis |
| | Severe forms cause a destructive arthritis mutilans |
| Erythroderma | See page 315 |

- Hypothyroidism
- Diabetes mellitus
- Pregnancy (last trimester)
- Hodgkin's disease
- Leukaemia
- Lymphoma
- Polycythaemia
- Iron deficiency anaemia
- Opiate drugs
- Carcinoid syndrome
- Tabes dorsalis
- Multiple sclerosis

- Dermatitis herpetiformis
- Miliaria rubra (prickly heat)
- Mastocytosis
- Mycosis fungoides

### *Variable itching*
- Psoriasis
- Impetigo
- Tinea
- Pretibial myxoedema

# Skin conditions causing pruritus

## *Always itch*
- Dermatitis
- Urticaria
- Insect bites
- Parasitic infection
- Lichen planus

# Disorders of pigmentation

## Causes of hyperpigmentation

### *Postinflammatory*
- Light exposure

- Post varicella infection
- Erythroderma
- Impetigo
- Dermatitis
- Lichen planus

### Endocrine
- Hypoadrenalism
- Cushing's syndrome
- Hypothyroidism
- Hyperthyroidism
- Nelson's syndrome
- Phaeochromocytoma
- Diabetes mellitus
- Acromegaly

### Metabolic
- Pellagra
- Chronic renal failure
- Pernicious anaemia
- Porphyria cutanea tarda
- Wilson's disease

### Gastrointestinal
- Chronic liver disease
- Malabsorption

### Drugs
- Arsenic, busulphan, psoralens, chlorpromazine, amiodarone, minocycline, chloroquine, gold, combined oral contraceptive pill, silver, ACTH, oestrogen

### Connective tissue disease
- Scleroderma
- Dermatomyositis
- SLE

### Miscellaneous
- Pregnancy
- UV radiation

### Chronic sepsis
- Malaria
- Kala-azar
- Tuberculosis

- HIV

# Causes of hypopigmentation

### Postinflammatory
- Pityriasis alba
- Dermatitis
- Disseminated lupus erythematosus (DLE)
- Burns
- Herpes zoster virus

### Immunological
- Vitiligo
- Amelanotic malignant melanoma

### Infection
- Pityriasis versicolor
- Leprosy
- Pinta

### Congenital
- Albinism
- Piebaldism
- Tuberous sclerosis
- Chédiak–Higashi syndrome
- Waardenburg's syndrome
- Cross syndrome
- Vogt–Koyanagi–Harada syndrome
- Phenylketonuria

### Chemical depigmentation
- Hydroxyquinones
- Phenolic germicides

### Miscellaneous
- Hypopituitarism

# Vascular disorders

## Causes of erythema nodosum

### Bacterial infection
- Streptococcal infection
- Tuberculosis
- Leprosy
- Diptheria
- Cat-scratch disease
- Yersinia

### Drugs
- Sulphonamides
- Combined oral contraceptive pill
- Tetracyclines
- Salazopyrin

### Inflammatory bowel disease
- Ulcerative colitis
- Crohn's disease

### Fungal infection
- Histoplasmosis
- Blastomycosis
- Coccidiodomycosis
- *Trichophyton verrucosum*

### Rickettsiae
- *Chlamydia trachomatis*
- *Chlamydia psittaci*

### Viral infection
- Herpes simplex virus
- EBV

### Malignancy
- Leukaemia
- Hodgkin's disease

### Miscellaneous
- Sarcoidosis
- Pregnancy
- SLE

# Causes of erythema multiforme

### Bacterial infection
- Mycoplasma
- Streptococcus
- Typhoid
- Diptheria

### Drugs
- Sulphonamides
- Penicillin
- Barbiturates
- Salicylates
- Sulphonylureas

### Inflammatory bowel disease
- Ulcerative colitis

### Viral infection
- *Herpes simplex virus*
- Orf

### Malignancy

### Miscellaneous
- Idiopathic
- Collagen vascular disease
- Pregnancy
- Radiotherapy

# Nail disorders

## Causes of clubbing

- Familial
- Idiopathic
- Carcinoma of the bronchus
- Chronic pulmonary infection
- Cyanotic congenital heart disease
- Infective endocarditis
- Hyperthyroidism
- Hepatic cirrhosis
- Inflammatory bowel disease
- Mesothelioma

- Cryptogenic fibrosing alveolitis
- Asbestosis
- Atrial myxoma
- Hypertrophic pulmonary osteoarthropathy
- Coeliac disease

# Disorders of hair growth

- Hirsuitism (hair growth in male distribution)
- Hypertrichosis (excessive hair growth at any site)
- Alpopecia: scarring (cicatricial) non-scarring (non-cicatricial)

**Table 14.4:  Causes of nail discolouration**

| Colour | Causes |
| --- | --- |
| White | Hypoalbuminaemia |
| | Anaemia |
| Blue-black | Cyanosis |
| | Subungual haematoma |
| | Cytotoxic drugs |
| | Minocycline |
| | *Pseudomonas* infection |
| | Subungual malignant melanoma |
| | Wilson's disease |
| | Ochronosis |
| Red | Polycythaemia |
| | CO poisoning |
| Green | Pseudomonal infection |
| Brown | Cigarette smoking |
| | Chronic renal disease |
| | Splinter haemorrhages |
| Yellow | Fungal infection |
| | Nailbed ischaemia |
| | Psoriasis |
| | Yellow nail syndrome |
| Red half-moon | Congestive cardiac failure |

# Causes of hirsutism

## *Idiopathic*

## *Ovarian disease*
- Polycystic ovary syndrome
- Ovarian tumours (androgen secreting)
- Turner's syndrome

## *Adrenal disease*
- Congenital adrenal hyperplasia
- Cushing's syndrome

## *Drugs*
- Long-term corticosteroid therapy
- Androgens
- Phenytoin
- Progesterone

## *Miscellaneous*
- Acromegaly
- Hypothyroidism

# Causes of hypertrichosis

## *Drugs*
- Minoxidil
- Phenytoin
- Corticosteroids
- Diazoxide
- Cyclosporin
- Penicillamine

## *Miscellaneous*
- Malnutrition
- Anorexia nervosa
- Spina bifida
- Hairy pigmented naevi
- Porphyria cutanea tarda
- Hypertrichosis lanuginosa
- Dermatomyositis
- Scleroderma
- Hurler's syndrome
- Epidermolysis bullosa
- Cornelia de Lange syndrome

# Causes of scarring alopecia

## *Idiopathic*

## *Skin disease*
- Discoid lupus erythematosus
- Herpes zoster infection
- Tinea
- Lupus vulgaris
- Lichen planus
- Tertiary syphilis
- Chronic staphylococcal folliculitis
- Psoriasis

## *Chemical*
- Chemical burns
- Radiation

## *Miscellaneous*
- Thermal burns
- HIV infection

# Causes of non-scarring alopecia

## *Physiological*
- Male pattern baldness (androgenic alopecia)
- Alopecia areata
- Childbirth
- Emotional stress

## *Endocrine*
- Hypothyroidism
- Hypopituitarism
- Hypoadrenalism

## *Drugs*
- Anticoagulants
- Antithyroid drugs
- Synthetic retinoids
- Cyclophosphamide
- Oral contraceptive pills
- Anticonvulsants (phenytoin, sodium valproate)

## *Miscellaneous*
- Severe acute infections
- Crash dieting, malnutrition
- Hypervitaminosis A
- Severe iron deficiency
- Trichotillomania

# Infections of the skin

## Bacterial diseases

### *Staphylococcus aureus*
- Impetigo
- Ecthyma
- Folliculitis
- Boils
- Carbuncles
- Scalded skin syndrome
- Toxic shock syndrome
- Erysipelas
- Cellulitis

### *Streptococcus pyogenes*
- Impetigo
- Ecthyma
- Erysipelas
- Cellulitis
- Necrotising fasciitis
- Scarlet fever
- Erythema nodosum
- Erythema multiforme

### *Tuberculosis*
- Lupus vulgaris
- Warty tuberculosis
- Scrofuloderma
- Erythema nodosum
- Erythema induratum (Bazin's disease)

### *Miscellaneous*
- *Pseudomonas aeruginosa*: nailfold infection, folliculitis
- *Erysipelothrix insidiosa*: erysipeloid

- *Corynebacterium minutissimum*: erythrasma
- *Bacillus anthracis*: anthrax
- *Mycobacterium marinum*: fishtank granuloma
- Secondary syphilis: diffuse maculopapular rash
- *Haemophilus ducreyi*: chancroid
- *Corynebacterium diphtheriae*: erythema nodosum, erythema multiforme
- *Yersinia enterocolitica*: erythema nodosum
- *Mycoplasma pneumoniae*: erythema multiforme
- *Salmonella typhimurium*: erythema multiforme
- Cat-scratch disease: erythema nodosum

# Viral infections

- Varicella zoster: chicken pox
- Measles
- Rubella
- Herpes zoster: shingles
- Herpes simplex: gingivostomatitis, vulvovaginitis, eczema herpeticum, erythema nodosum, erythema multiforme
- Molluscum contagiosum
- Human papilloma viruses: warts
- Coxsackie A16: hand, foot and mouth disease
- Pityriasis rosea
- Orf: erythema multiforme
- Parvovirus B19: erythema infectiosum
- Human herpes virus 6: roseola infantum
- HIV infection (Box 14.4)

# Parasitic infections

- *Sarcoptes scabiei hominis*: scabies
- Pediculosis: *pediculosis capitis* (head, hairy body skin)
  *Pediculosis corporis* (body)
  *Pthirus pubis* (head, hairy body skin)
- Insect bites: fleas
  *Cimex lecticularis* (bedbugs)
  Cockroaches
  Sandflies
  Horseflies
  Mosquitoes
  Midges

# Fungal infections

## *Superficial*

- Tinea: three genera – *Trichophyton, Microsporum, Epidermophyton*

  tinea pedis (feet): *Epidermophyton floccosum, Trichophyton rubrum*
  tinea cruris (groins): *Epidermophyton*

**Box 14.5: Patterns of candidiasis**

Oral thrush
Angular stomatitis/cheilitis
Balanoposthitis
Vulvovaginitis
Intertrigo
Onychia
Erosio interdigitalis
Chronic paronychia
Pruritus ani
Oesophageal candidiasis
Endocarditis
Meningitis
Pneumonia

floccosum, *Trichophyton rubrum*
tinea corporis (body): *Trichophyton*
tinea capitis (head): *Microsporum
   audouini, Microsporum canis,
   Trichophyton*
tinea manuum (hands): *Trichophyton
   rubrum*
tinea facei (face): *Trichophyton rubrum,
   Trichophyton mentagrophytes*
tinea unguium (nails): *Trichophyton
   rubrum, Trichophyton interdigitale*
tinea barbae (beard): *Trichophyton
   verrucosum, Trichophyton
   mentagrophytes*

- Candidiasis (Box 14.5)
  *Malassezia furfur*: pityriasis versicolor

## Deep (systemic)
- *Actinomyces israelii*: actinomycosis
- *Sporotrichum schenckii*: sporotrichosis
- *Blastomyces dermatitidis*: blastomycosis
- *Basidiobolus meristosporus*: phycomycosis
- *Coccidioides immitis*: coccidioidomycosis
- *Madurella*: maduramycosis
- *Nocardia*: maduramycosis
- *Phialophora*: chromoblastomycosis
- *Cladosporum*: chromoblastomycosis

# Malignancy

## Benign skin tumours

- Seborrhoeic keratoses
- Pilar cysts (wens)
- Cherry angioma (Campbell de Morgan spot)
- Milia
- Clear-cell acanthoma
- Epidermoid cyst
- Squamous papilloma
- Histiocytoma
- Pyogenic granuloma
- Haemangioma

## Pre-malignant skin lesions

- Lentigo maligna
- Actinic keratoses
- Leukoplakia
- Keratoacanthoma
- Bowen's disease
- Thermal keratoses
- Radiation keratoses
- Arsenical keratoses
- Hydrocarbon keratoses
- Congenital giant melanocyte naevus
- Dysplastic naevus syndrome
- Erythroplasia of Queyrat
- Paget's disease of the breast

**Box 14.6: Features suggesting malignant transformation of pigmented lesion**

Irregularity of contour
Irregularity of profile
Irregularity of pigmentation
Rapid growth
Change in colour
Presence of erosion or ulceration
Bleeding
Pruritus
Absent hair follicles

**Table 14.5: Cutaneous manifestations of malignant disease**

| Skin lesion | Commonly associated malignancy |
| --- | --- |
| Tylosis | Oesophagus |
| Paget's disease of the breast | Ductule breast carcinoma |
| Acanthosis nigricans | Gastrointestinal tract |
| Erythema gyratum repens | Bronchus |
| Necrolytic migratory erythema | Glucagonoma |
| Acquired hypertrichosis lanuginosa | Hodgkin's disease |
| Dermatomyositis | Bronchus |
| Thrombophlebitis migrans | Carcinoma of the pancreas |
| Acquired ichthyosis | Lymphoma |
| Palmar keratoses | Bladder/lung |

# Malignant skin tumours

- Basal cell carcinoma
- Squamous cell carcinoma
- Malignant melanoma
- Secondary deposits
- Kaposi's sarcoma
- Angiosarcoma
- Lymphangiosarcoma
- Cutaneous lymphoma

**Box 14.7: Poor prognostic factors in malignant melanoma**

Male gender
Large diameter
High Breslow thickness
Amelanosis
Regional lymphadenopathy
Involvement of the trunk
Metastatic spread

# Disorders of sweat production

## Causes of hyperhidrosis

- Idiopathic
- Heat
- Exercise
- Fever
- Fear
- Anxiety
- Thyrotoxicosis
- Acromegaly
- Diabetes mellitus
- Lymphoma
- Systemic malignancy
- Hypoglycaemia
- Alcohol intoxication

- Nausea
- Gustation
- Phaeochromocytoma
- Pontomedullary lesions
- Cervical lesions

## Causes of hypohidrosis

- Congenital
- Hypohidrotic ectodermal dysplasia
- Dermatitis
- Erythroderma
- Leprosy
- Diabetes mellitus
- Hypothyroidism
- Addison's disease
- Sjögren's syndrome
- Psoriasis
- Topical formaldehyde

# Sunlight and the skin

## Effects of light on the skin

### Immediate
- Thermal vasodilation
- Pigmentation
- Vitamin D synthesis

### Short-term
- Erythema (sunburn)
- Delayed pigmentation
- Epidermal hyperplasia
- Immunological suppression

### Long-term
- Elastosis
- Keratosis
- Dermal atrophy
- Senile purpura
- Epidermal atrophy
- Actinic lentigo
- Basal cell carcinoma
- Squamous cell carcinoma
- Malignant melanoma
- Keratoacanthoma
- Bowen's disease

# Drug induced photosensitivity

### Antibiotics
- Sulphonamides
- Tetracycline
- Griseofulvin

### Diuretics
- Chlorothiazide
- Frusemide

### Antidiabetic
- Sulphonylureas

> **Box 14.8: Light-aggravated metabolic diseases**
>
> Porphyria
> Pellagra
> Hartnup's disease
> Carcinoid syndrome
> SLE
> Darier's disease
> Herpes simplex virus
> Scleroderma
> Erythema multiforme
> Lichen planus
> Lymphocytoma
> Psoriasis
> Rosacea

### Antimalarials
- Chloroquine

### Antiarrhythmics
- Amiodarone

### Psychotropics
- Phenothiazines
- Chlordiazepoxide

### Miscellaneous
- Isoniazid
- Psoralens
- Methylene blue
- Rose bengal
- Nalidixic acid

# Inherited skin disorders

## Autosomal dominant disorders

- Neurofibromatosis
- Tuberous sclerosis
- Ehlers–Danlos syndrome

- Epidermolysis bullosa
- Ichthyosis vulgaris
- Tylosis
- Benign familial pemphigus
- Darier's disease
- Peutz–Jegher syndrome
- Hereditary haemorrhagic telangiectasia
- Gardner's syndrome
- Hidrotic ectodermal dysplasia
- Bullous ichthyosiforme hyperkeratosis
- Incontinentia pigmenti
- Epidermolysis bullosa simplex
- Epidermolysis bullosa dystrophica
- Pseudoxanthoma elasticum

## Autosomal recessive disorders

- Albinism
- Ichthyosiform erythroderma
- Dystrophic epidermolysis bullosa
- Phenylketonuria
- Werner's syndrome
- Acrodermatitis enteropathica
- Chondroectodermal dysplasia
- Xeroderma pigmentosa
- Ataxia telangiectasia
- Bloom's syndrome
- Pseudoxanthoma elasticum
- Refsum's syndrome
- Epidermolysis bullosa dystrophica

## X-linked disorders

- Ichthyosis
- Anhidrotic ectodermal dysplasia
- Keratosis pilaris atrophica
- Menke's syndrome
- Aldrich syndrome
- X-linked ichthyosis
- Anderson–Fabry disease

# Miscellaneous skin conditions

## Causes of hyperkeratosis of the palms and soles

- Barefoot walking
- Secondary syphilis
- Keratoderma blenorrhagicum (Reiter's disease)
- Hypovitaminosis A
- Chronic inorganic arsenic poisoning
- Carcinoma of bladder
- Carcinoma of lung

## Causes of lichen planus

### Drugs
- Gold
- Organic arsenic
- Antituberculous therapy
- Chlorpromazine
- Methyldopa
- Chloroquine
- Thiazide diuretics
- Frusemide
- β-Blockers
- Penicillamine
- Chlorpropramide

### Miscellaneous
- Graft-versus-host disease
- Colour photograph developing fluids

## Causes of pyoderma gangrenosum

- Ulcerative colitis
- Crohn's disease
- Rheumatoid arthritis
- Seronegative arthritis
- Paraproteinaemia
- Wegener's granulomatosis

- Myeloma
- Leukaemia
- Primary thrombocythaemia
- Myelofibrosis

## Causes of acneiform eruptions

- Cushing's syndrome
- Drugs: corticosteroids, isoniazid, lithium, bromides, iodides, halogens, anticonvulsants
- Greasy cosmetics
- Mineral oils
- Tars
- Halogenated hydrocarbons

## Causes of urticaria

### Trauma
- Dermographism
- Prolonged pressure

### Environmental
- Cold exposure
- Heat (cholinergic urticaria)
- Water (aquagenic urticaria)
- Light

### Drugs
- Opiates
- Aspirin
- Penicillin
- Serum toxoids
- Imipramine

### Food additives
- Azo dyes (tartrazine)
- Preservatives (sodium benzoate)
- Nuts
- Shellfish
- Fruit

### Emotional stress

### Chemicals
- Nettle rash
- Jellyfish stings
- Flea bites
- Bee or wasp stings
- Insect bites

### Infections
- Viral
- Scabies
- Intestinal parasites

### Physical disease
- Cold agglutinins
- Cryoglobulins
- Systemic disease
- Polyarteritis nodosa
- SLE
- Lymphoma
- Hepatitis B

## Causes of leg ulcers

### Vascular disease
- Atherosclerosis
- Venous hypertension
- Vasculitis

### Trauma
- Burns
- Mechanical
- Chemical
- Self-inflicted
- Venomous bites

### Infections
- Viral
- Bacterial (streptococcus, tuberculosis)
- Deep fungal infection
- Spirochaetes (yaws, syphilis)
- Protozoa (leishmaniasis)

### Neuropathy
- Diabetes mellitus
- Leprosy

- Syringomyelia
- Alcohol
- Tabes dorsalis

### Haematological disorders
- Disseminated intravascular coagulation
- Sickle cell anaemia
- Spherocytosis
- Thrombocythaemia
- Polycythaemia

### Plasma protein disorders
- Dysglobulinaemia
- Myeloma

### Neoplasia
- Basal cell carcinoma
- Squamous cell carcinoma
- Kaposi's sarcoma
- Malignant melanoma

### Skin lesions
- Necrobiosis lipoidica
- Erythema nodosum
- Pyoderma gangrenosum

### Lymphatic obstruction
- Milroy's disease
- Filariasis
- Lymphoedema

# Erythroderma

## Causes of erythroderma

- Idiopathic
- Dermatitis
- Psoriasis
- Drugs: sulphonamides
  Sulphonylureas
  Indomethacin
  Allopurinol
  Gold
  Phenylbutazone

**Box 14.9: Metabolic sequelae of erythroderma**

Disturbed thermoregulation
  (hypothermia/hyperthermia)
Hypovolaemia
High-output cardiac failure
Renal failure
Hypernatraemia
Hypocalcaemia
Hypoalbuminaemia
Folate deficiency
Anaemia
Intestinal malabsorption
Skin sepsis
Thrombophlebitis

  Phenytoin
  Para-aminosalicylic acid
  Captopril
- Pityriasis rubra pilaris
- Erythema gyratum repens
- Cutaneous lymphomas
- HIV infection

## Management of erythroderma

- Admit to hospital
- Identify and treat underlying cause
- Maintain normal body temperature
- Careful fluid balance and monitoring of renal function and electrolytes
- Correction of anaemia
- Prompt treatment of sepsis
- Apply: topical oil-based corticosteroid and emollients
- Oral steroids may be required for severe cases

# Clinical case scenarios

## Psoriasis

Psoriasis typically presents with circular plaques with well-defined edges which are red with a silvery scaly surface. Note pattern of skin involvement and type of psoriasis. Do not forget to look for nail pitting and arthropathy. If asked to examine a patient's hands, be sure to roll up their sleeves and look for psoriatic plaques on the arms and elbows.

* Other feature to look for:
  Koebner's phenomenon

## Erythema nodosum

* Patient is usually female
* Typically produces bilateral tender painful erythematous nodular lesions over both shins
* Residual bruising may occur after healing

## Necrobiosis lipoidica

* Patients are usually young
* Typically appears as a solitary patch of indurated erythema which spreads slowly
* Lesions have a shiny atrophic surface with a waxy yellow centre and brownish red edges
* There is usually telangiectasia over the surface of the lesion
* Lesions are almost always found on the shins
* Lesions are not tender and there are no constitutional symptoms as in erythema nodosum

## Clubbing

In typical clubbing there is thickening of the nailbed and loss of the obtuse angle between the nail and dorsum of the finger. There is increased curvature of the nailbed both sideways and lengthwise, with associated increased fluctuation of the nailbed. The finger may have a drumstick appearance.

* Other features to look for:
  Nicotine staining
  Weight loss (carcinoma of the bronchus)
  Basal fibrotic crackles (fibrosing alveolitis)
  Cyanosis
  Thoracotomy scars (cyanotic congenital heart disease)
  Features of bronchiectasis
  Features of cirrhosis
  Features of infective endocarditis
  Thyroid status
  Abdominal scars (surgery for inflammatory bowel disease)

## Peutz–Jeghers syndrome

* This typically produces small brownish-black macules on the lips and around the mouth, and sometimes in the buccal mucosa
* There are no lesions on the tongue
* Lesions may also be seen on the hands and fingers

* Other features to look for:
  Abdominal scars secondary to a laparotomy for intestinal obstruction or gastrointestinal haemorrhage

# Lupus pernio

- Patient is often female
- Characteristic rash is a diffuse purple red rash which predominantly affects the nose, cheeks, ears, hands and feet
- Associated with chronic pulmonary sarcoidosis

- Other features to look for:
  Facial palsy
  Parotid enlargement
  Peripheral neuropathy
  Cardiomyopathy
  Arthropathy
  Hepatomegaly
  Uveitis
  Pulmonary fibrosis

# Purpura

- The purpura will be obviously apparent

- Other features to look for:
  Age of the patient (senile purpura)
  Cushingoid features with thin skin
  Evidence of steroid-treated disease (rheumatoid arthritis, asthma, fibrosing alveolitis)
  Splenomegaly (idiopathic thrombocytopenic purpura)
  Hepatosplenomegaly (myelo- or lymphoproliferative disorder)
  Typical distribution of purpura over extensor surfaces in child or young adult with associated arthropathy indicative of Henoch-Schönlein purpura

# Xanthomata/xanthelasma

- *Tendon xanthomata*: typically found in extensor tendons on the back of the hand, Achilles and patellar tendons

There may also be tuberous xanthomata over the extensor surfaces of joints and buttocks
- *Eruptive xanthomatosis*: produces small yellow papules on the extensor surfaces of the joints, limbs, buttocks and back
- *Xanthelasma*: typically produces yellow plaques around both eyes

- Other features to look for:
  Features of secondary hyperlipidaemia:
    diabetes mellitus
    nephrotic syndrome
    myxoedema
  Consequences of hyperlipidaemia:
    previous stroke
    heart disease
    corneal arcus

# SLE

- Patient is typically female
- The typical rash is a red papular butterfly rash on the face
- It may occur on other light-exposed areas and there may be scaling, follicular plugging and scarring
- Healing of lesions may leave residual atrophy, telangiectasia, hyperpigmentation or vitiligo

- Other features to look for:
  Buccal mucosa involvement
  Scalp involvement leading to scarring alopecia
  Arthropathy
  Evidence of vasculitis
  Pulmonary involvement (pleural effusions, fibrosis)
  Features of nephrotic syndrome
  Cardiomyopathy
  Proximal muscle weakness
  Dry eyes
  Dry mouth

# Vasculitis

- This may present as a purpuric rash
- There may be small nailfold and nail-edge infarcts, and in severe cases digital gangrene
- There may be chronic leg ulcers

- Other features to look for:
  Features of peripheral neuropathy
  Features of underlying conditions:
    rheumatoid arthritis
    SLE
    Wegener's granulomatosis
    systemic sclerosis
    infective endocarditis
    lymphoproliferative disorders
    Henoch–Schönlein purpura
    temporal arteritis
    erythema nodosum
    erythema multiforme
    livedo reticularis

# Erythema ab igne

This typically produces a reticular pigmented rash on the lateral aspects of one leg.

- Other feature to look for:
  Evidence of hypothyroidism

# Pretibial myxoedema

- This typically produces symmetrical lesions over both shins and feet.
- The lesions are elevated, coarse, purple-red in colour with well-defined edges.
- The lesions are often tender and associated with pruritus

- Other features to look for:
  Thyroid status (associated with Graves' thyrotoxicosis, but

patient may be euthyroid or hypothyroid if treated. Even then there may be residual eye signs)
Thyroidectomy scar

# Vitiligo

- Areas of depigmentation
- Common sites are around eyes, mouth, knees, hands, feet, groins and axillae.
- Lesions are usually symmetrical but may be unilateral

- Other features to look for:
  Koebner's phenomenon
  Thyroid status (features of hypo- or hyperthyroidism)
  Splenomegaly (pernicious anaemia)
  Fundi (diabetes mellitus)
  Pulmonary fibrosis (cryptogenic fibrosing alveolitis)
  Portal hypertension (primary biliary cirrhosis, chronic active hepatitis)
  Scleroderma
  Telangiectasia (CREST syndrome)
  Pigmentation (Addison's disease)
  Tetany (hypoparathyroidism)

# Dermatomyositis

- Produces a heliotropic (purple/violet) rash around the eyes and on the back of the hands
- May affect the extensor surfaces of the elbows and knees
- There is usually proximal muscle weakness

- Other features to look for:
  Raynaud's phenomenon
  Arthralgia
  Thinning of skin and purpura (long-term steroid treatment)
  Features of internal malignancy

# Pemphigus vulgaris/Bullous pemphigoid

- Both conditions may produce widespread blistering lesions, but differentiation is possible (see Table 14.1)
- Note age of patient, site of blisters and stability of blisters
- Note also whether there is mucosal involvement

# Pseudoxanthoma elasticum

- Typically produces loose skin in the axillae, neck, antecubital fossae and groins
- Within these areas of loose skin are small yellow pseudoxanthomatous plaques: often described as a 'chicken skin' appearance

- Other features to look for:
  Angioid streaks in retina
  Blue sclerae
  Hypermobile joints
  Weak or absent peripheral pulses
    (peripheral vascular disease)
  Mitral regurgitation
  Features of hypothyroidism

# Radiation burns

- Usually found on the thorax.
- Indicative of radiotherapy for intrathoracic malignancy (usually carcinoma of the bronchus)

- Other features to look for:
  Signs of carcinoma of the bronchus
  Signs of superior vena caval
    obstruction

# Herpes zoster

- The patient is usually middle-aged or elderly
- Typically produces a rash localised to one dermatome
- The rash consists of lesions at different stages of development (papule → vesicle → pustule → crusting → scarring)
- There is usually regional lymphadenopathy
- The commonest site affected is the thorax
- The commonest cranial nerve affected is the opthalmic division of the trigeminal nerve

- Other features to look for:
  Ear involvement and seventh
    cranial nerve palsy (Ramsay
    Hunt syndrome)
  Lower motor neuron lesions of
    limbs
  Eye damage
  Other cranial nerve lesions
  Cerebellar signs (rare)

# Lichen planus

- The patient is usually young or middle-aged
- Typically there are flat-topped shiny, violaceous papules on the wrists and other flexor surfaces (may affect any part of the skin)
- Fine white streaks (Wickham's striae) may be seen on the papules
- There may also be central umbilication of the papules

- Other features to look for:
  Koebner's phenomenon
  Buccal mucosal lesions
  Excoriations (due to intense
    pruritus)

Alopecia (scalp involvement)
Nail dystrophy (nail involvement)

## Mycosis fungoides

- The patient is usually middle-aged or elderly
- There are erythematous, thickened, indurated plaques
- They may occur at any site
- Ulceration of the plaques may occur

- Other features to look for:
    Excoriations (due to pruritus)
    Lymphadenopathy (suggests extracutaneous spread)

## Dermatitis herpetiformis

- The patient is usually middle-aged or elderly
- The typical lesions consist of erythematous papules found on extensor surfaces (elbows, knees, buttocks)
- There may be vesicles, which may have ruptured because of scratching

- Other features to look for:
    Excoriations (due to pruritus, which is usually intense)
    Mucosal involvement uncommon (unlike pemphigus vulgaris)

## Urticaria pigmentosa (mastocytosis)

- There are multiple small, discrete, round, pigmented macules and/or papules
- Skin friction leads to urticarial weals (Darier's sign) due to histamine release

## Pyoderma gangrenosum

- This produces large necrotic ulcers with ragged bluish edges, together with erythematous plaques and pustules
- The lesions may be found anywhere

- Other features to look for:
    Erythema nodosum
    Erythema multiforme
    Thinning skin and purpura (long-term steroid therapy)
    Ileostomy/colostomy
    Abdominal scars (post bowel resection)

## Raynaud's phenomenon

- Fingers are cold and cyanosed
- There is atrophy of the finger pulps and there may be digital gangrene

- Other features to look for:
    Age and gender (young female indicative of Raynaud's disease)
    Collagen vascular disease (especially rheumatoid arthritis, SLE and scleroderma)
    Cervical rib (diminished radial pulse, supraclavicular bruit, wasting of the small muscles of the hand, sensory loss C8/T1)
    Thyroid status

## Scleroderma

- The skin over the face and fingers is smooth, shiny and tight
- This gives a facial appearance of a pinched nose and pursed lips
- There is sclerodactyly and the nails are atrophic

- Other features to look for:

Raynaud's phenomenon
Telangiectasia
Nailfold infarcts
Digital gangrene
Subcutaneous calcified nodules in
the fingers
Alopecia
Hyperpigmentation
Vitiligo
Skin ulcers
Pulmonary fibrosis
Features of chronic liver disease
(primary biliary cirrhosis)

# Nail–patella syndrome

- Autosomal dominant condition
- The nails are absent or rudimentary
- The patellae are absent or rudimentary

# 15 Ophthalmology

## Contents

## Visual pathways

### Normal visual pathway

Anatomy of the normal visual pathway is illustrated in Fig. 15.1. Lesions are shown in Fig. 15.2.

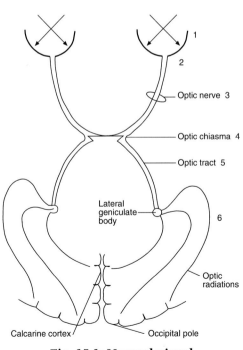

**Fig. 15.1: Normal visual pathway**

## Lesions of the visual pathways

### *Causes of sudden blindness*

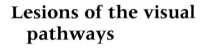

- Vitreous haemorrhage
- Retinal detachment
- Retinal artery emboli
- Cerebral infarction

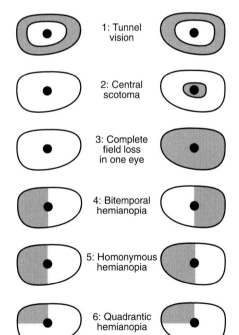

**Fig. 15.2: Lesions of the visual pathways**

- Retinal vein thrombosis
- Trauma
- Welding lights
- Acute glaucoma
- Optic neuritis
- Malignant hypertension
- Migraine
- Acute hydrocephalus
- Vasovagal attack
- Hysteria

## Causes of tunnel vision
- Retinitis pigmentosa
- Choroidoretinitis
- Acute ischaemia
- Glaucoma
- Papilloedema
- Tabes dorsalis
- Migraine
- Hysteria

## Causes of central scotoma
- Macular disease
- Retrobulbar neuritis
- Optic atrophy
- Trauma

## Causes of bitemporal hemianopia
- Pituitary tumour
- Internal carotid artery aneurysm
- Craniopharyngioma

## Causes of homonymous hemianopia
- Stroke
- Space-occupying lesion
- Occipital cortex lesion

## Causes of optic neuritis
### Ischaemia
- Giant cell arteritis
- Systemic vasculitis

### Demyelination
- Multiple sclerosis
- Leukodystrophies

### Infection
- Meningitis
- Retinitis
- Syphilis
- Toxoplasmosis
- Typhoid

### Toxins
- Methyl alcohol, lead, benzene, tobacco, arsenic, ethambutol, quinine

### Metabolic
- Diabetes mellitus
- Vitamin $B_{12}$ deficiency
- Cassava diet
- Anaemia

### Hereditary
- Leber's optic atrophy
- Friedreich's ataxia

### Miscellaneous
- Behçet's disease

## Causes of optic atrophy
- Glaucoma
- Optic neuritis
- Optic nerve compression (pituitary tumour)
- Choroidoretinitis
- Chronic papilloedema
- Retinitis pigmentosa
- Senile macular degeneration
- Central retinal artery occlusion
- Optic nerve trauma (surgery)
- Orbital fractures
- Internal carotid artery aneurysm
- Meningioma
- Paget's disease

# Control of eye movement

## Innervation

### Third cranial nerve
- Arises from nucleus in midbrain
- Runs close to posterior communicating artery and uncus of temporal lobe
- Passes through lateral wall of cavernous sinus
- Enters orbit through superior orbital fissure
- Supplies all extra ocular muscles except lateral rectus and superior oblique
- Also supplies motor parasympathetic fibres arising from oculomotor nucleus
- Parasympathetic fibres pass to ciliary ganglion and thence to ciliary and sphincter papillae muscles
- Parasympathetic stimulation leads to pupillary constriction

### Fourth cranial nerve
- Arises from nucleus in midbrain at level of inferior colliculus
- Follows similar course to third nerve
- Supplies superior oblique

### Sixth cranial nerve
- Arises from nucleus in upper pons
- Also runs in lateral wall of cavernous sinus
- Enters orbit through superior orbital fissure
- Supplies lateral rectus

## Conjugate eye movements

- Conjugate eye movements are both reflex and voluntary
- Voluntary conjugate gaze is the ability to gaze in a particular direction on command
- Involuntary conjugate gaze is the ability to follow an object with the eyes without command
- Responsible for doll's eyes movements
- Conjugate gaze controlled by pons
- Pons receives inputs from visual cortex, frontal cortex, vestibular system and cerebellum
- Efferents pass to medial longitudinal fasciculus

### Disorders of conjugate gaze
- Destructive lesion in frontal lobe leads to deviation of eyes towards the side of the lesion
- Irritative lesions in frontal lobe lead to deviation of eyes away from side of lesion
- Doll's eyes movements indicative of brainstem death

## Intranuclear ophthalmoplegia

- Caused by a lesion of the medial longitudinal fasciculus (usually demyelination)
- Ipsilateral medial rectus is affected, leading to defective adduction
- On contralateral gaze there is a nystagmus greater in the abducting eye (ataxia nystagmus)
- Pontine lesions affecting medial longitudinal fasciculus lead to skew deviation with one eye higher than the other
- Sixth-nerve nuclear lesion leads to paralysis of the ipsilateral lateral rectus and conjugate gaze palsy to ipsilateral side

## Causes of third-nerve palsy

- Posterior communicating artery aneurysm

- Brainstem stroke
- Subarachnoid haemorrhage
- Vasculitis
- Sphenoid wing meningioma
- Parasellar meningioma
- Syphilis
- Encephalitis
- Orbital tumours
- Diabetes mellitus
- Amyloid
- Sarcoid
- Toxins
- Metabolic
- Internal carotid artery aneurysm

## Causes of sixth-nerve palsy

- Sarcoid
- Raised intracranial pressure
- Meningitis (especially tuberculous)
- Nasopharyngeal carcinoma
- Gradanego's syndrome
- Intranuclear ophthalmoplegia
- Internal carotid artery aneurysm
- Toxic
- Metabolic
- Orbital tumours
- Vasculitis

## Causes of nystagmus

### Labyrinthine lesions
- Benign positional vertigo
- Inflammatory labyrinthitis
- Menière's disease
- Idiopathic
- Herpes zoster infection
- Trauma
- Labyrinthine ischaemia
- Alcohol
- Aminoglycosides

### Cerebellum and brainstem
- Anticonvulsants

- Multiple sclerosis
- Vascular lesions
- Wernicke–Korsakoff's syndrome
- Trauma
- Degenerative disorders
- Encephalitis
- Tumours
- Vertebrobasilar insufficiency

### Eighth nerve
- Acoustic neuroma

### Congenital
- Albinism
- Cataracts
- Retinal lesions

### Miscellaneous
- Physiological (optokinetic)
- Refractory errors
- Macular lesions
- Ocular muscle palsy
- High cervical cord lesions

# Pupillary abnormalities

## Normal pupillary reflexes

Normal pupillary reflexes follow set neural pathways, as shown in Fig. 15.3.

### Causes of impaired pupillary reflexes
- Cataracts
- Corneal opacities
- Retinal denervation
- Optic nerve lesions
- Optic chiasma lesions
- Optic tract lesions
- Iridocyclitis
- Third-nerve nucleus lesions

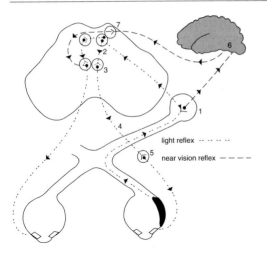

**Fig 15.3: Normal pupillary reflexes**
*1: Lateral geniculate body*
*2: Pretectal nucleus in midbrain*
*3: Edinger–Westphal nucleus*
*4: Oculomotor nerve*
*5: Ciliary ganglion*
*6: Occipital cortex*
*7: Superior colliculus*

- Ciliary ganglion lesions
- Holmes–Adie pupil
- Argyll Robertson pupil

# Causes of mydriasis

- Third nerve lesions
- Sympathetic stimulation
- Brain death
- Parasympathetic paralysis
- Optic nerve lesions
- Iritis
- Cataracts
- Vitreous haemorrhage
- Coma
- Holmes–Adie pupil

# Causes of meiosis

- Horner's syndrome
- Opiates
- Pontine lesions
- Argyll Robertson pupil
- Basal skull tumours

# Anterior eye disease

## Causes of dry eyes

- Sjögren's syndrome
- Trachoma
- Chronic staphylococcal infection
- Chemical burns
- Cyclophosphamide
- Erythema multiforme
- Sarcoid
- Graves' disease
- Pemphigoid

## Causes of uveitis/iritis

### Systemic disease
- Ankylosing spondylitis
- Reiter's disease
- Sarcoid
- Inflammatory bowel disease
- Rheumatoid arthritis
- Behçet's disease
- Juvenile chronic arthritis
- Whipple's disease
- Multiple sclerosis

### Infection
- Tuberculosis
- Herpes zoster virus
- Syphilis
- Leptospirosis
- HIV
- Histoplasmosis
- Malaria
- Toxoplasmosis

**Table 15.1: Distinction between iritis and conjunctivitis**

| Feature | Conjunctivitis | Iritis |
|---|---|---|
| Pain | Grittiness | Moderate/severe |
| Discharge | Purulent | No |
| Photophobia | Mild | Severe |
| Cornea | Bright and clear | Keratinic precipitates |
| Pupil | Normal | Fixed, small, irregular |
| Iris | Normal | Muddy |
| Tension | Normal | Normal (tender) |

- Toxocara
- *Neisseria gonorrhoeae*
- Brucellosis

### Ocular disease
- Ophthalmitis
- Trauma

### Miscellaneous
- Idiopathic
- Vogt–Koyanagi–Harada syndrome

# Causes of conjunctivitis

- *Staphylococcus aureus*
- *Streptococcus pneumoniae*
- *Haemophilus influenzae*
- *Neisseria gonorrhoeae*
- *Chlamydia trachomatis*
- Adenovirus
- Drug sensitivity
- Allergic (spring catarrh)

# Causes of cataracts

### Endocrine
- Diabetes mellitus
- Hypoparathyroidism
- Pseudohypoparathyroidism
- Corticosteroids
- Cretinism

### Hereditary
- Rubella

- Down's syndrome
- Wilson's disease
- Galactosaemia
- Dystrophia myotonica
- Lowe's syndrome
- Lawrence–Moon–Biedel syndrome
- Homocystinuria
- Refsum's disease

### Ocular disease
- Glaucoma
- Myopia
- Retinal detachment
- Ophthalmitis
- Trauma

### Miscellaneous
- Advanced age
- Heat
- Irradiation
- Anorexia nervosa

# Posterior eye disease

## Causes of papilloedema

### Raised intracranial pressure
- Cerebral tumour
- Benign intracranial hypertension
- Hydrocephalus
- Intracranial haemorrhage

**Table 15.2: Distinction between papilloedema and papillitis**

| Feature | Papilloedema | Papillitis |
|---|---|---|
| Visual field defect | Large blind spot | Central scotoma |
| Visual acuity | Normal | Impaired |
| Pain | No | Yes |
| Afferent pupillary defect | No | Yes |

- Cerebral abscess
- Malignant hypertension
- Venous sinus thrombosis
- Meningitis
- Encephalitis
- $CO_2$ retention
- Trauma
- Stroke
- Combined oral contraceptive pill
- Vitamin A poisoning
- Retinoids
- Tetracycline

## Venous obstruction
- Central retinal vein thrombosis
- Cavernous sinus thrombosis
- Caroticocavernous fistula
- SVC obstruction
- Orbital cellulitis
- Orbital tumours
- Thyroid tumours

## Metabolic
- Renal failure
- Arsenic
- Hypocalcaemia

## Blood disease
- Severe anaemia
- Polycythaemia rubra vera
- Disseminated intravascular coagulation
- Idiopathic
- Thrombocytopenic purpura
- Leukaemia
- Sickle cell disease

## Miscellaneous
- Optic neuritis

- Central retinal artery occlusion
- Optic nerve tumours
- Guillain--Barré syndrome
- Spinal cord tumours

# Causes of angioid streaks

- Pseudoxanthoma elasticum
- Idiopathic
- Sickle cell disease
- Ehlers–Danlos syndrome
- Paget's disease

# Causes of retinal haemorrhage

- Diabetes mellitus
- Hypertension
- Raised intracranial pressure
- Retinal vein thrombosis
- Trauma
- Retinal detachment
- Arteritis
- Subarachnoid haemorrhage
- Severe anaemia
- Coagulation disorders

# Causes of Roth spots

- Subacute bacterial endocarditis
- Leukaemia
- Severe anaemia
- Hypoxia

**Box 15.1: Ophthalmic manifestations in HIV infection**

CMV retinitis
Kaposi's sarcoma
Herpes zoster virus
Herpes simplex virus
Toxoplasmosis
Cryptococcus
*Mycobacterium avium intracellulare*

## Causes of retinitis pigmentosa

- X-linked
- Kerns–Sayer syndrome
- Usher's syndrome
- Lawrence–Moon–Biedel syndrome
- Refsum's disease
- Batten's disease
- Abetalipoproteinaemia
- Cockayne's syndrome

## Causes of a cherry red macula

- Tay–Sachs disease
- Neimann–Pick's disease
- Sandhoff's disease
- Sialidoses
- Gangliosidosis
- Central retinal artery occlusion

# Miscellaneous conditions

## Causes of Horner's syndrome

- Posterior inferior cerebellar artery infarction
- Pancoast tumours
- Cervical cord lesions
- Idiopathic
- Thyroidectomy
- Aortic aneurysm
- Syringomyelia
- Brainstem lesions

## Causes of ptosis

- Congenital
- Third-nerve lesion
- Horner's syndrome
- Myasthenia gravis
- Myopathy
- Tabes dorsalis
- Hysteria

# Clinical case scenarios

## Third-nerve palsy

- There is ptosis, which may be complete or partial
- With the patient looking forward there is a divergent squint
- With the eye fixed in the down and out position diplopia is produced on looking down and out
- The pupil may be dilated and unreactive to light or may be normal
- In a complete third-nerve palsy there

is complete ptosis and pupillary dilatation
- In a partial third-nerve palsy the ptosis is incomplete and the pupil may be spared

## Fourth-nerve palsy

The eye is deviated down and medially, and the patient is unable to look down and out.

## Sixth-nerve palsy

With the patient looking forward, there is a convergent squint with the eye deviated medially, There is impaired lateral movement of the eye with diplopia on attempting this movement.

## Visual field defects

- Visual field should be examined by direct confrontation
- The use of a finger to map out the fields is usually sufficient, but in order to detect a central scotoma the use of coloured pins is necessary
- Commonest cases encountered are homonymous hemianopia, bitemporal hemianopia, central scotoma, tunnel vision

## Hypertensive retinopathy

The following features are found according to the grade of retinopathy:
- Grade 1: mild narrowing of retinal arteries
- Grade 2: moderate narrowing of retinal arteries
  Increased light reflex (silver wiring)
  AV nipping

- Grade 3: grade 2 features, plus cotton-wool spots and flame-shaped haemorrhages
- Grade 4: as above, plus papilloedema

## Ptosis

- Ptosis will be obviously apparent

- Other features to look for:
  Other signs of third-nerve lesion
  Features of Horner's syndrome
  Myasthenic fatiguability
  Features of dystrophia myotonica
  Argyll Robertson pupil (tabes dorsalis)
  Wasting of the hands (syringomyelia)

## Diabetic retinopathy

### Background retinopathy
- Characterised by the presence of microaneurysms, blot haemorrhages and hard exudates (owing to lipid deposition)
- Lesions are most numerous in the macula area

### Proliferative retinopathy
- Characterised by the presence of soft exudates (cotton-wool spots caused by ischaemia), flame-shaped haemorrhages, circulate rings of hard exudates indicating oedema, and new vessel formation
- Photocoagulation scars may be seen

- Other features to look for:
  Cataract formation
  AV nipping in the presence of coexistent hypertension
  Vitreous haemorrhage
  Vitreous scar
  Retinal detachment

# Retinitis pigmentosa

- There is black pigmentation in the periphery of the fundus
- There is tunnel vision

- Other features to look for:
   Lawrence–Moon–Biedel syndrome:
      (Optic atrophy
      Obesity
      Hypogonadism)
   Refsum's syndrome
      (Dwarfism
      Cognitive impairment
      Polydactyly
      Cerebellar signs
      Ichthyosis
      Cardiomyopathy)
   Cockayne's syndrome
      (Peripheral neuropathy
      Deafness
      Premature ageing)

# Papilloedema

- There is bilateral blurring of optic disc margins

- Other features to look for:
   Hypertension
      (Haemorrhages,
      Exudates
      AV nipping)
   Benign intracranial hypertension
      (Obesity
      Female
      Young)
   Respiratory failure (raised $P_{CO_2}$)
   Thyroid status (Graves' disease)
   Pagetic appearance

# Old choroiditis

In the fundus there is a patch of white indicating exposed sclera due to choroidoretinal atrophy due to old choroidoretinitis.

# Nystagmus

- Nystagmus will usually be obvious.
- Direction of the fast phase indicates:
   towards the side of the lesion – labyrinthine lesions
   away from the side of the lesion – cerebellar disorders
- Direction of the nystagmus indicates:
   horizontal – labyrinthine and cerebellar lesions
   vertical or rotatory – brainstem lesions

- Other features to look for:
   Cerebellar signs
   Divergent squint
   Ataxic nystagmus (internuclear ophthalmoplegia)
   Fifth, sixth and seventh cranial nerve lesions (acoustic neuroma),
   Positive Hallpike's test (benign positional vertigo)

# Horner's syndrome

- There is meiosis, enophthalamos and ptosis

- Other features to look for:
   Ipsilateral anhidrosis in the neck
   Lymphadenopathy
   Aneurysms
   Thyroidectomy
   Cerebellar signs
   Pyramidal signs indicative of brainstem lesions
   Signs of carcinoma of the bronchus
   Bilateral wasting of the hands with dissociated sensory loss (syringomyelia)

# Retinal vein thrombosis

- The veins are tortuous and engorged
- There are numerous haemorrhages throughout the retina
- There may be papilloedema and soft exudates

- Other features to look for:
  Hepatosplenomegaly
  Lymphadenopathy
  Excessive bruising (indicative of myeloproliferative disorders, paraproteinaemia and hyperviscosity syndromes)

# Myelinated nerve fibres

- There are bright white streaky irregular patches with frayed margins seen at the end of the optic disc
- Visual acuity is normal

# Cataracts

- The cataracts should be obviously visible
- Other features to look for:
  Presence of diabetic retinopathy
  Retinitis pigmentosa
  Frontal balding, myotonia, myotonic facies and ptosis (dystrophia myotonica)
  Down's syndrome
  Advanced age: senile cataracts
  Youth: glycogen-storage disease

# Pupillary abnormalities

## *Anisocoria*
- Pupils are unequal in size but no other abnormalities are found

## *Holmes–Adie pupil*
- There is a unilaterally large pupil which fails to react to light
- Convergence is normal
- There is no ptosis and eye movements are normal (i.e. not third-nerve palsy)
- This is usually due to a lesion of the ciliary ganglion

## *Argyll Robertson pupil*
- Both pupils are small and irregular
- The light reflex is poor or absent but convergence is normal

- Other features to look for:
  Diabetic retinopathy
  Positive Romberg's, impaired joint position sense and vibration sense, absent ankle jerks and aortic regurgitation (tabes dorsalis)

# Optic atrophy

- The optic discs are pale and sharply defined

- Other features to look for:
  Loss of direct light reflex and intact consensual light reflex (optic neuritis)
  Cerebellar signs (multiple sclerosis, Friedreich's ataxia),
  Visual field defects (pituitary carcinoma)
  Pathological cupping (glaucoma)
  Pagetic appearance
  Argyll Robertson pupils (tabes dorsalis)

# Renal artery occlusion

- Visual acuity in the affected eye is nil
- Retinal arterioles are thin and scanty
- There may be a cherry-red spot at the macula

- Other features to look for:
    Source of emboli (atrial fibrillation, cardiac murmur, carotid bruits)

# 16 Psychiatry

## Contents

## Definitions

*Agitation*: a state of increased motility with accompanying tension. May comprise poorly organised but purposeful activities or repetitive activities

*Automatism*: a simple or complex motor act often inappropriate to the circumstances carried out while unaware of the environment and without conscious motivation. Associated with organic cerebral disorders and hysteria

*Blunting of affect*: loss of usual mood modulation

*Compulsions*: repetitive acts which the patient is unable to prevent. Patient knows the actions are their own and based on their own will

*Depersonalisation*: perception of change in mental functions or body image

*Derealisation*: external world seems altered and unfamiliar

*Delusions*: mistaken beliefs that are held with conviction, despite all the evidence to the contrary, and not shared by others

*Flight of ideas*: the way in which speech moves rapidly from one subject to another

*Fugue*: a disturbance of behaviour characterised by wandering without conscious motivation in a state of altered or diminished consciousness, with subsequent amnesia for the event

*Hallucinations*: perceptions which are not based on external stimuli

*Hypnagogic hallucinations*: hallucinations occurring as the patient falls asleep. Usually of no pathological significance but may occur in narcolepsy

*Hypnocampic hallucinations*: similar hallucinations occurring as the patient awakes

*Illusions*: misinterpretations of external stimuli

*Incongruous affect*: a display of affect inappropriate to the patient's subjective mood state

*Labile mood*: uncontrollable and rapid fluctuations in mood

*Mannerisms*: habitual and meaningless motor movements

*Mutism*: absence of speech

*Neologisms*: made-up words

*Obsessions*: repetitive thoughts which cannot be inhibited. Patient is aware that they are their own thoughts and originate in their own mind

*Passivity*: a belief that one's body is under the control of other people or forces

*Perseveration*: the repetition of a response when it is no longer appropriate

*Phobias*: fears of specific objects or situations not generally regarded as dangerous

*Pressure of speech*: a rapid outpouring of ideas accompanied by an increase in quantity of speech, and often volume. Continuity of thinking may be affected

*Reference*: belief that events in the environment have special meaning for the subject and refer particularly to them

*Thought block*: an interruption in the flow of thinking

*Thought broadcasting*: a delusion that one's private thoughts are being made known to others

*Volition*: a state of energy and drive which directs purposeful activity

# Psychological defence mechanisms

*Repression*: the exclusion from awareness of impulses or emotions that would otherwise cause distress

*Denial*: the mechanism by which experiences or feelings that might cause distress are prevented from entering conscious awareness

*Projection*: the process by which one's feelings or impulses are attributed to others

*Introjection*: the process by which aspects of another person may be incorporated into the subject's self perception

*Idealisation*: the way in which ambivalent feelings towards another person may be split, such that bad feelings are denied or introjected: the person is then regarded as perfect

*Somatisation*: a term used to describe a psychological disorder presenting primarily with physical symptoms

*Conversion*: this refers to the process by which the affect caused by a conflict is replaced by a physical symptom

*Dissociation*: a defence mechanism which involves splitting of two or more mental processes which would otherwise be integrated, one then becoming unconscious

**Table 16.1: Distinction between neurosis and psychosis**

| Feature | Neurosis | Psychosis |
|---|---|---|
| Relation to reality | Intact | Loss of contact |
| Relation to normality | Represents extremes of normal difficulties | Clear distinction between normal and psychotic experiences |
| Hallucinations | No | Yes |
| Delusions | No | Yes |
| Insight | Usually present | Often absent |

**Table 16.2: Hierarchical model of diagnosis**

| Level | Disorder | Diagnosis |
|---|---|---|
| 1 | Organic | Acute brain syndrome (delirium) |
| | | Chronic brain syndrome (dementia) |
| 2 | Functional psychosis | Mania |
| | | Schizophrenia |
| | | Psychotic depression |
| 3 | Non-psychotic disorders | Depressive illness |
| | | Anxiety disorders: anxiety |
| | | phobias |
| | | panic disorder |
| | | Maladaptive behaviours: obsession |
| | | compulsion |
| | | alcohol abuse |
| | | drug dependence |
| | | anorexia |
| | | bulimia |
| | | self poisoning |
| | | self mutilation |
| | | Abnormal illness behaviour: hypochondriasis |
| | | hysteria |
| | | malingering |
| | | factitious illness |
| 4 | Personality disorders | Schizoid |
| | | Cyclothymic |
| | | Sensitive |
| | | Depressive |
| | | Passive dependent |
| | | Obsessional |
| | | Histrionic |
| | | Antisocial |

# Physical disease and psychiatric illness

There are five kinds of relationship between psychiatric disorders and physical symptoms:

1 Psychiatric disorder may provoke or release physical disease (most commonly depression)
2 Psychiatric symptoms may present with symptoms of physical disease
3 Psychiatric illness may be a direct consequence of physical disease
4 Psychiatric disorder may exacerbate a physical disease
5 Psychiatric illness may present with physical symptoms that have no organic basis (somatisation)

# Psychiatric presentations of physical disease

## *Depression*
### *Endocrine*
- Hypothyroidism

- Cushing's syndrome
- Hypopituitarism
- Hypoadrenalism
- Acromegaly
- Hypoparathyroidism
- Hyperparathyroidism

*Metabolic*
- Hypomagnesaemia
- Renal failure
- Renal dialysis
- Hyponatraemia
- Hypokalaemia
- Thiamine deficiency
- Alkalosis
- Acidosis
- Vitamin B$_{12}$ deficiency
- Folate deficiency
- Pellagra
- Hepatic failure

*Neurological*
- Parkinson's disease
- Multiple sclerosis
- Epilepsy
- Chronic pain

*Anxiety*
*Endocrine*
- Hyperthyroidism
- Phaeochromocytoma

*Metabolic*
- Hypoglycaemia
- Pellagra

*Neurological*
- Temporal lobe epilepsy
- Multiple sclerosis
- Frontal lobe lesions

*Drugs*
- SSRI antidepressants
- Amphetamines
- Caffeine
- Alcohol withdrawal
- Benzodiazepine

withdrawal
- Barbiturate withdrawal

# Schizophrenia

## Symptoms of schizophrenia

### Positive (acute)
- Disorders of thought possession
- Passivity phenomenon
- Hallucinations
- Delusions
- Incongruous affect

### Negative (chronic)
- Poverty of speech
- Slowness of thought and movement
- Emotional flatness
- Loss of volition
- Social withdrawal

## Poor prognostic features

- Family history of schizophrenia
- Schizoid personality

---

**Box 16.1: Schneider's first-rank symptoms**

**Disorders of thought possession**
Thought insertion or withdrawal
Thought broadcasting

**Passivity phenomenon**
Emotions, impulses, sensations, acts

**Auditory hallucinations**
Patient's thoughts echoed out aloud
Two or more people talking about patient in the third person
A running commentary on patient's behaviour

**Delusions**

Box 16.2: Differential diagnosis of schizophrenia

Amphetamine intoxication
Temporal lobe epilepsy
Huntington's chorea
Cerebral tumours
Alcohol hallucinosis
Hallucinogenic drugs (LSD, magic mushrooms, cannabis)
Morbid jealousy
Erotomania
Schizoaffective disorder

Box 16.3: Differential diagnosis of mania

**Cerebral lesions**
Frontal lobe lesions
Encephalitis

**Metabolic**
Renal failure
Hyperthyroidism

**Psychiatric**
Schizophrenia
Manic depression
Cyclothymic personality

**Drugs**
Sympathomimetics
Steroids
Isoniazid
Levodopa
Amphetamine
Hallucinogens

- Stressful home environment
- Poor previous work record
- Gradual onset
- No clear precipitating cause
- Absence of prominent affective symptoms
- Pronounced negative symptoms

# Mania

## Symptoms of mania

### Elevation in mood
- Euphoria
- Elation
- Irritability
- Disinhibition

### Increased activity
- Motor activity
- Pressure of speech
- Thoughts are speeded up
- Flight of ideas
- Reduced sleep
- Easy distractibility

### Schneiderian first-rank symptoms
- Delusions (typically grandiose, congruent with mood)
- Hallucinations

# Depression

## Symptoms of depression

### Emotional changes
- Anhedonia
- Low mood
- Loss of sense of humour
- Dwelling on past and present feelings
- Hopelessness about the future
- Inability to show affection
- Loss of religious beliefs

### Cognitive changes
- Self-dislike, self-blame
- Dislike of body image
- Ideas of reference
- Difficulty in making decisions/ thinking
- Lack of confidence
- Feelings of guilt/worthlessness
- Nihilistic/suicidal ideas
- Psychosis

**Table 16.3: Distinction between neurotic and psychotic depression**

| Feature | Neurotic | Psychotic |
| --- | --- | --- |
| Severity of depression | Less severe | More severe |
| Delusions /Hallucinations | No | Yes |
| Sleep disturbance | Difficulty initiating | Early morning waking |
| Neurovegetative symptoms | Yes/no | Prominent |
| Diurnal mood variation | No/worse later in day | Worse on waking |
| Family history | No | Yes |
| Response to ECT | No | Yes |

## Motivational changes
- Low energy, fatigue, apathy
- Inability to concentrate
- Unwillingness to accept responsibility
- Loss of interest in hobbies

## Neurovegetative symptoms
- Poor appetite (increased appetite may occur less commonly)
- Weight loss (weight gain may occur less commonly)
- Loss of libido
- Disturbed sleep
- Non-specific complaints (e.g. headache, pain)
- Psychomotor retardation (may be agitation in some)

---

**The CAGE questionnaire**

Have you ever felt that you should **C**ut down your drinking?

Are you **A**nnoyed by criticism of your drinking?

Have you ever felt **G**uilty about your drinking?

Have you ever had a drink first thing in the morning to steady your nerves (an **E**ye opener)?

*A positive reply to two or more of the above questions suggests possible dependence*

---

# Drug and alcohol dependence

## Complications of alcohol abuse

### Physical
**Gastro-intestinal**
- Liver cirrhosis
- Acute alcohol-induced hepatitis
- Precipitation of encephalopathy
- Pancreatitis
- Peptic ulcer disease

**Haematological**
- Megaloblastic anaemia
- Haemolytic anaemia

**Cardiological**
- Ischaemic heart disease
- Dilated cardiomyopathy

---

**Box 16.4: Edward's criteria for physical alcohol dependence**

Compulsion to drink
Increased tolerance
Withdrawal symptoms relieved by alcohol
Restricted drinking repertoire
Alcohol takes salience over other activities

---

**Table 16.4 Illicit drug abuse**

| Drug | Features of intoxication | Features of withdrawal |
|---|---|---|
| Heroin | Initial rush<br>Decreased appetite<br>Decreased libido<br>Constipation | Rhinorrhoea, lacrimation, yawning, sweating, nausea, vomiting, diarrhoea, abdominal cramps, mydriasis, tachycardia, hypertension, flushing, involuntary movements |
| Amphetamine/Ecstasy | Increased energy, awareness, speech<br>Reduced appetite and sleep<br>Sweating, mydriasis, tachycardia, hypertension, cardiac arrhythmias, hyperreflexia, seizures, renal failure | Depression<br>Anxiety<br>Irritability<br>Anergia |
| Cocaine | Similar to amphetamine<br>Formication | Similar to amphetamine |
| Hallucinogens | Distorted sensations (synaesthesia)<br>Distorted body image<br>Exaggeration of existing mood<br>Schizophreniform symptoms<br>Mania | None |
| Cannabis | Wellbeing<br>Relaxation<br>Exaggeration of existing moods<br>Perceptual disturbances<br>Psychosis | None |
| Solvents | Initial euphoria, then stupor<br>Disorientation, ataxia<br>Renal failure<br>Cardiac arrhythmias<br>Polyneuropathy<br>Aplastic anaemia<br>Hepatitis | |

- Atrial fibrillation

*Neurological*
- Ischaemic stroke
- Subdural haematoma
- Peripheral neuropathy
- Cerebellar degeneration
- Myopathy
- Wernicke–Korsakoff syndrome

*Miscellaneous*
- Trauma
- Hyperlipidaemia
- Fetal alcohol syndrome

*Psychological*
- Depression
- Anxiety
- Morbid jealousy
- Alcoholic hallucinosis
- Sociopathic personality
- Retrograde amnesia
- Dementia

*Social*
- Marital problems
- Work problems
- Vagrancy
- Forensic problems
- Financial problems

# Eating disorders

## Features of anorexia nervosa

*History*
- Self-induced weight loss
- Distorted body image
- Fear of fatness
- Intense desire to be thin
- Amenorrhoea
- Loss of libido
- Purgative abuse
- Diuretic abuse

- Avoidance of situations where food is present
- Selective exclusion of carbohydrate
- Vigorous exercise
- Vomiting after meals
- Mood disturbances

*Examination*
- Cold blue extremities
- Lanugo hair
- Bradycardia
- Hypotension
- Low body temperature
- Muscular weakness
- Dental caries (repeated vomiting)
- Lack of insight

*Investigations*
- Reduced $LH/FSH/T_4/T_3/BMR$
- Raised GH/cortisol/urea

## Features of bulimia

- Uncontrollable binge eating (often in secret)
- Binges typically involve high-calorie food
- Self-induced vomiting or purgative abuse after binge
- Rigorous dieting between binges
- Normal body weight
- Normal insight
- Menstrual disorders (50%)
- Dental caries common

# Personality disorders

*Personality traits*: individual characteristics exhibited by people.
*Personality disorders*: exist when those personality traits are sufficient to cause the patient or society to suffer.

# Schizoid personality

- Leads to withdrawal from social and interpersonal contacts
- Associated with emotional coldness and introspection
- May have few friends outside immediate family and difficulties with personal relationships
- Associated with an increased risk of developing frank schizophrenia

# Cyclothymic personality

- A tendency to experience periods of pronounced mood disorder
- Characterised by fluctuations between periods of elation and periods of depression
- Associated with an increased risk of developing mania and manic depression

# Sensitive personality (paranoid personality)

- Patients displays excessive sensitivity to humiliations and rebuffs
- Neutral or friendly actions by others are often misconstrued as hostile
- May be associated with jealousy and excessive self-importance
- Associated with an increased risk of developing persecutory symptoms during depressive illness

# Passive dependent personality

- Difficulty in making decisions and inability to admit disagreement
- Often associated with a fear of abandonment and constantly seeking reassurance from others

- Associated with an increased risk of developing depression

# Depressive personality

- A personality associated with low self-esteem and negative outlook on life
- Associated with an increased risk of development of depression

# Obsessional personality

- Feelings of personal insecurity, doubt and incompleteness, leading to excessive conscientiousness, checking and caution, with perfectionism and meticulous accuracy
- Associated with increased risk of developing obsessional symptoms during a depressive illness

# Histrionic personality

- The patient is usually female
- Descriptions of symptoms and circumstances are exaggerated, dramatised and romanticised
- Associated with excessive displays of emotion
- Behaviour may be manipulative and demanding
- Attention-seeking and sexual provocativeness are common features
- Associated with an increased risk of developing conversion phenomena and parasuicide attempts

# Antisocial personality (psychopathic or sociopathic personality)

- Inability to conform to social obligations

- Often an unstable work record and a repeated failure to honour financial obligations
- Patients are normally aggressive and impulsive, which may be associated with a significant forensic history and other evidence of aggressiveness such as repeated involvement in fights
- There is a failure to learn from adverse experiences and a failure to accept responsibility or exhibit remorse for such offences
- There is often a failure to maintain a monogamous sexual relationship for a long period
- Associated with a high risk of development of alcoholism and drug dependence

# Bereavement

## Features of a normal bereavement reaction

There is an initial state of shock and numbness lasting about a week. This is followed by realisation of loss, an acute grief reaction gradually resolving over several months and characterised by:
- Intense pining for the lost person
- Preoccupation with thoughts of the deceased
- Dreams of the deceased
- Illusions
- Visual or auditory pseudohallucinations
- Sense of presence of the deceased
- Depression
- Anxiety and restlessness
- Guilt
- Hostility towards others

---

**Box 16.5: Risk factors for atypical grief reaction**

Female gender
The death was sudden and unexpected
Inability to view the body of the deceased
Inability to express grief at an early stage
Previous poor relationship with deceased
The loss involves a child
The person experienced the loss of a parent as a child
Lack of social support/relatives

---

## Features of atypical grief reaction

- Prolonged grief reaction
- More severe reaction: social withdrawal, inability to work, suicidal ideas
- Delayed grief reaction
- Denial of grief

# Psychiatric emergencies

## Management of noisy and aggressive patients

- Identify and treat accordingly the cause of aggression: frustration, inability to communicate, anxiety, fear, delirium, resentment, psychosis, intoxication, sensory impairment, pain
- Stay calm
- Give the patient space
- Avoid distracting activity
- Make sure room is well lit
- Listen to the patient
- Communicate clearly with the patient
- Show understanding and sympathy
- Do not argue with patient
- Sedation (as a last resort): may

**Table 16.5: Important sections of the Mental Health Act**

| Section | Description | Signatures needed | Patient in | Duration of order |
|---|---|---|---|---|
| 2 | Assessment order | 2 doctors (1 approved), nearest relative or approved social worker | Unspecified | 28 days |
| 3 | Treatment order | As for Section 2 | Unspecified | 6 months |
| 5 (2) | Admission order | 1 doctor | Hospital | 72 hours |
| 5 (4) | Holding order | Qualified nurse | Hospital | 6 hours |
| 37 | Hospital order | 2 doctors, magistrates or Crown Court | Unspecified (often prison) | 6 months |
| 41 | Restriction order | Crown Court | Unspecified | Indefinite |
| 136 | Admission order | Police | Public place | 72 hours |

exacerbate delirium and sensory impairment

# Management of confused and wandering patients

- Identify cause of confusion and treat accordingly
- Ensure a calm, well-lit environment
- Maintain a familiar routine (named nurse)
- Redirect wandering patients rather than restrict:
    Map out environment
    Warning signs
    Distraction behaviour
    Security systems
- Sedation (as a last resort)

# Psychiatric drug treatment

## Classification of neuroleptics

### Tricyclic neuroleptics
- Phenothiazines:
  with aliphatic side chain
  (Chlorpromazine)
  with piperidine side chain
  (Thioridazine)
  with piperazine side chain
  (Trifluoperazine)
- Thioxanthines:
  dibenzoxapines (Loxapine),
  dibenzodiazepenes
  (Clozapine)

### Butylperidines
- Butyrophenones (Haloperidol)
- Diphenylbutylperidines
  (Pimozide)

### Heterocyclic compounds
- Indoles (Oxypertine)
- Substituted benzamines
  (Sulpiride)

### Rauwolfia alkaloids
- Reserpine

## Side effects of neuroleptics

### Extrapyramidal syndromes
- Parkinsonism
- Akathisia
- Acute dystonia
- Tardive dyskinesia
- Neuroleptic malignant syndrome

**Box 16.6:  Signs of neuroleptic malignant syndrome**

Muscle rigidity
Hyperpyrexia
Decreased consciousness
Renal failure: dehydration, rhabdomyolysis
Rhabdomyolysis: raised creatinine kinase,
  myoglobinuria
Pneumonia

## *Lowering of seizure threshold*

## *Autonomic side effects*
- Thermoregulatory failure
- Postural hypotension
- Anticholinergic effects

## *Endocrine complications*
- Hyperprolactinaemia
- Reduced gonadotrophins, oestrogens,
  progesterone

## *Psychiatric complications*
- Apathy, lassitude, lack of initiative
- Disturbed sleep, depression, acute
  psychosis

## *Hypersensitivity reactions*
- Cholestatic jaundice,
  agranulocytosis

## *Skin reactions*
- Contact dermatitis, photosensitivity
- Hyperpigmentation, urticaria

# Agents causing neuroleptic malignant syndrome

- Neuroleptics
- Tricyclic antidepressants
- Tricyclic-related antidepressants:
  trimipramine
  maprotiline
  mianserin

viloxazine
trazadone
- SSRI antidepressants
- Antiemetics: prochlorperazine
  metoclopramide

# Guidelines for the use of neuroleptics

## *Appropriate for:*
- Psychotic disorders
- Organic brain syndromes with
  behaviours that present a danger to
  the patient or others, or that interfere
  with the provision of care
- Tourette's syndrome
- Short-term treatment of hiccoughs,
  nausea
- Pruritus

## *Inappropriate for:*
- Wandering
- Poor self-care
- Restlessness
- Memory impairment
- Anxiety
- Insomnia
- Unsociability
- Fidgeting
- Nervousness
- Agitation that is not dangerous
- Uncooperativeness
- Neurotic depression

# Side effects of tricyclic antidepressants

## *Neurological*
- Tremor
- Convulsions
- Anticholinergic effects

## *Cardiovascular*
- Tachycardia
- Postural hypotension

- Cardiac arrhythmias
- Reduced cardiac output

### Psychiatric

- Hypomania
- Paranoid hallucinatory state
- Acute psychosis

### Hypersensitivity reactions

- Cholestatic jaundice
- Blood dyscrasias
- Allergic dermatitis

# Side effects of monoamine oxidase inhibitors (MAOIs)

- Excessive central stimulation (agitation, hypomania, convulsions)
- Postural hypotension
- Hepatocellular jaundice
- Hypertensive crisis (cheese reaction):
  Cream cheese
  Broad beans
  Pickled herrings
  Avocados
  Marmite
  Chianti
  Chocolate
- Potentiation of drugs:
  Opiates
  Hypoglycaemics
  Phenytoin
  Tricyclic antidepressants
  Centrally acting anticholinergics
  Alcohol
  Barbiturates

# Side effects of lithium therapy

### Gastrointestinal

- Nausea
- Vomiting

- Dyspepsia
- Altered taste
- Diarrhoea

### Neurological

- Tremor
- Ataxia
- Fasciculations
- Hyperreflexia

### Metabolic

- Nephrogenic diabetes insipidus
- Water retention
- Endocrine
- Hypothyroidism

# Contraindications to lithium therapy

- Renal failure
- Cardiac failure
- Addison's disease
- Hypothyroidism
- Pregnancy

# Electroconvulsive therapy (ECT)

## Indications for ECT

- Depressive illness which fails to respond to antidepressant drug therapy
- Psychotic delusions (especially if depressive delusions)

---

**Box 16.7: Features predicting good response to ECT**

Severe weight loss
Pronounced early-morning waking
Psychomotor retardation
Psychotic features

- Depressive stupor
- Catatonic stupor
- Puerperal psychosis
- Acute schizophrenia
- Schizophrenia with depressive features
- Mania which has failed to respond to drug therapy

# Side effects of ECT

- Myocardial infarction
- Cardiac arrhythmias
- Pulmonary embolism
- Pneumonia
- Joint dislocations
- Fractures
- Cerebral haemorrhage
- Mania
- Acute confusional state
- Retrograde and anterograde amnesia

## *Methods of reducing psychological side effects of ECT*

- Unilateral shock to non-dominant hemisphere
- Low number of treatments
- Low frequency of treatments
- Good preoperative oxygenation
- Low voltage shocks

# Contraindications to ECT

- Cerebral and aortic aneurysms
- Recent cerebral haemorrhage
- Myocardial infarction
- Cardiac arrhythmias
- Raised intracranial pressure
- Contraindications to general anaesthetic

# 17 Neurology

## Contents

## Anatomy of the CNS

### Cerebral cortex

The anatomy of the cerebral cortex is shown in Fig. 17.1.

### Brainstem (Fig. 17.2)

- *Midbrain*: connects pons and cerebellum to diencephalon (hypothalamus and thalamus) Contains cerebral peduncles, red

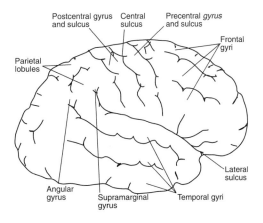
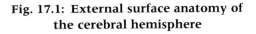

**Fig. 17.1: External surface anatomy of the cerebral hemisphere**

**Table 17.1: Lesions of the cerebral cortex**

| Lobe | Function | Effect of lesion |
|------|----------|------------------|
| Frontal | Motor cortex (precentral gyrus)<br>Broca's area<br>(dominant inferior frontal gyrus)<br>Particularly involved with emotional<br>and behavioural aspects of<br>motor function | Contralateral hemiparesis<br>Expressive dysphasia<br>Emotional lability<br>Disinhibited behaviour<br>Loss of insight<br>Primitive reflexes |
| Parietal | Sensory cortex (postcentral gyrus)<br>Control of visuospatial awareness<br>(non-dominant hemisphere)<br>Control of motor movement | Impaired cortical sensation<br>Motor apraxia<br>Dyscalculia (dominant hemisphere)<br>Dysgraphia (dominant hemisphere)<br>Agnosia (non-dominant hemisphere)<br>Homonymous hemianopia<br>Sensory inattention |
| Temporal | Wernicke's area<br>(posterior dominant inferior<br>frontal gyrus)<br>Receives auditory input from ears<br>Memory | Receptive dysphasia<br>Nominal aphasia<br>Auditory hallucinations<br>Amnesia<br>Upper homonymous quadrantopia<br>Temporal lobe epilepsy |
| Occipital | Primary visual cortex | Homonymous hemianopia<br>Cortical blindness |

nucleus, cranial nerve nuclei III
and IV
- *Pons*: lies between midbrain and
  medulla
  Contains cranial nerve nuclei V, VI,
  VII, VIII
- *Medulla*: continuous with the pons
  above and spinal cord below
  Contains cranial nerve nuclei XI, X,
  XI, XII, respiratory and
  cardiovascular centres, as well as
  chemoreceptor trigger zone and
  vomiting centre

### Brainstem reflexes
- Pupillary
- Control of conjugate gaze
- Corneal reflex
- Gag reflex
- Control of respiration

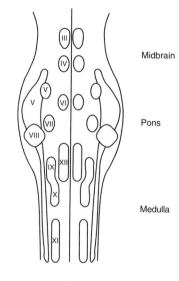

**Fig. 17.2: Longitudinal section through
the brainstem showing sites of cranial
nerve nuclei**

## Lesions of the brainstem
### Intrinsic
- Lead to focal abnormalities of brainstem reflexes and cranial nerve abnormalities which are present from the onset of coma and persistent
- Also produce bilateral pyramidal tract signs and irregular breathing patterns (most commonly Cheyne–Stokes respiration)

### Compressive
- Produce brainstem signs as above that are progressive
- There is also papilloedema

### Lesions of cranial nerves IX, X and XII
- *Bulbar palsy*: lower motor neuron lesions
- *Pseudobulbar palsy*: upper motor neuron lesions

# Cerebellum

- Lies in posterior fossa above brainstem
- Composed of two hemispheres and central vermis
- Involved in control of motor function (coordination)
- Receives afferents from muscles, joint receptors via spinocerebellar tracts, cutaneous afferents, vestibular afferents and visual afferents

### Effects of hemispheric lesion
- Ipsilateral limb incoordination leading to past pointing and intention tremor
- Hypotonia (may be normal)
- Dysarthria
- Staccato speech
- Nystagmus (away from the side of the lesion)
- Dysdiadochokinesia

### Effects of vermis lesion
- Truncal ataxia
- Wide-based ataxic gait

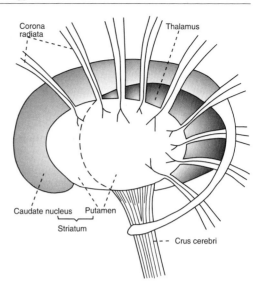

**Fig. 17.3: Lateral view of basal ganglia anatomy**

# Basal ganglia

The basal ganglia are concerned with control of motor function.

### Lesions of the basal ganglia
- Parkinsonism
- Hemiballismus (contralateral subthalamic nucleus)
- Chorea

# Cranial nerves

### Causes of bilateral seventh-nerve palsy
- Motor neuron disease
- Sarcoid
- Multiple sclerosis
- Guillain–Barré syndrome
- Poliomyelitis
- Bilateral acoustic neuroma
- Cephalic tetanus
- Meningitis

### Table 17.2: Cranial nerves

| Nerve | Function | Effect of lesion |
|---|---|---|
| I | Sense of smell | Anosmia |
| II, III, IV, VI | see Ophthalmology (Chapter 15) | |
| V | Motor to muscles of mastication (masseter, temporalis and pterygoid) Sensory to face (ophthalmic, maxillary, mandibular divisions) Corneal reflex | Weakness of jaw movement Absent corneal reflex Facial numbness Brisk jaw jerk |
| VII | Motor to muscles of facial expression Taste to anterior two-thirds of tongue (chorda tympani) Hearing (stapedius muscle) | Facial muscle weakness, dysarthria (LMN: all muscles UMN: lower facial muscles) Loss of taste, hyperacusis |
| VIII | Hearing (cochlear division) Balance (vestibular division) | Deafness Vertigo |
| IX | Motor to stylopharyngeus muscle Taste to posterior third of tongue Sensory to pharynx Secretomotor fibres to parotid | Impaired taste Absent gag reflex |
| X | Motor to intrinsic muscles of larynx and pharynx Motor to cricopharyngeus Sensory to pharynx, larynx, base of tongue, epiglottis Parasympathetic fibres to thoracic and abdominal viscera | Dysarthria Dysphonia Dysphagia |
| XI | Motor to sternomastoid and trapezius muscles | Weakness of head turning and shoulder shrugging |
| XII | Motor to tongue muscles | LMN: ipsilateral wasting, weakness, fasciculation, deviation to weak side on protrusion UMN: spastic immobile tongue |

## Blood supply to the CNS

The supply of blood to the central nervous system is illustrated in Fig. 17.4.

# Neurological signs

## Causes of coma

### *Primary cerebral disease*
- Meningitis
- Encephalitis
- Haemorrhage
- Infarction
- Tumour
- Abscess

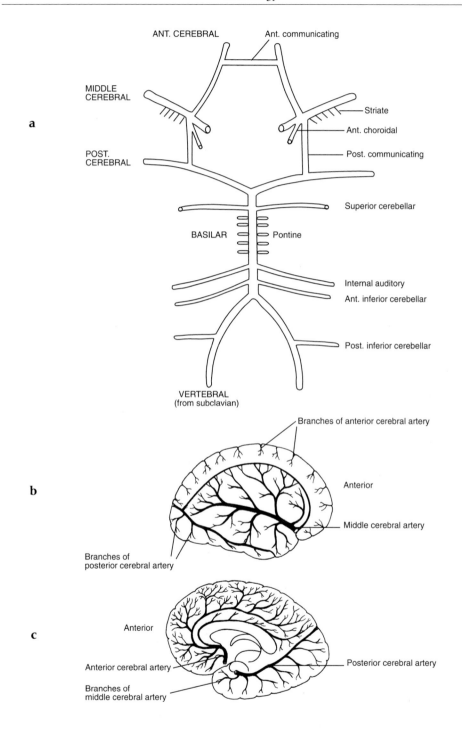

Fig. 17.4: (a) The circle of Willis; (b) Supply to the external surface of the cerebral hemisphere; (c) Internal supply to the cerebral hemisphere

- Venous thrombosis
- Epilepsy
- Hypertensive encephalopathy
- Head injury

## Miscellaneous
- Systemic sepsis
- Psychogenic

## Metabolic disturbance
- Drug overdose
- Hypoglycaemia
- Diabetic ketoacidosis
- Hyperosmolar non-ketotic coma
- Hyponatraemia
- Hypernatraemia
- Hypercalcaemia
- Renal failure
- Hepatic encephalopathy
- Hypothyroidism
- Hypoadrenalism
- Hypopituitarism
- Respiratory failure
- Severe cardiac failure
- Hyperpyrexia
- Hypothermia
- Porphyria

| Box 17.1: Glasgow coma scale | |
| --- | --- |
| **Feature** | **Score** |
| **Eye opening** | |
| Spontaneously | 4 |
| To verbal command | 3 |
| To pain | 2 |
| None | 1 |
| **Best motor response** | |
| Spontaneously | 5 |
| Localises to pain | 4 |
| Flexion to pain(decorticate rigidity) | 3 |
| Extension to pain (decerebrate rigidity) | 2 |
| None | 1 |
| **Best verbal response** | |
| Normal | 5 |
| Confused | 4 |
| Inappropriate | 3 |
| Incomprehensible | 2 |
| None | 1 |
| **Total** | 3–14 |

Cerebellar dysfunction
Vestibular dysfunction or sensory ataxia (impaired joint position sense)

## Festinant gait
- Stooped posture, difficulty initiating movement, short shuffling steps
- Typical of parkinsonism

## Marche à petits pas
- Upright posture, stiff-legged gait, short steps
- Typical of diffuse cerebrovascular disease

## Hemiplegic gait
- Dragging and weakness and spasticity of one leg
- Usually indicative of previous stroke

## Waddling gait
- Produced by proximal weakness in the

# Gait abnormalities

## Station
- The ability to stand and posture of stance
- Stooped posture typical of parkinsonism
- Wide-based stance typical of cerebellar disease or impaired sensory input

## Apraxic gait
- Patient able to stand but unable to walk
- Usually indicative of parietal lobe lesion

## Tandem gait
- The ability to walk heel to toe
- Impaired if: lower limb weakness

hip girdle
- Inability to tilt pelvis normally when swinging leg through
- Leads to compensatory exaggerated lateral movement of the trunk

### Steppage gait
- As a result of footdrop, patient has to flex leg at hip more than normal to avoid catching toes on floor. Has appearance of trying to step up
- May be associated with stamping if impaired joint position sense

### Ataxic gait
- Broad-based stance, gait unsteady akin to being drunk
- Caused by:
  Cerebellar lesions (negative Romberg's)
  Impaired joint position sense (positive Romberg's)
  Brainstem lesions
  Leg weakness
  Sensory impairment

## Speech abnormalities

### Receptive dysphasia
- Caused by a lesion to Wernicke's area
- Difficulty with comprehension of language
- Patient does not understand what is said or written
- Speech usually fluent and inappropriate, with jargon

### Expressive dysphasia
- Due to a lesion of Broca's area
- Difficulty with expression of language
- Patient understands what is said or written and knows what he/she wants to say but is unable to find the right words
- Speech usually hesitant and associated with extreme frustration

### Nominal aphasia
- Patient has difficulty naming objects
- Patient is able to recognise objects correctly when asked to point them out but is unable to name them verbally

### Mixed aphasia
- Patient has receptive and expressive difficulties

### Global aphasia
- Impairment of all modalities of speech and language

### Dysarthria
- Caused by lesions of the muscles of articulation, or local defects of oral construction
  Seventh-nerve lesion
  Pseudobulbar palsy
  Bulbar palsy
  Basal ganglia lesions
  Cerebellar lesions
  Myopathy
  False teeth
  Cleft palate
- Leads to impaired articulation of speech
- Comprehension and expression are normal

### Dysphonia
- Defect in voice production
- May be caused by vocal cord lesions (sepsis, tumour), hysteria or lesions of recurrent laryngeal nerve (carcinoma of bronchus, aortic aneurysm)

### Aphonia
- Loss of voice
- Causes as for dysphonia

## Deafness

### Rinne's test
- Normally air conduction greater than

bone conduction
- In conductive hearing loss bone conduction is greater than air conduction
- In sensorineural hearing loss both air conduction and bone conduction are diminished but air conduction remains greater than bone conduction

### Weber's test
- Normally sound is heard centrally
- In conductive hearing loss, sound heard on the affected side
- In sensorineural hearing loss, sound heard on the unaffected side

### Causes of deafness
#### Conductive loss
- Wax
- Foreign body
- Eustachian tube obstruction
- Otitis media
- Otosclerosis
- Paget's disease
- Klippel–Feil deformity

#### Sensorineural impairment
- Degenerative (presbyacusis)
- Trauma:
  Chronic loud noise
  Fracture of petrous temporal bone
- Infection:
  Congenital syphilis
  Rubella
  Mumps
  Influenza
  Meningococcal meningitis
- Toxic:
  Quinine
  Aspirin
  Streptomycin
  Neomycin
  Tobacco
  Alcohol
  Frusemide
- Miscellaneous:
  Acoustic neuroma

Brainstem lesions
Alport's syndrome

# Memory

- Memory has three components:
- Immediate recall
- Short-term memory
- Long-term memory

### Causes of chronic amnesia
#### Vascular
- Bilateral thalamic infarcts
- Posterior cerebellar artery occlusion

#### Metabolic
- Thiamine deficiency
- Hypoglycaemia
- Severe epilepsy
- Chronic sedative abuse

#### Infection
- Meningitis (especially TB)
- Encephalitis (especially HSV)

#### Miscellaneous
- Dementia
- Tumour
- Trauma
- Transient global amnesia

# Miscellaneous signs

### Causes of raised intracranial pressure
- Cerebral tumours
- Hydrocephalus
- Benign intracranial hypertension
- Intracranial haemorrhage
- Cerebral abscess
- Encephalitis
- Meningitis
- Pituitary tumours
- Trauma (cerebral oedema)
- Malignant hypertension

**Table 17.3: Upper or lower motor neuron lesions**

| Feature | Upper | Lower |
|---|---|---|
| Tone | Increased | Decreased |
| Power | Reduced | Reduced |
| Reflexes | Increased | Reduced/absent |
| Wasting | Yes | Yes |
| Fasciculations | No | Yes |
| Plantar response | Extensor | Flexor |

- Venous sinus thrombosis
- $CO_2$ retention
- Oral contraceptive pill
- Vitamin A intoxication
- Retinoids
- Tetracycline

### Causes of absent ankle jerks and extensor plantar response

- Subacute combined degeneration of the cord
- Tabes dorsalis
- Friedreich's ataxia
- Motor neuron disease
- Diabetes mellitus
- Conus medullaris lesion

# Headache

## Causes of headache

### Tension headache

### Trauma

### Vascular disorders
- Migraine
- Intracranial haemorrhage
- Hypertensive encephalopathy
- Arteritis

### Skull disease
- Sinusitis
- Fracture
- Mastoiditis

- Tumour
- Paget's disease

### Toxic
- Sepsis
- $CO_2$ retention
- Hypoxia
- Hypoglycaemia
- Alcohol withdrawal

### Raised intracranial pressure

### Meningeal irritation
- Meningitis
- Subarachnoid haemorrhage

### Ear disease
- Otitis media

### Ocular disease
- Glaucoma
- Iritis
- Orbital tumours

### Haematological
- Anaemia
- Polycythaemia

### Miscellaneous
- Postictal
- Psychogenic
- Coital cephalgia

## Migraine

- Most have first attack of migraine

before 30 years of age
- Usually reduce in frequency by the age of 50

## Pathophysiology of migraines
- Aura and other features prior to headache: vasoconstriction of cerebral arteries
- Headache: release of vasoactive amines (substance P and neurokinin), leading to vasodilatation

## Classification of migraine
### Classic migraine
- Prodrome for up to 24 hours before attack (mood change, increased energy, lethargy, food craving or avoidance)
- Aura may take many forms (flashing dots, scotomas, fragmentation, teichopsia) and lasts about 30 minutes
- Other features may occur during or just after visual aura (paraesthesia, limb weakness, dysphasia), all of which develop over a period of a few minutes
- Headache is often unilateral
- Associated features include photophobia, nausea, syncope, diarrhoea and vomiting
- Whole attack may last 6–24 hours
- Usually less than 1 attack per month

### Common migraine
- No aura
- Other features similar to classic migraine

### Hemiplegic migraine
- Hemiplegia, dysphasia, hemianopia, usually preceding headache
- Usually resolves quickly

### Basilar migraine
- Brainstem dysfunction leading to coma, vertigo, dysarthria, diplopia or limb weakness

---

> **Box 17.2: Factors provoking migraine**
>
> Stress
> Altered sleep pattern
> Alcohol
> Combined oral contraceptive pill
> Exercise
> Bright lights
> Hunger
> Menses
> Food sensitivity (chocolate, wine, cheese)

---

### Ophthalmoplegic migraine
- Headache followed by unilateral ophthalmoplegia and ptosis

## Treatment of migraine
- *Acute attack*: analgesia, antiemetic, sumatriptan, ergotamine
- *Prophylaxis*: if attacks frequent, pizotifen, propranolol
  Other options include calcium antagonists, amitriptyline, cyproheptadine and methysergide

# Facial pain

## Causes of facial pain

### Local disease
- Teeth problems
- Sinusitis
- Temporomandibular joint disease
- Nasopharyngeal tumour
- Salivary gland disease
- Glaucoma
- Iritis
- Optic neuritis
- Giant cell arteritis

### Central lesions
- Thalamic infarcts
- Brainstem glioma

- Posterior inferior cerebellar artery infarction
- Syringobulbia
- Tabes dorsalis

## Cavernous sinus and pons
- Acoustic neuroma
- Meningioma
- Basal meningeal granuloma or tumour
- Herpes zoster virus
- Skull fracture

## Facial neuralgia
- Trigeminal neuralgia
- Post-herpetic neuralgia
- Migrainous neuralgia (cluster headache)
- Atypical facial pain

## Others
- Myocardial ischaemia
- Aneurysm of the posterior communicating artery
- Cranial arteritis

# Facial neuralgias

## Trigeminal neuralgia (tic douloureux)
- Gender: women to men 3:1
- Onset usually over 50 years of age
- May be associated with multiple sclerosis
- Aetiology unknown
- No nocturnal symptoms
- No trigeminal sensory impairment
- Usually affects maxillary or mandibular division
- Always unilateral
- Severe lancinating pain lasting 10–60 seconds
- Pain triggered by movement of face, eating, drinking, touching of face, cold wind blowing on face
- Patient usually has episodic bouts of

attacks lasting weeks to months
- Asymptomatic in between attacks
- Treatment with carbamazepine, phenytoin, amitriptyline or nerve thermocoagulation

## Post-herpetic neuralgia
- Shingles affecting trigeminal nerve almost always involves ophthalmic division only
- Produces cutaneous hyperaesthesia
- May disturb sleep
- Difficult to treat
- Development not related to treatment of shingles itself

## Migrainous neuralgia
- Gender: men to women 7:1
- Characterised by bouts of daily pain for a few weeks to months, with long periods of remission
- Pain unilateral around eye and cheek
- Characteristically pain occurs once a day usually early hours of morning
- Pain lasts 20–60 minutes
- May be associated with facial flushing, rhinorrhoea, conjunctival hyperaemia, ipsilateral Horner's
- Prophylactic treatment with ergotamine

# Epilepsy

## Classification of epilepsy

### Generalised seizures
Petit mal
- Brief, 10–15-second absence attacks
- Characteristic 3-second spike and wave discharge on EEG
- Always starts in childhood
- Only occasionally continues into adulthood
- 50% go on to develop grand mal seizures later

### Myoclonic seizures
- Single or repetitive sudden convulsive movements of limbs or trunk
- May be hereditary (Lafora body disease)

### Tonic–clonic seizures (grand mal)
- Often preceded by aura
- Sudden loss of consciousness
- Tonic phase leads to sustained muscle contractions
- Clonic phase leads to violent jerking movements of limbs and trunk
- May be associated tongue biting, urinary incontinence
- Postictal phase consists of drowsiness, confusion, irritability and headache

### Infantile spasms
- Brief sudden head flexion (salaam attacks)

### Febrile convulsions
- Only occur in children aged 6 months to 6 years
- Small increased risk of later epilepsy

### Tonic seizures
- No clonic phase

### Atonic seizures
- No tonic phase

## Partial seizures
### Simple
- No loss of consciousness
- May be motor, sensory, aphasic, cognitive, affective, amnesic, olfactory, jacksonian
- Paroxysmal discharges develop in one part of the brain (focal discharges) leading to focal abnormalities according to the region of the brain involved
- Temporal lobe most commonly involved

### Jacksonian epilepsy (march epilepsy)
Focal progressive motor fits
Usually affects limbs

### Temporal lobe epilepsy
May be simple or complex
Olfactory or psychic phenomenon (déjà vu/jamais vu)
Repetitive motor acts (lip smacking, chewing and grimacing)
Amnesia may occur for part or all of the attack
May be associated with violent outbursts and aggression
May be confused with acute schizophrenia

### Complex
- Impairment of consciousness

### Partial seizures with secondary generalisation
- Activity may spread and become generalised, giving rise to a grand mal seizure

# Aetiology of epilepsy

## Hereditary
- Lipidoses
- Down's syndrome
- Aminoacidurias
- Tuberous sclerosis
- Temporal lobe epilepsy
- Petit mal epilepsy

## Developmental defects
- Congenital rubella
- CMV
- Toxoplasmosis

## Birth trauma
- Perinatal anoxia
- Cerebral contusion or haemorrhage

## Primary or secondary tumours

### Metabolic
- Renal failure
- Hyponatraemia
- Hypoglycaemia
- Hypocalcaemia
- Hypomagnesaemia
- Water intoxication
- Hepatic encephalopathy

### Degenerative
- Alzheimer's disease
- Creutzfeldt–Jakob disease
- Huntington's chorea

### Vascular
- Cerebral infarction/haemorrhage
- AV malformation

### Inflammatory
- SLE
- Polyarteritis nodosa (PAN)
- Multiple sclerosis

### Sepsis
- Febrile convulsions
- Encephalitis
- Meningitis
- Cerebral abscess
- Cystercicosis
- Neurosyphilis
- Hydatid disease
- Toxocara
- Toxoplasmosis

### Toxic
- Alcohol
- Amphetamine
- Barbiturates
- Lignocaine
- Tricyclic antidepressants
- Lead
- Phenothiazines
- Cocaine

---

**Box 17.3: Reasons to investigate first fit**

Late-onset seizure
Atypical neurological signs
Persistent neurological signs
Atypical seizure
Abnormal clinical examination

---

### Miscellaneous
- Idiopathic
- Head injury
- Anoxia in infancy and childhood

# Diagnosis of epilepsy

- CT scan may show gross structural abnormalities
- MRI able to show more subtle structural changes (especially temporal lobe)
- EEG: normal EEG does not exclude epilepsy
  Abnormal EEG does not confirm epilepsy
  24-hour monitoring may be useful

# Emergency management of status epilepticus

- This is a series of fits with no regain of consciousness in between
- Patient should be placed if possible in a suitable safe environment
- Initial treatment consists of diazepam rectally or diazemuls intravenously
- Chlormethiazole infusion may be effective, with rapid onset of action (especially in seizures caused by alcohol withdrawal)
- Paraldehyde intramuscularly or intravenous phenytoin are alternatives
- Avoid paralysing patient as this removes observable manifestations of convulsive activity and makes

assessment of treatment efficacy difficult
- In such cases, continuous EEG monitoring is required
- Identify causes and treat appropriately

# Syncope and dizziness

## Causes of vertigo

### Peripheral
**Labyrinthine**
- Labyrinthitis (vestibular neuronitis)
- Motion sickness
- Benign positional vertigo
- Menière's disease
- Traumatic vestibular damage
- Quinine
- Salicylates
- Labyrinthine ischaemia
- Middle ear disease
- Alcohol excess

**Eighth-nerve palsy**
- Ototoxic drugs (streptomycin, gentamicin, frusemide)
- Acoustic neuroma
- Herpes zoster virus (Ramsay–Hunt syndrome)

### Central
**Brainstem**
- Multiple sclerosis
- Vertebrobasilar ischaemia
- Migraine
- Encephalitis
- Tumours
- Posterior inferior cerebellar artery (PICA)
- Syringobulbia

**Cerebral**
- Temporal lobe epilepsy

# Other causes of dizziness

### Cardiovascular
- Vasovagal
- Postural hypotension
- Aortic stenosis
- Cardiac arrhythmias
- Hypertrophic cardiomyopathy
- Cardiac failure

### Ocular
- Poor acuity
- Diplopia
- Oscillipsia

### Others
- Migraine
- Epileptic aura
- Psychogenic

### Haematological
- Anaemia
- Polycythaemia

### Metabolic
- Hypoglycaemia
- Hyperventilation

### Drugs
- Benzodiazepines
- Tricyclic antidepressants
- Anticonvulsants
- Diuretics
- ACE inhibitors
- Anti hypertensive drugs

## Clinical points regarding dizziness

- In most patients the cause is a peripheral labyrinthine lesion or syncope
- Acute vertigo with no other neurological signs is usually due to peripheral labyrinthine lesions
- Peripheral labyrinthine lesions are

more likely to be associated with tinnitus or deafness
- Caloric testing may help in distinguishing between peripheral and central labyrinthine lesions
- Romberg's test detects peripheral labyrinthine lesions

## Causes of syncope

- Vasovagal attack
- Postural hypotension
- Cardiac dysrhythmias
- Aortic stenosis
- Low-output cardiac failure
- Coughing
- Micturition
- Defecation
- Hypoxia
- Carotid sinus syndrome

## Causes of postural hypotension

### Idiopathic

### Autonomic neuropathy
- Diabetes mellitus
- Guillain–Barré syndrome
- Surgical sympathectomy
- Syringomyelia
- Tabes dorsalis
- Familial dysautonomia
- Shy–Drager's syndrome

### Steroid deficiency
- Addison's disease
- Hypopituitarism

### Drugs
- Antihypertensives
- Phenothiazines
- Tricyclic antidepressants
- L-Dopa

### Venous pooling
- Prolonged standing
- Varicose veins

### Reduced vascular tone
- Prolonged bed rest
- Hypokalaemia

## Distinction between syncope and epilepsy

- Nocturnal attacks while patient is recumbent are unlikely to be syncopal
- Syncopal attacks may occur during the night on getting up to micturate
- Syncopal attacks usually preceded by a feeling of impending loss of consciousness
- Epilepsy often has no aura, but if there is it is different from that preceding syncope
- In syncopal attacks the loss of consciousness is brief (less than 1 minute)
- In epilepsy loss of consciousness usually lasts for more than 1 minute
- No postictal phase occurs in syncopal attacks
- Syncope is usually postural. Urinary incontinence may occur in both

# Cerebral haemorrhage

## Causes of intracranial haemorrhage

- Subarachnoid haemorrhage (berry aneurysms)
- Hypertension (Charcot–Bouchard aneurysms)
- Subdural haematoma

- Extradural haematoma
- AV malformation
- Haemorrhage into cerebral tumour
- Haematological disease (thrombocytopenia, clotting defects)
- Hereditary haemorrhagic telangiectasia
- Haemangioblastoma (Von Hippel–Lindau syndrome)
- Cavernous haemangiomas
- Amyloid angiopathy
- Mycotic aneurysms

## Causes of aneurysms

- Idiopathic (congenital)
- Polycystic kidney disease
- Ehlers–Danlos syndrome
- Coarctation of the aorta
- Fibromuscular dysplasia
- Pseudoxanthoma elasticum

## Subarachnoid haemorrhage

- Commonest sites for aneurysms: anterior/posterior communicating arteries
  Bifurcation of the middle cerebral artery
- Subhyaloid haemorrhage is unique to subarachnoid haemorrhage
- CT may be normal if bleed is small
- Lumbar puncture if within 8 hours may not contain blood
- Xanthochromia seen only after 24 hours

### Treatment
Bed rest until headache subsides
Intravenous normal saline to maintain adequate blood pressure
Nimodipine prevents vasospasm
Continue for 10–14 days, after which risk of vasospasm falls substantially
Consider surgery if little neurological deficit

## Extradural haemorrhage

- Due to traumatic rupture of meningeal arteries, most commonly middle meningeal

## Subdural haemorrhage

- Due to rupture of cortical veins
- May present acutely with neurological deficit, raised intracranial pressure, or coma
- May present chronically with insidious features such as confusion, dementia, recurrent falls
- Increased risk in the elderly, alcoholics and malnourished

# Intracranial venous thrombosis

## Causes of intracranial venous thrombosis

### Infection
- Scalp
- Skull
- Face
- Middle ear
- Mastoiditis
- Meningitis
- Septicaemia

### Others
- Postpartum
- Dehydration
- Diabetes mellitus
- Trauma
- Catheterisation of jugular veins
- Blood dyscrasias (especially leukaemia)
- Cardiac failure
- Malignant infiltration of sinuses

- Nonmetastatic effect of malignancy
- Combined oral contraceptive pill
- Hypercoagulable states

# Cerebral tumours

- *Children*: usually posterior fossa (gliomas and meningiomas rare)
- *Adults*: usually supratentorial
- 60% of metastases originate from a bronchial primary

## Presentation of cerebral tumours

- Focal neurological deficit
- Epilepsy (generalised if supratentorial)
- Raised intracranial pressure
- Endocrine effects (pituitary tumours)

# Infections of the CNS

## Bacterial meningitis

### Common causes of bacterial meningitis (Fig. 17.6)

**Neonates**
- *Escherichia coli*
- Group B streptococci
- *Listeria*

**Children/young adults**
- Haemophilus B
- *Neisseria meningitidis*
- *Streptococcus pneumoniae*

**Older adults/elderly**
- *Neisseria meningitidis*
- *Streptococcus pneumoniae*

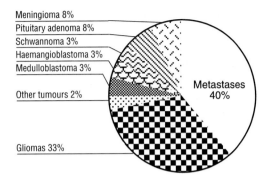

**Fig. 17.5: Classification of cerebral tumours**

## Causes of viral meningitis

- Echovirus
- Coxsackie virus
- Polio virus
- Mumps
- Lymphocytic choriomeningitis virus

## Causes of aseptic meningitis

- Partially treated bacterial meningitis
- Viral infection
- Sarcoid
- Polyarteritis nodosa
- Whipple's disease
- Mollaret's meningitis
- Vogt–Koyanagi–Harada syndrome

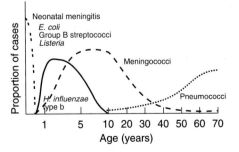

**Fig. 17.6: Age-related incidence of the major types of bacterial meningitis**

### Table 17.4: CSF findings in meningitis

| Finding | Bacterial meningitis | Viral meningitis | Tuberculous meningitis |
| --- | --- | --- | --- |
| Colour | Turbid | Clear | Clear |
| Cells | Neutrophils | Lymphocytes | Early neutrophils |
|  |  |  | Later lymphocytes |
| Protein | High | High | High |
| Glucose | Low | Normal (rarely low) | Low |

- Lyme disease
- *Rickettsia*
- Meningovascular syphilis
- Leptospirosis
- SLE
- Behçet's disease
- Carcinomatous meningitis
- Lead
- Post vaccination
- Fungal infection
- Malaria
- Amoeba
- Trypanosomiasis
- *Strongyloides*
- Schistosomiasis

- *Bacillus* spp.
- Fusobacterium
- Anaerobic cocci
- Cryptococcus
- *Blastomyces*
- *Naegleria fowleri*
- Acanthamoeba
- *Yersinia*
- *Pseudomonas*
- *Brucella*

# Rare causes of meningitis

- Tuberculosis
- Leptospirosis
- *Branhamella*
- *Bacteroides* spp.

## Box 17.4: Complications of meningitis

Cranial nerve palsies
Deafness
Cerebral abscess
Venous sinus thrombosis
Hydrocephalus
Stroke
Subdural empyema
Epidural abscess
Spinal cord compression
Cognitive impairment
SIADH

# Management of acute bacterial meningitis

- Have a high index of suspicion
- Commence high-dose penicillin or cephalosporin immediately (before investigations if necessary)
- Conduct brain CT: (if possibility of raised intracranial pressure)
  In meningitis, fundi may not be adequately visualised owing to photophobia
  Acute raised intracranial pressure may not cause papilloedema

## Box 17.5: Conditions leading to low CSF glucose

Bacterial meningitis
Tuberculous meningitis
Carcinomatous meningitis
Subarachnoid haemorrhage
Malignant hypertension
Viral meningitis
Fungal meningitis
Sarcoid

**Box 17.6: Organisms causing cerebral abscess**

*Streptococcus viridans*
*Staphylococcus aureus*
*Klebsiella*
*Streptococcus pneumoniae*
*Bacteroides*
*Fusobacterium*
Anaerobic cocci
Actinomyces
*Nocardia*
Amoeba
Cystercicosis

Investigations:
　(Many centres routinely perform CT prior to lumbar puncture as a consequence of the difficulty in excluding raised intracranial pressure on clinical examination.)
　Lumbar puncture (definitive test)
　Blood cultures
　Serology for bacteria
　Polymerase chain reaction (PCR) is an alternative

* Continue intravenous antibiotics for 1 week
* Supportive treatment
* Treatment of contacts with rifampicin, ciproxin or ceftriaxone

# Causes of cerebral abscess

* Middle ear infection
* Frontal sinusitis
* Septicaemia
* Hydatid disease
* Penetrating skull trauma

# Causes of encephalitis

* Herpes simplex virus
* Mumps
* Measles
* Polio virus
* Varicella zoster virus
* Glandular fever
* Coxsackie virus
* Echovirus
* Rabies
* Influenza virus
* Togavirus
* Bunyavirus
* Kuru
* Creutzfeldt–Jakob disease
* Papovavirus
* Toxoplasma
* Malaria
* Trypanosomiasis
* Syphilis

# Neurological manifestations of HIV

## *Cerebral lesions*
* Progressive multifocal leukoencephalopathy
* Toxoplasmosis
* Cerebral abscess
* Lymphoma
* CMV retinitis
* Dementia
* Encephalitis
* Infective meningitis
* Aseptic meningitis
* Hydrocephalus
* Vasculitis
* Cerebral infarction
* Cerebral haemorrhage
* Optic atrophy

## *Myelopathy*
* Herpes zoster virus
* CMV
* Abscess

- Lymphoma
- Plasmacytoma

### Radiculopathy
- Herpes zoster virus
- CMV

### Peripheral neuropathy
- Guillain–Barré syndrome
- Distal sensory neuropathy
- Mononeuropathies
- Mononeuritis multiplex

### Myopathy
- Polymyositis
- Dermatomyositis
- Zidovudine-induced myopathy

# Cerebellar disorders

## Causes of cerebellar dysfunction

### Toxic
- Alcohol
- Phenytoin
- Carbamazepine
- Solvent abuse

### Degenerative
- Senile cerebellar ataxia

### Hereditary
- Friedreich's ataxia
- Ataxia telangiectasia
- Wilson's disease
- Refsum's disease
- Mitochondrial cytopathy
- Cerebellar dysgenesis
- Dandy –Walker syndrome
- Arnold–Chiari malformation

### Inflammatory
- Multiple sclerosis
- Viral encephalitis

> **Box 17.7: Common sites and manifestations of demyelination in multiple sclerosis**
>
> **Optic nerve**
> Optic neuritis
> Papillitis
> Optic atrophy
>
> **Cervical cord**
> Sensory symptoms in limbs
> L'Hermitte phenomenon (tingling paraesthesia in legs induced by neck flexion)
> Spastic paraparesis
> Tetraparesis
> Bladder dysfunction (urgency, frequency and incontinence)
> Impotence
> Constipation
>
> **Brainstem**
> Diplopia (VIth nerve palsy, internuclear ophthalmoplegia)
> Vertigo
> Facial numbness
> Facial neuralgia
> Dysarthria
> Dysphagia
> Ataxia
>
> **Cerebral hemispheres**
> Altered mood (euphoria and depression)
> Dementia
> Seizures

- HIV
- Tuberculosis
- Cerebral abscess

### Malignancy
- Medulloblastoma
- Astrocytoma
- Hemangioblastoma
- Cerebral metastases
- Oat cell carcinoma of the lung

*Vascular*
- Cerebellar infarction
- Brainstem infarction
- Cerebellar haemorrhage

*Metabolic*
- Hypothyroidism

# Demyelination

## Causes of demyelination

- Multiple sclerosis
- Peripheral neuropathy
- Guillain–Barré syndrome
- Sphingolipidoses
- Postviral encephalomyelitis
- Postvaccinial encephalomyelitis

## Multiple sclerosis

- Unknown cause
- Increased incidence in temperate climates
- Characterised by acute episodes of demyelination in central white matter

## Other causes of l'Hermitte phenomenon

- Cervical cord trauma
- Cervical spondylosis
- Subacute combined degeneration of the cord
- Cervical cord tumours

## Causes of oligoclonal bands in CSF

- Multiple sclerosis
- Neurosyphilis

**Box 17.8: Poor prognosis features of MS**

Advanced age at onset (leads to chronic progressive course)
Dementia
Early development of ataxia
No remissions
Brainstem involvement

- Sarcoid
- Subacute sclerosing panencephalitis
- SLE

# Movement disorders

## Causes of tremor

*Rest tremor*
- Parkinsonism

*Postural tremor*
- Essential tremor
- Anxiety
- Thyrotoxicosis
- Drugs: tricyclic antidepressants, lithium, sympathomimetics

*Intention tremor*
- Cerebellar disease
- Brainstem disease

*Flapping tremor*
- Respiratory failure
- Hepatic failure
- Renal failure

## Causes of chorea

- Huntington's chorea
- Drugs: combined oral contraceptive pill, neuroleptics, phenytoin, alcohol,

L-dopa
- Rheumatic fever (Sydenham's chorea)
- Chorea gravidarum
- Space-occupying lesions
- Cerebral infarction
- Thyrotoxicosis
- Polycythaemia rubra vera
- Encephalitis lethargica
- SLE
- Hypocalcaemia
- Hypernatraemia
- Advanced age (senile chorea)
- Carbon monoxide poisoning

## Causes of hemiballismus

- Infarction of contralateral subthalamic nucleus
- Space-occupying lesions
- Head injury

## Causes of dystonia

### Focal
- Writer's cramp
- Spasmodic torticollis
- Cranial dystonia (blepharospasm, oromandibular)
- Hemiplegic dystonia

### Generalised
- Drugs: maxolon, stemetil, neuroleptics, L-dopa, dopamine agonists
- Torsion dystonia
- Gangliosidoses
- Metachromatic leukodystrophy
- Wilson's disease
- Huntington's chorea
- Homocystinuria
- Cerebral palsy
- Encephalitis lethargica
- Mitochondrial cytopathy

## Causes of myoclonus

### Generalised
- Essential familial myoclonus
- Myoclonus and epilepsy
- Encephalopathies: Lafora body disease
  Gangliosidoses
  Hereditary ataxia
  Encephalitis lethargica
  Subacute sclerosing panencephalitis
  Creutzfeldt–Jakob disease
  Renal failure
  Hepatic failure
  Hyponatraemia
  Respiratory failure
  Alcohol withdrawal
  Post traumatic
  Hypoxia

### Focal
- Cortical or cerebral hemisphere lesions
- Brainstem degeneration or infarction
- Spinal cord lesion

# Cerebral palsy

## Causes of cerebral palsy

### Antenatal
- Development abnormalities
- Intrauterine infection
- Fetal hypoxia (maternal hypotension, placenta praevia, placenta haemorrhage)
- Pre-eclampsia
- Multiple pregnancies

### Natal
- Trauma
- Breech
- Prolonged or precipitous delivery
- Prematurity
- Postmaturity

### Postnatal (preterm)
- Cerebral ischaemia/Haemorrhage

> **Box 17.9: Classification of cerebral palsy**
>
> **Spastic cerebral palsy**
> Hemiplegia
> Paraplegia
> Tetraplegia
>
> **Ataxic cerebral palsy**
> Cerebellar signs
>
> **Athetoid cerebral palsy**
> Athetoid movements
> Dystonia
>
> **Mixed cerebral palsy**
> Mixed features of above

- Hypoxia (respiratory distress syndrome)
- Acidosis
- Hypothermia
- Hypoglycaemia

### Postnatal (term)
- Encephalitis
- Meningitis
- Hypoxia
- Kernicterus
- Trauma

# Miscellaneous CNS disorders

## Narcolepsy

- Irresistible desire to sleep in inappropriate circumstances
- Associated with abnormal EEG pattern of REM sleep
- Due to abnormalities of mono-aminergic pathways in brainstem and reticular formation
- Associated with the following:
  1 *Cataplexy*: abrupt reduction in muscle tone leading to collapse to ground Consciousness preserved
  2 *Sleep paralysis*: episodes of complete paralysis (except respiratory muscles) Occurs transiently on waking
  3 *Hypnagogic hallucinations*: hallucinations that occur as patient falls asleep

## Benign intracranial hypertension

- Raised intracranial pressure with no mass or hydrocephalus
- Due to increased cerebral blood volume leading to reduced CSF absorption
- Clinically: papilloedema
  Impaired visual acuity
  Reduced colour vision
  Sixth-nerve palsy
  CT shows normal or small ventricles
  CSF opening pressure markedly raised
  Permanent loss of vision may occur

### Causes of benign intracranial hypertension
- Idiopathic
- Obesity
- Empty sella
- Dural sinus thrombosis
- Hypervitaminosis A
- Tetracycline
- Nitrofurantoin
- Steroids

## Causes of Wernicke–Korsakoff syndrome

- Alcohol abuse
- Thiamine deficiency
- Prolonged vomiting
- Head injury
- Cerebral anoxia
- Cerebral tumours (primary and secondary)

# Causes of intracerebral calcification

- Pineal gland (normal)
- Congenital toxoplasmosis
- Tuberous sclerosis
- Sturge–Weber syndrome
- Craniopharyngioma
- Tuberculosis
- Old haematoma
- Old abscess
- Hyperparathyroidism
- Pseudohypoparathyroidism
- Cystercicosis
- Hydatid cyst

# Causes of hydrocephalus

- Cerebral atrophy
- Non-communicating (obstructed CSF outflow)
  Space-occupying lesion
  Aqueduct stenosis
  Dandy–Walker syndrome
  Arnold–Chiari malformation
- Communicating (impaired CSF absorption)
  Subarachnoid haemorrhage
  Meningitis
- Excess CSF production
  Choroid plexus papilloma

- Normal-pressure hydrocephalus
- Cerebral dysgenesis

# Spinal cord and peripheral nervous system

## Anatomy of the spinal cord

- Average length 45 cm
- Extends from foramen magnus to lower border of L1
- Below L1, nerve roots form the cauda equina

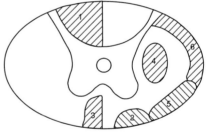

Uncrossed       Crossed

**Fig. 17.7: Cross-section of cord showing major pathways (see Table 17.5)**

Table 17.5: Spinal cord pathways (see Fig. 17.7)

| Number | Name | Function |
|--------|------|----------|
| 1 | Dorsal column | Joint position sense |
|   |   | Vibration sense |
|   |   | 2-point discrimination |
| 2 | Spinothalamic | Pain |
|   |   | Temperature |
|   |   | Touch |
| 3 | Anterior corticospinal | Head movement |
| 4 | Lateral corticospinal | Limb motor function |
| 5 | Anterior spinocerebellar | Reflex arcs |
| 6 | Posterior spinocerebellar | Unconscious proprioception |

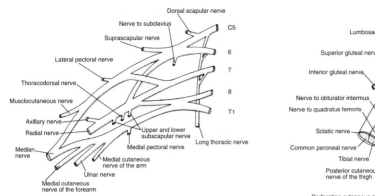

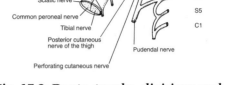

**Fig. 17.8: Roots, trunks, divisions, cords and terminal branches of the brachial plexus**

**Fig. 17.9: Roots, trunks, divisions and terminal branches of the sacral plexus**

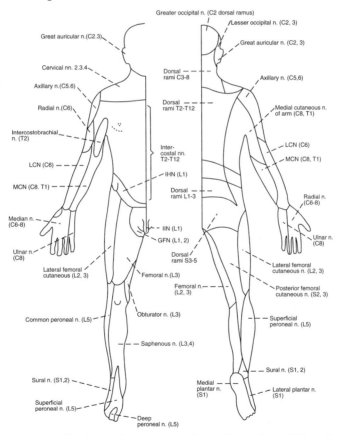

**Fig. 17.10: Distribution of cutaneous branches of peripheral nerves.**
**GFN: genitofemoral nerve; IIN: ilioinguinal nerve;**
**IHN: iliohypogastric nerve; LCN: lateral cutaneous nerve of the forearm;**
**MCN: medial cutaneous nerve of the forearm**

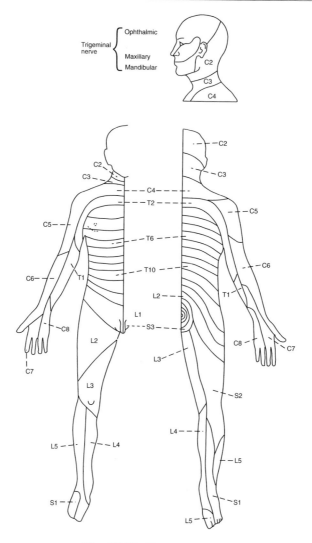

**Fig. 17.11: Dermatomes**

- Expansion of spinal cord at lower end is called the conus medullaris
- Blood supply comes from two anterior spinal arteries which supply the anterior of the cord (branches of vertebral artery)
- There are also two posterior spinal arteries (branches of vertebral or posterior cerebellar arteries) which supply the rest

### Spinal nerve roots

- Each segment of spinal cord gives off dorsal and ventral spinal nerve roots
- There are therefore a total of 31 nerve roots (8 cervical, 12 thoracic, 5 lumbar, 5 sacral, 1 coccygeal)

### Brachial plexus

- Formed by union of anterior rami of C5–T1 (Fig. 17.8)

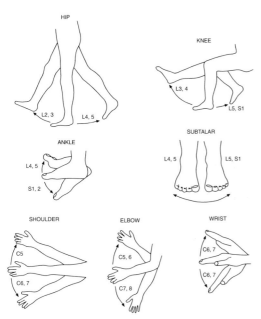

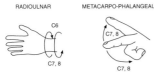

**Fig. 17.12: Spinal nerve roots that control limb movements**

## *Sacral plexus*
- Formed by union of anterior rami of L4–S4 (Fig. 17.9)

# Anatomy of the peripheral nerves

- Nerve fascicles are surrounded by connective tissue (perineurium)
- Maintains blood–nerve barrier to protect the endoneurium
- Nerves may be myelinated or unmyelinated
- Myelinated are large in size and convey rapid-conduction
- Myelin produced by Schwann cells
- Unmyelinated are small and convey slow conduction

## *Myotomes*
- C6: Biceps, brachioradialis, radial extensors of wrist
- C7: Triceps, finger extensors, ulnar extensors of wrist
- C8: Finger flexors
- T1: Intrinsic muscles of hand
- L4: Quadriceps femoris
- L5: Extensor hallucis longus
- S1: Hamstrings, calf muscles, small muscles of foot

## *Control of reflexes*
- Biceps: C5, C6
- Triceps: C7
- Brachioradialis: C5, C6
- Knee: L3, L4
- Ankle: S1
- Plantars: S1

# Spinal cord lesions

## Causes of acute or subacute paraplegia

### *Trauma*

### *Vertebral disease*
- Metastases
- Spondylosis
- Disc prolapse
- Paget's disease
- Rheumatoid arthritis
- Pott's disease

### *Infection*
- Epidural abscess
- TB abscess
- Syphilitic myelitis
- HIV

### *Inflammatory*
- Multiple sclerosis
- Idiopathic myelitis
- SLE

- Sarcoid

## Tumours
- Extradural
- Intradural
- Carcinoma
- Lymphoma
- Myeloma
- Leukaemia
- Meningioma
- Neurofibroma

## Haematological
- Epidural or intramedullary haemorrhage

## Vascular
- Anterior spinal artery occlusion
- Aortic dissection
- Vasculitis
- AV malformation

## Metabolic
- Subacute combined degeneration

# Causes of chronic progressive paraplegia

## Vertebral disease
- Spondylosis
- Disc prolapse
- Paget's disease
- Rheumatoid arthritis
- Pott's disease
- Ankylosing spondylitis

## Syringomyelia
- Trauma
- Arnold–Chiari malformation
- Spinal cord tumours
- Klippel–Feil deformity

## Inflammatory
- Multiple sclerosis
- Sarcoid

- Radiation
- Arachnoiditis

## Primary spinal cord tumours

## Infection
- Syphilis
- Human T-cell lymphotropic virus (HTLV-1)

## Vascular
- AV malformation

## Metabolic
- Subacute combined degeneration

## Hereditary
- Hereditary spastic paraplegia
- Cerebral palsy

## Degenerative
- Motor neuron disease

# Features of spinal cord lesions

- Progressive leg weakness and bladder symptoms should be considered to be due to spinal cord compression until proven otherwise
- Total loss of bladder control for more than 24 hours is likely to be permanent
- Urgency of investigations depends on speed of progression of symptoms
- Development of bladder symptoms indicates need for urgent investigation
- Commonest causes of cervical cord lesions are demyelination and cervical spondylosis
- Compressive lesions tend to produce dorsal column impairment
- Intrinsic lesions tend to produce spinothalamic disturbance
- Above site of lesion, lower motor neuron signs are found

- Below site of lesion, upper motor neuron signs are found
- Sensory level may indicate site of lesion

# Developmental abnormalities of spinal cord

## Spina bifida
- Cause unknown
- Increased risk in females and in patients taking sodium valproate or carbamazepine
- Folate supplements in early pregnancy reduces risk
- Most commonly affects lumbar region
- Defect may affect one isolated vertebra
- If many segments are affected the following may occur: tuft of hair overlying defect
  Low tethered spinal cord
  Dermal sinus
  Intraspinal lipoma
  Diasternatomyelia (splitting of cord)

## Spina bifida cystica
- Severe form with prolapse of meninges through bony defect
  *Meningocele*: only meninges prolapse
  *Meningomyelocele*: neural tissue and meninges prolapse
  *Rachischisis*: wide-open defect
- Usually associated with Arnold–Chiari malformation type 2 and hydrocephalus

## Spina bifida occulta
- Partial cauda equina syndrome
- May be asymptomatic
- May be a long history of bladder difficulties
- No intervention usually needed

## Arnold–Chiari malformations
### Type 1
- Cerebellar tonsillar herniation through foramen magnum, often with syringomyelia
- Presents with features of syringomyelia, ataxia, nystagmus, cranial nerve palsies, tetraparesis

### Type 2
- Cerebellar tonsils and vermis and lower brainstem herniate through foramen magnum, leading to hydrocephalus
- Often associated with platybasia (upward displacement of skull base)

## Dandy–Walker syndrome
- Hypoplasia of cerebellar vermis
- Cystic dilatation of fourth ventricle
- Expansion of posterior fossa
- Hydrocephalus

## Klippel–Feil deformity
- Fusion of two or more cervical vertebrae
- Abnormal unstable joints in cervical spine
- Short neck
- Low hairline
- Associated with platybasia, syringomyelia and conductive hearing loss

# Anterior horn cell diseases

- Motor neurone disease
- Werdnig–Hoffman disease
- Kugelberg–Welander syndrome
- Poliomyelitis

## Motor neuron disease

- Unknown aetiology
- Cognitive function usually intact
- Gradually progressive condition (no remission)
- No sensory signs or bladder problems
- Presents with a mixture of lower and upper motor neuron signs
- Supportive treatment only

# Peripheral neuropathy

## Pathophysiology

### Axonal degeneration
- Lesion of axon and cell body
- Regeneration may occur after a period of Wallerian degeneration
- Regeneration proceeds at 1–2 mm/day

### Demyelination
- If severe may lead to axonal degeneration
- Remyelination occurs in short distinct intervals
- Characteristic findings of greatly reduced conduction velocities

## Clinical classification

- *Mononeuropathy*: one nerve affected
- *Mononeuritis multiplex*: more than one nerve affected
- *Polyneuropathy*: diffuse symmetrical involvement of peripheral nerves

## Clinical features

### Motor involvement
- Weakness, wasting, fasciculation, hyporeflexia
- In polyneuropathy signs are usually more marked distally

### Sensory involvement
- Negative symptoms consist of numbness and sensory loss
- Positive symptoms include hyperaesthesia and pain
- Neuropathy affecting large fibres leads to impairment of touch, pressure, two-point discrimination and joint position sense
- Neuropathy affecting small fibres leads to impairment of pain and temperature
- In polyneuropathy sensory loss occurs in a stocking-and-glove distal distribution

### Autonomic involvement
- Causalgia (severe burning pain after damage to major limb nerves)
- Associated with reflex sympathetic discharge
- In a minority autonomic dysfunction is severe, leading to postural hypotension, impaired sweating and incontinence

## Causes of mononeuritis multiplex

### Diabetes mellitus

### Connective tissue disease
- SLE
- Vasculitis
- Rheumatoid arthritis

### Infection
- Leprosy
- Herpes zoster virus
- Lyme disease

### Familial entrapment neuropathy
- Tomaculous neuropathy

### Physical injury
- Radiotherapy
- Electrical
- Thermal
- Ischaemia

### Malignancy
- Carcinomatous infiltration
- Lymphoma
- Neurofibromatosis
- Malignant nerve tumours
- Paraproteinaemia

### Miscellaneous
- Sarcoid
- Post vaccination

# Causes of polyneuropathy

### Inflammatory
- Guillain–Barré syndrome
- Serum sickness
- Sarcoid
- SLE
- PAN

### Nutritional
- Vitamin B$_{12}$ deficiency
- Thiamine deficiency
- Pellagra

### Infection
- Leprosy
- Diphtheria
- Measles
- Mumps
- Glandular fever
- Brucellosis
- HIV

### Drugs
- Isoniazid
- Nitrofurantoin
- Vincristine
- Metronidazole
- Disulfiram

- Dapsone
- Sulphonamide
- Phenytoin
- Pyridoxine
- Amiodarone
- Tricyclic antidepressants

### Metabolic
- Diabetes mellitus
- Renal failure
- Porphyria
- Hypothyroidism
- Amyloid
- Metachromatic leukodystrophy

### Malignancy
- Non-metastatic manifestation
- Myeloma
- Paraproteinaemia

### Toxic
- Alcohol
- Mercury
- Lead
- Arsenic
- Gold
- Thallium
- Insecticides

### Hereditary
- Charcot–Marie–Tooth
- Hereditary sensory neuropathy
- Friedreich's ataxia
- Riley–Day syndrome
- Fabry's disease
- Refsum's disease

# Guillain–Barré syndrome

- Usually follows a viral illness (usually upper respiratory tract infection)
- Mainly presents with distal sensory symptoms (no objective sensory signs usually)
- Later develop ascending paralysis (no muscle wasting)

- Bladder dysfunction rare
- Bulbar weakness may occur leading to cranial nerve palsies (especially of the seventh nerve)
- Autonomic dysfunction may occur
- CSF protein markedly raised
- Vital capacity must be monitored to detect respiratory muscle involvement (arterial blood gases not sufficient: when $Po_2$ falls, patient is already severely compromised)
- Miller–Fisher syndrome is an ocular variant with good prognosis and requiring no treatment
  *Treatment*: ventilation if vital capacity falls, human immunoglobulin infusion, plasma exchange, steroids of no proven benefit

# Causes of brachial plexus lesions

### Non-birth trauma
- Most commonly motorcycle accidents

### Birth trauma
- Erb's palsy
- Klumpke's paralysis

### Structural abnormalities
- Cervical rib

### Neuralgic amyotrophy
- Post vaccination
- Connective tissue disorders

### Malignancy
- Carcinoma of the lung
- Carcinoma of the breast
- Lymphoma
- Neurofibroma

### Radiation

# Erb's palsy

- Damage to C5 and C6 resulting from birth trauma
- Leads to paralysis of deltoid, biceps, brachioradialis
- Leads to winged scapula and sensory loss over the lateral aspect of the shoulder/upper arm

# Klumpke's paralysis

- Damage to T1 resulting from birth trauma
- Leads to paralysis of the intrinsic muscles of the hand
- Leads to the development of claw hand, Horner's syndrome and sensory loss over the medial border of the forearm and medial two fingers

# Causes of lumbosacral plexus lesions

- Disc prolapse
- Malignancy (cervix, rectum, uterus, bladder, prostate, lymphoma)
- Pelvic fracture
- Fetal head during childbirth

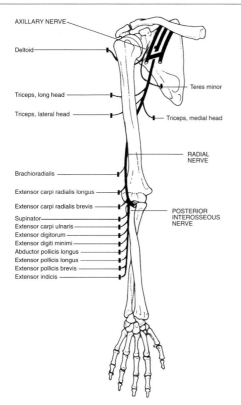

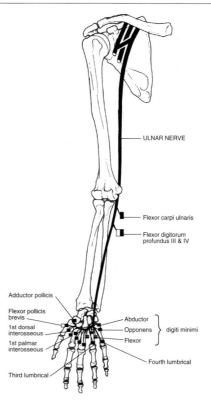

**Fig. 17.13: Diagram of the axillary and radial nerves, and the muscles they supply**

**Fig. 17.14: Diagram of the ulnar nerve and the muscles it supplies**

# Radial nerve lesions

### *Causes of radial nerve lesions*
- Pressure palsy (Saturday night palsy)
- Fractured humerus
- Axillary trauma

# Ulnar nerve lesions

### *Causes of ulnar nerve lesions*

> **Box 17.10: Features of radial nerve lesions**
>
> Wrist drop
> Sensory loss over the dorsum of the hand

- Fracture/dislocation of elbow
- Laceration of the wrist
- Pressure palsy
- Carpal tunnel syndrome
- Vibrating tools

# Median nerve lesions

### *Causes of median nerve lesions*
- Carpal tunnel syndrome
- Trauma

# Sciatic nerve lesions

### *Causes of sciatic nerve lesions*
- Lumbar disc prolapse

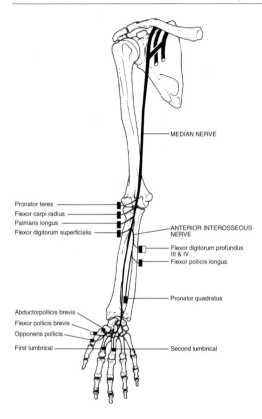

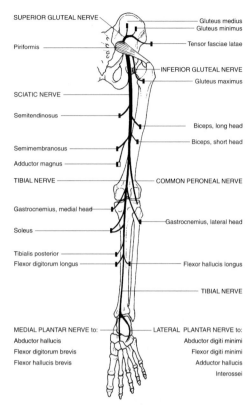

**Fig. 17.15: Diagram of the median nerve and the muscles it supplies**

**Fig. 17.16: Diagram of nerves on the posterior aspect of the lower limb and the muscles they supply**

- Penetrating injuries

- Fractures of pelvis/femur/tibia/fibula
- Posterior dislocation of the hip
- Pressure palsy
- Baker's cyst

**Box 17.11: Features of ulnar nerve lesions**

**Above elbow**
Weakness of finger flexion

**At elbow**
Radial deviation of the wrist
Weakness of finger abduction
Claw hand
Sensory loss over dorsum and medial palm of the hand

**At wrist**
Claw hand
Sensory loss over the medial half of the palm of the hand

**Box 17.12: Features of median nerve lesions**

**At elbow**
Impaired pronation
Weak wrist flexion
Ulnar deviation

**At wrist**
Weakness and wasting of thenar eminence
Sensory loss over the lateral 2½ fingers of the palm of the hand

## Box 17.13: Features of sciatic nerve lesions

**Lesion of main sciatic nerve**
Paralysis of knee flexion
Foot drop
Sensory loss below knee
Absent ankle jerks
Plantar response

**Lesion of tibial nerve**
Impaired plantar flexion
Inversion of foot
Toe flexion
Claw deformity of toes
Sensory loss on the sole of the foot

**Lesion of common peroneal nerve**
Foot drop
Impaired eversion of the foot
Toe extension
Sensory loss anterolateral aspect of lower leg/dorsum of the foot

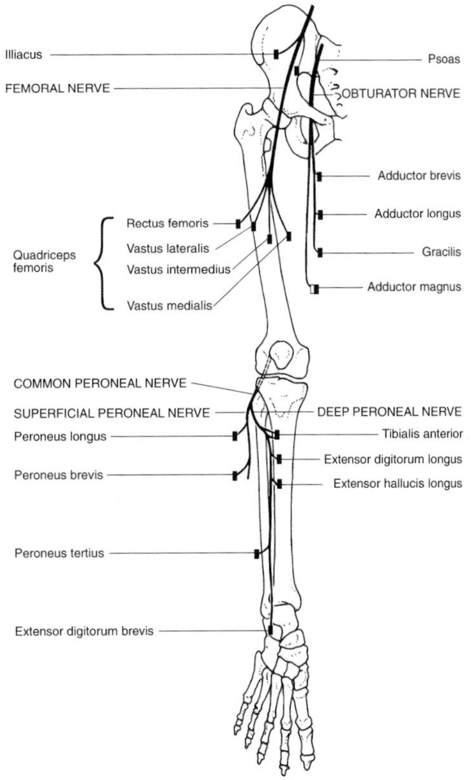

# Femoral nerve lesions

## Causes of femoral nerve lesions
- Fractured pelvis
- Fractured femur
- Posterior dislocation of the hip
- Psoas abscess
- Psoas haematoma

## Box 17.14: Features of femoral nerve lesions

Impaired knee extension
Absent knee reflex
Sensory loss of the anterolateral aspect of the thigh

**Fig. 17.17: Diagram of nerves on the anterior aspect of the lower limb and the muscles they supply**

# Neuromuscular disease

## Disease of neuromuscular transmission

- Myasthenia gravis
- Eaton–Lambert syndrome
- *Clostridium botulinum*
- SLE
- Polymyositis
- Anticholinesterase poisons (nerve gas)
- Venoms
- Magnesium poisoning
- Aminoglycosides

- Suxamethonium
- Anticonvulsants

## Myasthenia gravis
- Characterised by fatiguable weakness of striated muscle
- May be localised or generalised
- Due to defects of neurotransmitter release at neuromuscular junction
- In young patients associated with thymic hyperplasia
- In older patients associated with thymic tumours, which may be benign or malignant
- Also associated with other autoimmune diseases (especially Graves' thyrotoxicosis)
- In 90% of patients acetylcholine receptor antibodies are found (titre not related to disease severity)
- Usually affects external ocular muscles initially
- Bulbar muscle weakness may occur
- Reflexes normal
- Wasting of affected muscles may occur in advanced disease

### Tensilon test
- Give test dose edrophonium (Tensilon) to ensure no major adverse effects
- Give full dose and check for fatiguability
- Give control injection and check fatiguability
- Both doctor and patient should be blinded if possible
- Useful to have two doctors perform the test to strengthen subjective assessment of response

### Treatment
- Avoid aminoglycosides, anticonvulsants, suxamethonium
- Long-acting anticholinesterase (pyridostigmine)
- Thymectomy useful if thymoma

- Immunosuppression with prednisolone or azathioprine may be useful in those not responding
- Plasma exchange useful in life-threatening situations

## Eaton–Lambert syndrome
- Prejunctional defect leading to failure of release of acetylcholine
- No bulbar involvement
- Tendon reflexes usually absent
- 50% associated with small cell carcinoma of the lung, 50% idiopathic

# Muscle disease

## Classification of myopathy

### Muscular dystrophy
- Duchenne
- Becker
- Limb girdle
- Childhood
- Facioscapulohumeral

### Infective
- Clostridium perfringens
- *Staphylococcus aureus*
- Influenza virus
- Coxsackie virus
- Echovirus
- Cystercicosis
- Trichinosis
- Toxoplasmosis
- Trypanosomiasis

### Toxic
- Corticosteroids
- Chloroquine
- Amiodarone
- Penicillamine
- Alcohol
- Zidovudine
- Clofibrate

**Box 17.15: Clinical features of myopathy**

Weakness, wasting, hypotonia
Pain: inflammatory disorders
Fatiguability: myasthenia gravis
Myotonia: delayed muscle relaxation, seen in myotonic disorders
Tendon reflexes usually preserved until wasting severe
Most acquired myopathy affects proximal limb muscles

### Myotonic disorders
- Dystrophia myotonica
- Myotonia congenita (Thomsen's disease)

### Inflammatory
- Dermatopolymyositis
- Connective tissue disease
- Sarcoid
- Eosinophilic myositis
- Granulomatous myositis

### Endocrine disease
- Cushing's syndrome
- Hypothyroidism
- Hyperthyroidism
- Addison's disease
- Hyperparathyroidism
- Acromegaly

### Metabolic
- Glycogen storage disease
- Periodic paralysis
- Mitochondrial myopathy

## Dystrophia myotonica

- Presents at 30–50 years of age
- Initially produces distal myopathy and myotonia
- Later may cause proximal muscle involvement, including respiratory failure

- Other features: low IQ, dementia, frontal balding in males, cardiomyopathy, diabetes mellitus, gonadal atrophy, infertility, sleep apnoea, dysphagia

## Myotonia congenita

- Presents at birth
- No myopathy (may be hypertrophy)
- Improves with age and exercise. Exacerbated by cold, rest

# Autonomic nervous system

## Sympathetic trunk

- Originates in hypothalamus
- Extends whole length of spinal cord
- Ganglia are associated with each spinal segment except in the cervical cord, where there are three: the superior cervical ganglion (C2–C4); the middle cervical ganglion (C5–C6); the inferior cervical (stellate) ganglion (C7, C8, T1)

## Parasympathetic trunk

- Cranial outflow supplies viscera in head and neck via oculomotor, facial and glossopharyngeal nerves
- Supplies thoracic and upper abdominal viscera via vagus
- Sacral outflow supplies lower abdominal and pelvic viscera via S2–S4

## Box 17.16:  Features of autonomic neuropathy

Inability to sweat
Gustatory sweating
Impaired light reflex
Postural hypotension
Vomiting (gastric stasis)
Dysphagia (oesophageal spasm)
Diarrhoea (colonic atony)
Erectile impotence
Ejaculatory failure
Urinary retention
Overflow urinary incontinence
Sudden death

# Causes of autonomic dysfunction

- Idiopathic
- Multiple system atrophy
- Idiopathic Parkinson's disease
- Diabetes mellitus
- Alcohol
- Phenothiazines
- Tricyclic antidepressants
- Antihypertensive drugs
- Craniopharyngioma
- Cerebrovascular disease
- Tabes dorsalis
- Trypanosomiasis
- Familial dysautonomia
- Amyloid
- Fabry's disease
- Guillain–Barré syndrome
- Porphyria
- Spinal cord lesions

# Clinical case scenarios

## Spastic paraparesis

- There are bilateral lower limb upper motor neuron signs
- In patients with chronic immobility there may be muscle wasting
- In severe cases there may be flexion contractures

- Other features to look for:
    Signs of multiple sclerosis cerebellar signs and pes cavus (Friedreich's ataxia)
    Upper limb lower motor neuron signs and wasted hands (cervical spondylosis, syringomyelia or motor neuron disease)
    Horner's syndrome (syringomyelia)
    Posterior column loss (tabes dorsalis, subacute combined degeneration of the cord)
    Argyll Robertson pupils (tabes dorsalis)
    Raised intracranial pressure (parasagittal meningioma)
    Dissociated sensory loss (syringomyelia)
    Peripheral stocking sensory loss (subacute combined degeneration of the cord)

## Bulbar palsy

- The tongue is flaccid and fasciculating and poorly mobile
- Speech is indistinct and has a nasal quality
- Palatal movements are absent

- Other features to look for:
    Skeletal muscle fasciculation (motor neuron disease)

Nystagmus
Horner's syndrome and dissociated
  sensory loss (syringobulbia)
Peripheral neuropathy
  (Guillain–Barré syndrome)
Old polio
Argyll Robertson pupils
  (neurosyphilis)

# Pseudobulbar palsy

- The tongue is wasted, rigid and immobile
- The patient has dysarthria
- Palatal movements are absent
- The jaw jerk is exaggerated
- The patient may be emotionally labile
- Other features to look for:
  Hemiplegia (CVA)
  Signs of multiple sclerosis
  Skeletal muscle fasciculation (motor neuron disease)

# Motor neuron disease

- There is wasting, weakness and fasciculation of the upper limb muscles
- The upper limb reflexes may be increased, decreased or absent
- The patient has a spastic paraparesis
- The patient may have a bulbar palsy

- Other features to look for:
  Limited neck movement and generalised arthritis (cervical spondylosis)
  Horner's syndrome, dissociated sensory loss (syringomyelia)
  Old polio
  Young age, absent pyramidal and bulbar signs (spinal muscular atrophy)

# Cerebellar disease

- There is horizontal nystagmus, with the fast phase towards the side of the lesion
- In the upper limbs there is an intention tremor, past pointing and dysdiadochokinesia
- In the lower limbs there is impaired heel-to-shin test and the gait is ataxic
- There may be hypotonia
- Romberg's test is negative
- There may also be dysarthria and staccato speech
- In vermis lesions there are few or no abnormalities seen when examining the patient on the bed, but on standing the patient has a wide-based ataxic gait

- Other features to look for:
  Features of multiple sclerosis
  Clubbing, cachexia (paraneoplastic syndrome)
  Features of chronic alcohol abuse
  Gingival hypertrophy, hirsutism (phenytoin)
  Thyroid status
  Pes cavus (Friedreich's ataxia)
  Cranial nerve palsies (Arnold–Chiari malformation)

# Dystrophia myotonica

- The patient has typical myopathic facies (drooping mouth, sad, lifeless and sleepy expression)
- There is frontal balding (in males)
- There is ptosis (may be unilateral or bilateral)
- There is wasting of the facial muscles, sternomastoid, shoulder girdle and quadriceps
- Tendon reflexes are absent
- The patient may have cataracts
- The patient has myotonia (delayed grip release, difficulty opening eyes after firm closure)

- In advanced cases there may be limb muscle wasting and weakness

- Other features to look for:
    Evidence of cardiomyopathy
    Cognitive impairment
    Dysarthria
    Gonadal atrophy
    Features of diabetes mellitus

## Myotonia congenita

- The patient has myotonia but no other features of dystrophia myotonica

## Abnormal gait

- Review types of abnormal gait given earlier in the chapter and, having identified the type of gait, direct further examination to finding the cause
- Commonest gait abnormalities found are cerebellar ataxia, spastic paraplegia, sensory ataxia and Parkinson's disease

## Seventh lower motor neuron cranial nerve palsy

- There is paralysis of the upper and lower face as evidenced by inability to close eyes, raise eyebrows, smoothing of nasolabial folds and inability to puff out cheeks or bare teeth on affected side
- If bilateral may be difficult to recognise as there is no asymmetry

- Other features to look for:
    Evidence of herpes zoster on the external auditory meatus

    (Ramsay–Hunt syndrome)
    Parotid enlargement (tumour)
    Fifth, sixth and seventh cranial nerve palsies (acoustic neuroma)
    Hyperacusis (involvement of the nerve to the stapedius)
    Taste to anterior of tongue
    Brainstem signs
    Features of multiple sclerosis
    Features of motor neuron disease

## Friedreich's ataxia

- The young patient has bilateral cerebellar signs in the upper and lower limbs
- There is pes cavus and a high arched palate; there is also kyphoscoliosis
- The ankle jerks are absent and the plantars are extensor
- Joint position sense and vibration sense are reduced in both feet
- Romberg's test may be positive (if there is impaired joint position sense) or negative

- Other features to look for:
    Optic atrophy
    Cardiomyopathy
    Evidence of diabetes mellitus
    Cognitive impairment

## Charcot–Marie–Tooth

- There is distal wasting of the lower limb, with weakness
- The ankle jerks are absent and there is no plantar response
- In the feet there is pes cavus and clawing of the toes
- There may also be associated distal sensory impairment and posterior column signs
- In some cases there may be distal wasting of the upper limb, particularly

the hands
- The gait is high-stepping

PEG tube
Central line (plasmapheresis)

## Speech abnormalities

### Dysarthria
- Revise causes of dysarthria and direct examination to identify cause
- Be sure to examine patient's mouth
- Also look for other language disorders

### Dysphasia
- By asking the patient simple questions or to perform simple commands (touch your nose, lift your arm up, etc.) you will be able to identify problems with reception and/or expression
- Look for nominal aphasia by holding up a simple object and ask the patient to name it (patient will be unable to do this. but when you ask them to pick up the object they will be able to do so)

## Myasthenia gravis

- There is ptosis (may be unilaterial or bilateral)
- There may be strabismus and diplopia
- There is generalised facial weakness
- The patient snarls when attempting to smile and cannot whistle
- The voice may be weak and nasal in quality and there may be dysarthria
- There may also be proximal muscle limb weakness
- All of the above myopathies are exacerbated by repetitive movement (ask patient to count out loud from 20 down to 1)

- Other features to look for:
  Thymectomy scar
  Tracheostomy

## Syringomyelia

- The patient has wasting of the small muscles of the hand and lower motor neurone signs in both arms
- There is impaired pinprick and temperature sensation in both arms but joint position sense, vibration sense and two-point discrimination are normal (dissociated sensory loss)

- Other features to look for:
  Charcot joints and scars on arms (trauma secondary to sensory loss)
  Horner's syndrome (C8–T1 involvement)
  Kyphoscoliosis
  Ataxia, nystagmus, bulbar palsy (syringobulbia)

## Acoustic neuroma

- There is sensorineural hearing loss in one ear (Rinne's test shows air conduction greater than bone conduction but both are reduced. Weber's test is referred to the unaffected side)
- There are associated fifth, sixth and seventh cranial nerve palsies on the affected side
- There may be unilateral cerebellar signs
- There may be papilloedema with large tumours

## Subacute combined degeneration of the cord

- The patient presents with lower limb dorsal column signs (impaired joint

position sense, vibration sense and two-point discrimination)
- Romberg's test is positive
- The ankle jerks are absent and the plantar response is extensor
- There are no cerebellar signs or pes cavus (Friedreich's ataxia)
- The pupils are normal (no evidence of tabes dorsalis)
- The patient may not be anaemic

- Other features to look for:
    Multiple abdominal scars (Crohn's disease or previous gastrectomy)
    Splenomegaly (pernicious anaemia)
    Optic atrophy
    Cognitive impairment
    Oral aphthous ulcers (Crohn's disease)

# Wasting of the small muscles of the hand

- May have a number of causes which should be looked for
- Note distribution of wasting and weak movements

## Median nerve palsy
- There is wasting of the thenar eminence and weakness of opponens pollicis
- There is sensory loss of the lateral half of the palm

## Ulnar nerve palsy
- There is wasting of the hypothenar eminence and weakness of finger abduction
- In advanced cases there may be a claw hand and there is sensory loss over the medial half of the palm

## Brachial plexus lesions
- This produces sensory loss on the medial side of the palm and forearm

- Look for Reynaud's phenomenon (cervical rib) or Horner's syndrome, clubbing and lymphadenopathy (Pancoast tumour)

## Cervical spine lesions
- There is spastic paraparesis and lower motor neuron lesions in both arms

## Charcot–Marie–Tooth
- There is distal wasting and weakness, which may affect arms and legs, and pes cavus

## Motor neuron disease
- There may be visible fasciculation
- The patient may have a spastic paraparesis and bulbar palsy

## Syringomyelia
- There is disocciated sensory loss and upper limb lower motor neuron signs
- There may be Horner's syndrome, bulbar palsy and nystagmus

## Generalised cachexia
- Wasting of the hands may be part of a generalised cachectic syndrome secondary to malignancy, advanced cardiac or pulmonary disease, malabsorption, malnutrition

# Peripheral neuropathy

- There is loss of all sensory modalities in a glove and/or stocking distribution

- Other features to look for:
    Signs of diabetes mellitus
    Cachexia, clubbing and lymphadenopathy (carcinomatosis)
    Absent ankle jerks and extensor plantar responses (subacute combined degeneration of the cord)

Cerebellar signs and pes cavus
(Friedreich's ataxia)
Distal muscle wasting
(Charcot–Marie–Tooth)
Purpura (vasculitis)
Thyroid status
Acromegalic facies
Uraemic facies (renal failure)
Signs of alcohol induced liver
disease

# Muscular dystrophy

## *Facioscapulohumeral dystrophy*

- The patient has a dull, unlined, expressionless face (myopathic facies)
- The lips are open and slack
- There is wasting of the facial and shoulder girdle muscles
- The superior margins of the scapulae may be visible above the clavicles, from the front
- The movements of smiling, whistling and closing the eyes are impaired
- There is winging of the scapulae
- There may be weakness and wasting of the leg muscles (particularly foot drop)

## *Limb girdle (Erb's) muscular dystrophy*

- There is weakness and wasting of the limb girdle muscles
- There may be enlargement of the calf muscles
- The face is normal

## *Becker's muscular dystrophy*

The presentation of Becker's muscular dystrophy is very similar to that of Duchenne muscular dystrophy. However, the latter is usually more severe, leading to earlier disability (usually confined to a wheelchair by the age of 10) and earlier death (commonly around the age of 20). Duchenne muscular dystrophy is also associated with cardiomyopathy (not found in the other dystrophies).

- The patient is young (<50 years)
- There is enlargement of the calf and buttock muscles
- There is proximal limb weakness
- The gait is waddling (may be in a wheelchair)
- The face is normal

# 18 Geriatric medicine

## Contents

# Disability and handicap

## Disability

- May be defined as restriction or lack of ability to perform an activity
- Assessed by measuring activities of daily living (ADLs) and communication

### Primary ADL scores
- Concerned with basic activities (mobility, continence, dressing, washing, feeding, communication)
- Barthel ADL index most commonly used
- Lambeth disability screening questionnaire used to assess communication

### Barthel score (Box 18.1)
- Measures what patients actually do, not what they can do
- Well validated and reliable, especially among stroke patients
- Correlates well with mortality, length of stay and discharge destination
- Ceiling effect: only includes self-care tasks. Patients able to score highly despite marked disability
- Patients scoring highly should be assessed by a secondary ADL score

### Secondary ADL scores
- Instrumental/extended activities (shopping, cleaning, hobbies)
- May also give some indication of handicap
- Nottingham extended ADL scale, Frenchay activities index, modified Rankin scale (Oxford handicap scale) most commonly used

## Handicap

- May be defined as the disadvantage suffered by an individual as a result of ill health due to an inability to fulfil a role which is normal for someone of that age, sex and culture
- Usually results from impairment and disability, but is also dependent on society's view

### Example
Following a stroke (pathology), a man

**Box 18.1: Barthel index**

| | | |
|---|---|---|
| Bowels | 0 | Incontinent (or needs to be given enema) |
| | 1 | Occasional accident (once a week) |
| | 2 | Continent |
| Bladder | 0 | Incontinent (or catheterised and unable to manage) |
| | 1 | Occasional accident (max once per 24 hours) |
| | 2 | Continent |
| Grooming | 0 | Needs help with personal care (face, hair, teeth, shaving) |
| | 1 | Independent (implements provided) |
| Toilet use | 0 | Dependent |
| | 1 | Needs some help but can do something alone |
| | 2 | Independent (on and off, wiping, dressing) |
| Feeding | 0 | Unable |
| | 1 | Needs help with cutting and implements |
| | 2 | Independent (food within reach) |
| Transfer | 0 | Unable (no sitting balance) |
| | 1 | Major help (physical, one or two people), can sit |
| | 2 | Minor help (physical or verbal) |
| | 3 | Independent |
| Mobility | 0 | Immobile |
| | 1 | Wheelchair independent (including corners) |
| | 2 | Walks with the help of one person (physical or verbal) |
| | 3 | Independent |
| Dressing | 0 | Dependent |
| | 1 | Needs help but can do half unaided |
| | 2 | Independent (including buttons, laces etc) |
| Stairs | 0 | Unable |
| | 1 | Needs help (verbal, physical, carrying aid) |
| | 2 | Independent (up and down) |
| Bathing | 0 | Dependent |
| | 1 | Independent (bath: must get in and out unsupervised shower: unsupervised / unaided) |
| **Total** | **0–20** | |

developes a hemiplegia (impairment) and is unable to walk (disability). He goes to the cinema but cannot gain entry as there are no wheelchair ramps (handicap). However, if there were wheelchair ramps he would be able to go to the cinema and would suffer no handicap.

Handicap is more difficult to measure and is assessed by measuring quality of life (Philadelphia Geriatric Center Morale Scale (Box 18.2)), healthy active life expectancy (HALE), and quality-adjusted life years (QALYs). Such measures are currently underdeveloped and have limited clinical use

# Falls and immobility

• *Explained fall*: A simple trip, slip or

---

**Box 18.2: Philadelphia Geriatric Center Morale Scale (Anglicised version)**

| Question | Positive response *(score 1 point for each positive response)* |
|---|---|
| 1  Do things keep getting worse as you get older? | No |
| 2  Do you have as much energy as you did last year? | Yes |
| 3  Do you feel lonely much? | No |
| 4  Do you see enough of your friends and relatives? | Yes |
| 5  Do little things bother you more this year? | No |
| 6  As you get older do you feel less useful? | No |
| 7  Do you sometimes worry so much you can't sleep? | No |
| 8  As you get older are things better than expected? | Yes |
| 9  Do you sometimes feel that life isn't worth living? | No |
| 10  Are you as happy now as you were when you were younger? | Yes |
| 11  Do you have a lot to be sad about? | No |
| 12  Are you afraid of a lot of things? | No |
| 13  Do you get angry more than you used to? | No |
| 14  Is life hard for you most of the time? | No |
| 15  Are you satisfied with your life today? | Yes |
| 16  Do you take things hard? | No |
| 17  Do you get upset easily? | No |
|  | **Total 0–17** *(The higher the score the better the quality of life)* |

---

environmental hazard leading to the fall
- *Unexplained fall*: No apparent cause for the fall
- *Recurrent falls*: More than two falls per year

# Risk factors for falls

## Disease
- Gait/balance problems
- Previous falls
- Visual impairment
- Arthritis
- Cerebrovascular disease
- Malnourishment
- Cardiovascular disease
- Neuromuscular disease
- Hearing impairment

## Drugs
- Alcohol
- Antiparkinsonian drugs
- Antidepressants
- Diuretics
- Antihypertensives
- Benzodiazepines
- Tranquillisers

## Psychosocial
- Advanced age
- Cognitive impairment
- Low ADL
- F > M
- Anxiety/Depression
- Living alone
- Institutionalisation

## Environmental
- Hazards
- Seasonal: increased fall rate in winter

| Box 18.3: Consequences of falls | Box 18.4: Consequences of immobility |
|---|---|
| Soft tissue injury | Pressure sores |
| Fractures | Venous thromboembolism |
| Increased risk of further falls | Malnutrition |
| Immobility | Muscle wasting |
| Dependency | Osteoporosis |
| Institutionalisation | Stroke |
| Anxiety | Ischaemic heart disease |
| Depression | Renal failure |
| Social withdrawal | Constipation |
| Impaired quality of life | Urinary incontinence |
| Financial loss | Sepsis |
| Death | Depression |
| | Institutionalisation |
| | Impaired quality of life |

# Prevention of falls

## *Primary prevention*
- Screening: Falls risk score (Table 18.1) Age > 75 – yearly GP health check
- Treatment of medical illnesses
- Avoidance of toxic drugs
- Environmental modifications: OT home assessments
- Specialist hospital-based clinics for at-risk patients (Falls Clinic)

## *Secondary prevention*
- All of the above

### Table 18.1: Falls risk score

| Known previous fall | No |
| | Yes * |
| Medications | None |
| | Tranquillisers/sedatives * |
| | Diuretics * |
| | Antihypertensives * |
| | Antiparkinsonian drugs * |
| | Antidepressants * |
| | Other medications |
| Sensory deficits | None |
| | Visual impairment * |
| | Hearing impairment * |
| | Limbs (amputation, stroke, neuropathy) * |
| Mental state | Orientated |
| | Confused * |
| Gait | Normal |
| | Safe with walking aid |
| | Unsafe with walking aid * |
| | Unable * |

* Score one point each  (score >3 indicates a high risk of falling)

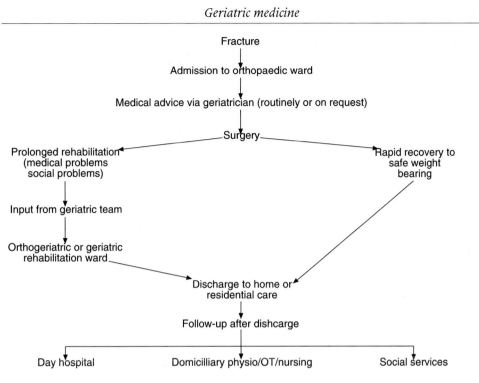

**Fig. 18.1: Guidelines for orthogeriatric liaison
(Royal College of Physicians, 1989)**

- Identification and correction of the causes of falls
- Orthogeriatric liaison (Fig. 18.1)
- Close liaison with A&E departments

# Pressure sores

## Aetiology of pressure sores

- Prolonged immobility
- Sensory impairment
- Anaemia
- Hypoproteinaemia
- Malnutrition
- Urinary incontinence
- Acute illness
- Diabetes mellitus
- Advanced age
- Corticosteroids

# Cognitive impairment

## Causes of delirium

- Drugs
- Alcohol
- Malignancy
- Trauma
- Epilepsy
- Vascular
- Sepsis
- Metabolic disturbance
- Endocrine disorders

## Clinical features of delirium

*Clouding of consciousness*
- Acute-onset, fluctuating course

## Table 18.2: Waterlow pressure sore risk assessment

| Feature | Score | Feature | Score | Feature | Score |
|---|---|---|---|---|---|
| *Body build* | | *Mobility* | | *Tissue malnutrition* | |
| Average | 0 | Fully | 0 | Terminal cachexia | 3 |
| Above average | 1 | Restless/fidgety | 1 | Cardiac failure | 5 |
| Obese | 2 | Apathetic | 2 | Peripheral vascular | 5 |
| Below average | 3 | Restricted | 3 | disease | |
| | | Inert/traction | 4 | Anaemia | 2 |
| | | Chairbound | 5 | Smoking | 1 |
| *Continence* | | *Appetite* | | *Neurological deficit* | |
| Complete/catheterised | 0 | Average | 0 | Diabetes, MS, CVA | 4–6 |
| Occasional | 1 | Poor | 1 | Motor/Paraplegia | 4–6 |
| incontinence | | NG tube | 1 | Sensory | 4–6 |
| Catheterised/ | 2 | Fluids only | 2 | | |
| incontinent of faeces | | NBM/anorexic | 3 | | |
| Doubly incontinent | 3 | | | | |
| *Skin type* | | *Sex/Age* | | *Major surgery/trauma* | |
| Healthy | 1 | Male | 1 | Orthopaedic | 5 |
| Tissue paper | 1 | Female | 2 | Below waist/spinal | 5 |
| Dry | 1 | 14–49 | 2 | On table > 2 hours | 5 |
| Oedematous | 1 | 50–64 | 2 | | |
| Clammy | 1 | 65–74 | 3 | *Medication* | |
| Discoloured | 2 | 75–80 | 4 | Steroids | 4 |
| Broken spot | 3 | > 81 | 5 | Cytotoxics | 4 |
| | | | | Anti-inflammatories | 4 |

**Total score: 10+ at risk**
**15+ high risk**
**20+ very high risk**

generally worse at night

## Disorientation
• In time, space and person

## Impaired thinking

## Impairment of short-term memory

## Perceptual abnormalities
• Illusions
• Hallucinations (particularly visual)

## Emotional changes
• Anxiety
• Irritability
• Depression

## Psychomotor changes
• Retardation or restless overactivity

## Disturbed sleep/wake cycle
• Insomnia and daytime sleeping

# Causes of dementia

## Degenerative
• Alzheimer's disease
• Multi-infarct dementia

- Pick's disease
- Huntington's chorea
- Creutzfeldt–Jakob disease
- Alcohol
- Parkinson's disease
- Progressive supranuclear palsy
- Multiple sclerosis
- Repeated head injury

## Cerebral lesions
- Tumours (primary/secondary)
- Subdural haematoma
- Normal-pressure hydrocephalus
- Neurosyphilis
- Chronic encephalitis

## Anoxia
- Anaemia
- Cardiac/respiratory failure
- Carbon monoxide poisoning
- Post cardiac arrest

## Metabolic
- Renal/hepatic failure

## Endocrine
- Hypothyroidism
- Addison's disease
- Recurrent hypoglycaemia
- Hypoparathyroidism

## Nutritional
- $B_{12}$/folate deficiency
- Thiamine/nicotinic acid deficiency

# Clinical features of dementia

## Progressive global memory impairment
- Short-term memory loss is the initial deficit
- Memory impairment gradually becomes global

## Personality deterioration
- Initially may cause exacerbation of personality traits
- Loss of manners, egocentricity, stubbornness, withdrawal,
- Deterioration in personal care and hygiene
- Incontinence

## Impaired thinking
- Perseveration, impaired concentration and judgement
- Ideas of reference and delusions may develop
- Speech may become impoverished with limited vocabulary

## Emotional changes
- Anxiety, irritability, depression, blunting of affect, emotional lability

## Abnormal perceptions
- Delusions, hallucinations

Note that in dementia there is no clouding of consciousness.

| Box 18.5: Abbreviated mental test score | |
|---|---|
| 1 | Age |
| 2 | Time (to nearest hour) |
| 3 | Address for recall at end of test |
| 4 | Year |
| 5 | Name of institution |
| 6 | Recognition of two persons |
| 7 | Date of birth (day and month sufficient) |
| 8 | Dates of Second World War |
| 9 | Name of present monarch |
| 10 | Count backwards from 20 to 1 |

Each correct answer scores 1 point

0–3: severe impairment
4–7: moderate impairment
8–10: normal

**Box 18.6:  Mini mental-state examination**

**Orientation**
*(1 point for each answer, maximum 10)*
> Name: year, month, day, date, time, country, town, district, hospital, ward

**Registration**
*(1 point for each answer, maximum 3)*
> Name three objects and ask patient to repeat

**Attention and calculation**
*(1 point for each answer, maximum 5)*
> Subtract 7 five times, starting at 100 (gives 93, 86, 79, 72, 65)

**Recall**
*(1 point for each answer, maximum 3)*
> Ask patient to repeat the three objects used in registration

**Language**
*(1 point for each, maximum 8)*
> Give the correct name for a pencil and a watch
> Ask patient to repeat 'no ifs, ands or buts'
> Give a three-stage command (e.g. 'Place the index finger of your right hand on your nose and then on your left ear'). Award one point for each stage successfully achieved
> Ask patient to read and obey a command written on a piece of paper, saying: 'Close your eyes'
> Ask patient to write a sentence. Award 1 point if it is sensible and has a subject and a verb

**Copying** *(maximum 1)*
> Ask patient to copy a drawing of a pair of intersecting hexagons

**Total out of 30:**      (< 24 indicates cognitive impairment)

# Idiopathic Parkinson's disease

Idiopathic Parkinson's disease is characterised by the presence of parkinsonism.

## Parkinsonism

### Upper body akinesia (akinesia complex)
- Slowness of movement (bradykinesia)
- Poverty of movement (impaired arm swing, facial amimia)
- Difficulty initiating movement
- Progressive fatiguing and reduced amplitude of repetitive alternating movements
- Difficulty with sequential or simultaneous motor acts
- Responsible for micrographia
- Essential for a diagnosis of parkinsonism

## Geriatric depression score (GDS-15 and GDS-30)

*Choose the best answer for how you felt over the past week*

| 1 | **Are you basically satisfied with your life?** | yes/**NO** |
| 2 | **Have you dropped many of your activities and interests?** | **YES**/no |
| 3 | **Do you feel that your life is empty?** | **YES**/no |
| 4 | **Do you often get bored?** | **YES**/no |
| 5 | Are you hopeful about the future? | yes/**NO** |
| 6 | Are you bothered by thoughts you can't get out of your head? | **YES**/no |
| 7 | **Are you in good spirits most of the time?** | yes/**NO** |
| 8 | **Are you afraid that something bad is going to happen to you?** | **YES**/no |
| 9 | **Do you feel happy most of the time?** | yes/**NO** |
| 10 | **Do you often feel helpless?** | **YES**/no |
| 11 | Do you often get restless and fidgety? | **YES**/no |
| 12 | **Do you prefer to stay at home, rather than going out?** | **YES**/no |
| 13 | Do you frequently worry about the future? | **YES**/no |
| 14 | **Do you feel you have problems with memory more than most?** | **YES**/no |
| 15 | **Do you think it is wonderful to be alive now?** | yes/**NO** |
| 16 | Do you often feel downhearted and blue? | **YES**/no |
| 17 | **Do you feel pretty worthless the way you are now?** | **YES**/no |
| 18 | Do you worry a lot about the past? | **YES**/no |
| 19 | Do you find life very exciting? | yes/**NO** |
| 20 | Is it hard for you to get started on new projects? | **YES**/no |
| 21 | **Do you feel full of energy?** | yes/**NO** |
| 22 | **Do you feel that your situation is hopeless?** | **YES**/no |
| 23 | **Do you think that most people are better off than you are?** | **YES**/no |
| 24 | Do you frequently get upset by little things? | **YES**/no |
| 25 | Do you frequently feel like crying? | **YES**/no |
| 26 | Do you have trouble concentrating? | **YES**/no |
| 27 | Do you enjoy getting up in the morning? | yes/**NO** |
| 28 | Do you prefer to avoid social gatherings? | **YES**/no |
| 29 | Is it easy for you to make decisions? | yes/**NO** |
| 30 | Is your mind as clear as it used to be? | yes/**NO** |

GDS-15 questions are in bold type
Patients should not see the scoring guidance
Answers indicating depression are in capitals (each scores one point)
GDS 30 > 11, GDS 15 > 5, indicate depression

---

**UK Parkinson's Disease Society Brain Bank (UK-PDSBB)
diagnostic criteria for idiopathic Parkinson's disease**

1  Presence of parkinsonism
2  Criteria supporting diagnosis:      Unilateral onset
                                       Rest tremor
                                       Progressive disorder
                                       Persistent asymmetry
                                       Good response to levodopa for 5 years or more
                                       Clinical course > 10 years
3  Features that exclude diagnosis:    History of repeated strokes
                                       History of repeated head injury
                                       History of encephalitis
                                       Oculogyric crises
                                       Neuroleptic treatment at onset
                                       > 1 affected relative
                                       Sustained remission
                                       Unilateral after 3 years
                                       Supranuclear palsy
                                       Cerebellar signs
                                       Early severe autonomic involvement
                                       Early severe dementia
                                       Babinski sign
                                       Cerebral tumour
                                       Hydrocephalus
                                       Negative response to levodopa
                                       MPTP exposure

---

## Rigidity

- Usually, but not always, present
- Lead pipe in the absence of tremor
- Cogwheel if coexistent tremor
- Affects predominantly flexor muscles

## Tremor

- Absent in 30% at presentation
- May never occur in some
- Intermittent resting tremor, usually of hands
- May be uncovered by wrist flexion or by asking patient to perform motor tasks
- May have intention or postural components

**Box 18.7:  Red flag signs against a diagnosis of IPD**

Early instability and falls
Rapid progression
Poor or transient response to levodopa
Lower-body parkinsonism
Autonomic failure
Pyramidal or cerebellar signs
Dementia
Downgaze palsy
Dysphonia, dysarthria
Inspiratory sighs
Groaning
Respiratory stridor
Myoclonic tremor
'Wheelchair sign'

**Table 18.3: Differential diagnosis of Parkinson's disease**

| Feature | Idiopathic Parkinson's disease | Essential tremor | Cerebro-vascular disease | Multisystem atrophy | Progressive supranuclear palsy |
|---|---|---|---|---|---|
| Parkinsonism | Yes | No | Lower body | Yes | Yes |
| Postural instability | Late | No | Early | Early | Early |
| Symmetry | No | Yes | No | No | Yes |
| Autonomic failure | Mild, late | No | Unusual | Severe, early | No |
| Impaired down gaze | No | No | No | No | Yes |
| Dementia | Late | No | Yes, stepwise | No | Yes, mild |
| Cerebellar signs | No | No | Yes/no | Yes | No |
| Pyramidal signs | No | No | Yes | Yes | No |
| Response to L-dopa | Good | None | None | None/ transient | None/ transient |
| Life expectancy | > 10 years | Normal | Variable | 9 years | 6–7 years |

# Causes of parkinsonism

- Idiopathic Parkinson's disease
- Multisystem atrophy
- Supranuclear palsy
- Antidopaminergic drugs (phenothiazines, Maxolon)
- Alzheimer's disease
- Wilson's disease
- Huntington's disease
- Pick's disease
- Postencephalitis lethargica
- Methyl-phenyl-tetrahydro-pyridine (MPTP) toxicity
- Space-occupying lesion
- Hydrocephalus
- CO poisoning

# Cerebrovascular disease

## Risk factors for cerebrovascular disease

- Hypertension (systolic pressure most predictive)
- Previous stroke/TIA
- Male gender
- Heart disease
- Atrial fibrillation
- Peripheral vascular disease
- Diabetes mellitus
- Smoking
- Obesity
- Alcohol abuse
- Combined oral contraceptive
- Hyperlipidaemia

# Oxford Community Stroke Project (OCSP) classification of stroke

## Total anterior circulation infarct (TACI)

- Extensive middle cerebral artery infarct
- Highest mortality with little chance of functional recovery
- New higher cerebral dysfunction (dysphasia, inattention)
- Contralateral motor and/or sensory deficit of at least two areas of the face, arm and leg
- Homonymous visual field defect

## Partial anterior circulation infarct (PACI)

- More restricted middle cerebral artery infarct, more distal occlusion of MCA
- Highest chance of early recurrence
- Only two of the three components of TACI
- Higher cerebral dysfunction alone

## Lacunar infarction (LACI)

- Infarction of basal ganglia, pons
- Often asymptomatic, consciousness preserved
- Low mortality
- Pure motor stroke
- Pure sensory stroke
- Sensorimotor strokes

**Box 18.8: Poor prognostic indicators following stroke**

Loss of consciousness at onset

Progression of deficit after admission

Drowsy or comatose on admission/after 24 hours

Conjugate gaze palsy

Complete limb paralysis (MRC 0 or 1)

Age > 65 years

Dysphagia

Urinary incontinence

- Ataxic hemiparesis

## Posterior circulation infarct (POCI)

- Infarction of brainstem, cerebellum, occipital lobes
- Low mortality, best chance of functional recovery
- High recurrence rate in first year
- Ipsilateral cranial nerve palsy with contralateral motor and/or sensory deficit

**Box 18.9: Orpington prognostic score**

| | | |
|---|---|---|
| Motor deficit in arm | MRC grade 5 | 0 |
| | MRC grade 4 | 0.4 |
| | MRC grade 3 | 0.8 |
| | MRC grade 1–2 | 1.2 |
| | MRC grade 0 | 1.6 |
| Proprioception (eyes closed ) | Locates affected thumb | |
| | Accurately | 0 |
| | Slight difficulty | 0.4 |
| | Via arm | 0.8 |
| | Unable | 1.2 |
| Balance | Walks 10 feet without help | 0 |
| | Maintains standing position | 0.4 |
| | Maintains sitting position | 0.8 |
| | No sitting balance | 1.2 |
| Cognition | MTS 10 | 0 |
| | MTS 8–9 | 0.4 |
| | MTS 5–7 | 0.8 |
| | MTS 0–4 | 1.2 |

**Total score = 1.6 + motor
+ proprioception
+ balance + cognition**

**Orpington prognosis: < 3.2: discharged
within 3 weeks
> 5.2: requires
long-term
nursing care**

- Bilateral motor and/or sensory deficit
- Disorder of conjugate eye movement
- Cerebellar dysfunction without hemiparesis
- Isolated homonymous visual field defect

# Predictors of outcome following stroke

## *Predictors of death/poor functional recovery*

- Loss of consciousness at onset
- Drowsiness after 24 hours
- Conjugate gaze palsy
- Urinary incontinence at 1 week
- Dysphagia
- Impaired pupillary reflexes
- Cheyne–Stokes respiration
- Advanced age
- Previous stroke
- Premorbid disability

## *Neurological recovery*

- Fastest recovery occurs in the first few weeks
- Most recovery occurs within 3 months
- Little recovery after 6 months
- If no movement in arm after 3 weeks, chances of full recovery poor

## *Predictors of early discharge*

- Good arm function
- Improvement in mobility
- Improvement in ADL
- Absence of sensory inattention
- Recovery of continence
- Orpington score (Box 18.9)

---

**Box 18.10:  Risk factors for self-neglect**

Dementia
Depression
Bereavement and isolation
Poverty
Disability
Alcohol
Previous psychiatric disorder
Educationally subnormal

---

# Social aspects of elderly care

## Aetiology of hypothermia

- Inadequate heating provision
- Inadequate clothing
- Social isolation
- Poor mobility
- Falls
- Inability to get up following fall
- Prolonged lying down
- Hypothyroidism
- Hypopituitarism
- Dementia
- Acute illness
- Phenothiazines
- Alcohol abuse
- Sedatives
- Poverty
- Increased ill health
- Polypharmacy
- Failed autonomic nervous system

## Clinical features of hypothermia

- Core temperature < 35°C
- Confusion
- Drowsiness
- Cold skin

- Absent shivering
- Increased skeletal muscle tone
- Bradycardia
- Prolonged PR interval on ECG
- J wave on ECG
- Shallow respiration
- Hypoxia
- Hypercapnia
- Renal failure
- Hyperglycaemia
- Raised transaminases
- Raised creatinine kinase
- Acute pancreatitis
- DIC
- Thrombocytopenia

# Diogenes syndrome

- Hoarding syndrome found in older people
- Patients usually not demented, but of high intellect
- Personality disorder
- Associated with frontal lobe abnormalities
- Patients usually suffer from chronic ill health related to poor hygiene

# Old age abuse

## Risk factors
- Resentful carer
- Carer with divided loyalties
- Carer with health problems of their own (especially alcoholism)
- An isolated carer
- Heavily dependent patient
- Communication problems
- Behaviour problems /Cognitive impairment

## Forms of old age abuse
- Physical
- Psychological
- Financial
- Emotional
- Neglect
- Sexual

## Recognition of old age abuse
- Repeated falls
- Multiple unusual injuries

# Legal aspects of elderly care

## Consent to treatment

The ability to participate autonomously in decisions regarding medical treatment depends on the capacity to understand and communicate information and to make reasoned decisions in the context of personal values and goals. In the absence of these abilities, decisional capacity cannot be presumed.

Essential features are:
1 Ability to comprehend the nature of an act being undertaken
2 Ability to make adequate judgements and reasoned decisions

## Joint report by BMA and Law Society 1995
To demonstrate sufficient mental capacity to give valid consent to treatment, an individual must be able to:
1 Understand in simple language

what the treatment is, its purpose and why it is being proposed

2  Understand its principal benefits, risks and alternatives

3  Understand, in broad terms, what the consequences would be of not receiving the proposed treatment

4  Retain the information long enough to make an effective decision

5  Make a free choice

# Attendance allowance

- Claimed by over 700,000 people
- Paid to the person that needs care
- Evidence that it is used to provide care not required
- May be claimed if attention is needed:
  1  Due to disability
  2  For help with bodily functions
  3  To avoid danger
- Only available to people of pensionable age (as of April 1992)
- Frequent respite care may disqualify a claim
- Claims made on form DS2 from DSS
- Medical examination required
- Disability must have been present for 6 months (unless terminally ill)
- Awarded for life
- Tax free
- If refused, appeals allowed within 3 months (72% successful)

# Power of Attorney

- If person becomes physically unable or simply chooses not to deal with his/her affairs they can set up a Power of Attorney
- This is a legal document whereby one person (the Grantor) enables another person of his/her choice (the Attorney) to act on his/her behalf
- Not endorsed or supervised by a court

- Private arrangement between parties involved
- Power may be general or limited to specific acts
- Power restricted to financial matters
- Grantor must be mentally competent
- Automatically ceases to be valid if the Grantor becomes mentally incompetent (except in Scotland, where an ordinary Power of Attorney remains valid if signed after January 1991)

## *Enduring Power of Attorney*

- Power of Attorney that continues to have effect when the Grantor becomes mentally incompetent
- Introduced into England and Wales in 1985
- Restricted to financial matters
- May be generalised or limited
- When the Grantor becomes mentally incompetent, the Attorney registers the enduring Power of Attorney with the Court of Protection (for a fee)
- Court of Protection does not routinely supervise the Attorney
- Court of Protection can terminate the enduring Power of Attorney if the Attorney becomes mentally incapable or is found to be dishonest
- May have more than one Attorney

# Court of Protection

- Office of the supreme Court of Judicature
- Judges nominated to it by Lord Chancellor
- Driven by statutory authority from Mental Health Act 1983

## *Function*

- To protect and control the administration of the affairs of people who become mentally incapable of

- doing so themselves
- Powers restricted to financial affairs (includes making wills )

### Court's procedures
- Referral made usually by nearest relative
- Doctor asked to certify mental incompetence
- Court obtains details of assets and financial commitments
- Receiver is appointed to manage the patient's affairs under the supervision of the court

### Drawbacks
- Procedures can be very lengthy
- Court charges fees

## Compulsory admission

- Section 47 National Assistance Act 1948 (amended 1951) allows admission of patients against their will if they are:
  1 Mentally competent
  2 Suffering from grave chronic disease or being aged, infirm or physically incapacitated, living in insanitary conditions
  3 Unable to devote to themselves, or are not receiving from others, proper care and attention

- Two doctors certify that in the interests of the person, or for preventing injury to the health of, or serious nuisance to, other persons, it is necessary to remove that person from the premises in which he/she is residing
- Application made to Court of Summary Jurisdiction or single justice
- Order removal to hospital or other place for not more than three weeks
- Renewable for further three weeks

- Used in around 200 cases per year
- Mentally incompetent patients: use Mental Health Act 1983

# Clinical case scenarios

## Hemiplegia

- There is unilateral seventh-nerve palsy
- There are ipsilateral upper or lower motor neuron signs in the arm and/or leg
- The ipsilateral plantar response is extensor
- There may be an homonymous hemianopia
- There may be associated sensory impairment in affected areas

- Other features to look for:
  Dysphasia/dysarthria
  Cerebellar signs
  Conjugate gaze palsy
  Sensory/visual inattention
  Contralateral third-nerve palsy
  (Weber's syndrome)

On visual field testing, a patient with an homonymous hemianopia will recognise they have a visual field defect and will turn their head to compensate. In contrast, a patient with visual inattention who does not acknowledge the affected side will not.

## Lateral medullary syndrome (Wallenberg's syndrome)

- Caused by infarction of the posterior inferior cerebellar artery (PICA)
- Patient usually presents with vertigo

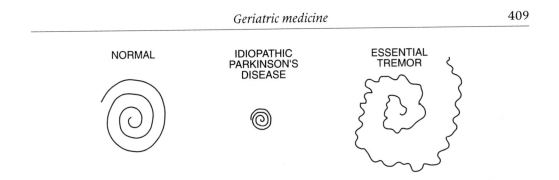

**Fig. 18.2: Spiral test: the patient draws a spiral without taking the pen off the paper. Typical spiral tests as seen in: normal individuals; idiopathic Parkinson's disease; essential tremor**

- Ipsilateral Horner's syndrome, cerebellar signs, palatal palsy, fifth-nerve sensory deficit
- Contralateral impaired pain and temperature sensation in limbs

## Idiopathic Parkinson's disease

- Patient has upper body akinesia, characterised by slow and delayed movement, fatiguability of fine, repetitive motor acts (ask patient to touch thumb successively with each finger)
- Patient also has an expressionless face
- The voice may be monotonous and low in volume
- There may be rigidity in the arms (lead-pipe or cogwheeling, if additional tremor)
- There may be a tremor which is resting in nature
- The signs are asymmetrical
- The gait is festinant (stooped posture, short shuffling steps, asymmetrical lack of arm swing)
- Patient has micrographia (ask them to do a spiral test, as shown in Fig. 18.2)

- Other features to look for:
    Impaired downgaze (supranuclear palsy)
    Cerebellar signs (multisystem atrophy)
    Orofacial dyskinesia, choreoathetosis (drug induced)

# Landmark geriatric studies

## Falls

**Province M, Hadley E, Hornbrook M et al for the FICSIT Group**
The effects of exercise on falls in elderly patients. A preplanned meta analysis of the FICSIT trials
*JAMA* 1995;273:1341

*The FICSIT series of randomised controlled trials looked at the effects of exercise on the rate of falls. The exercise interventions consisted of a variety of methods including balance training, resistance training, flexibility exercises and Tai Chi. The trials were performed in community and nursing-home-based patients. Overall, exercise significantly reduced the risk of falling by 10%.*

**Lauritzen JH, Petersen MM, Lund B**

Effects of external hip protectors on hip fractures
*Lancet 1993;341:11–13*

*This randomised controlled trial found that, in elderly residential-home-based patients, the use of hip protectors halved the risk of hip fracture, demonstrating a clear benefit for such an intervention in patients at high risk of falling*

# Thrombolysis in acute ischaemic stroke

### Multicentre Acute Stroke Trial – Italy (MAST-I) Group
Randomised controlled trial of streptokinase, aspirin and combinations of both in the treatment of acute ischaemic stroke
*Lancet 1995;346:1509–14*

### Multicentre Acute Stroke Trial – Europe (MAST-E) Group
Thrombolytic therapy with streptokinase in acute ischaemic stroke
*New Engl J Med 1996;335:145-150*

### Donnan G, Davis SM, Chambers BR et al for the Australian Streptokinase (ASK) Trial Study Group
Streptokinase for acute ischaemic stroke with relationship to the time of administration
*JAMA 1996;276:961–6*

*The above randomised controlled trials evaluated the potential benefits of standard-dose streptokinase given to patients within 6 hours of suffering an acute ischaemic stroke. All the trials were terminated early because, although there was reduced disability in survivors, there was an increase in early mortality.*

### Hacke W, Kaste M, Fieschi C et al for the ECASS Study Group
Intravenous thrombolysis with recombinent tissue plasminogen activator for acute hemispheric stroke

*JAMA 1995;274:1017–25*

### The National Institute of Neurological Disorders and Stroke r-tPa Stroke Study Group
Tissue plasminogen activator for acute ischaemic stroke
*New Engl J Med 1995;333:1581-7*

*The above two randomised controlled trials looked at the effects of r-tPa in acute ischaemic stroke. In the ECASS trial patients were randomised to receive thrombolysis within 6 hours of stroke onset, and in the NINDS trial patients received similar treatment within 3 hours of symptom onset. Both trials used the same doses of thrombolysis, which were lower than the doses of streptokinase used in previous trials. Neither of the r-tPa trials used other antithrombotic treatment, as was the case in the streptokinase trials*

*The ECASS trial results were negative. Although survivors had increased rates of recovery and shorter hospital stays, mortality was increased in the first 3 months.*

*The NINDS trial showed similar improved outcomes at 3 months, and although there was an increased risk of haemorrhage in the thrombolysis group, overall mortality was not increased compared to the placebo group. This therefore represents the first trial of thrombolysis in acute ischaemic stroke to show positive results.*

# Stroke units

### Stroke Unit Trialists' Collaboration
Collaborative systematic review of the randomised controlled trials of organised inpatient (stroke unit) care after stroke
*Br Med J 1997;314:1151–9*

*This meta-analysis looked at the randomised controlled trials of stroke unit care and concluded that it results in long-term reductions in death, dependency and the need for institutional care for all stroke types.*

# Carotid endarterectomy

## North American Symptomatic Carotid Endarterectomy Trial Collaborators (NASCET)
Beneficial effect of carotid endarterectomy in symptomatic patients with high grade stenosis
*New Engl J Med* 1991;325:445

## European Carotid Surgery Trial Collaborative Group (ECST)
MRC European carotid surgery trial: interim results for symptomatic patients with severe (60–99%) or with mild (0--29%) stenosis
*Lancet* 1999;337:1235

*These two randomised controlled trials demonstrated the benefits of carotid endarterectomy in patients suffering from TIA or non-disabling stroke in the presence of severe stenosis of the internal carotid artery. The results showed that carotid endarterectomy reduced the risk of stroke by 75% over 3 years, compared to best medical treatment. This equates to the need to perform four endarterectomies to prevent one stroke per year.*

## Asymptomatic Carotid Atherosclerosis Study Group (ACAS)
Carotid endarterectomy for patients with asymptomatic internal carotid artery stenosis
*JAMA* 1995;273:1421–8

*This randomised controlled trial looked at the benfits of carotid endarterectomy in patients with asymptomatic 60–99% stenosis of the internal carotid artery. The results showed a small but significant benefit, equating to the need to perform 85 endarterectomies to prevent one stroke per year.*

# Antiplatelets in stroke prevention

## CAST (Chinese Acute Stroke Trial) Collaborative Group
CAST: randomised placebo controlled trial of early aspirin use in 20,000 patients with acute ischaemic stroke
*Lancet* 1997;349:1641–9

## IST (International Stroke Trial) Collaborative Group
The International Stroke Trial (IST): a randomised trial of aspirin, subcutaneous heparin, both, or neither among 19,435 patients with acute ischaemic stroke
*Lancet* 1997;349:1569–81

*These two large randomised controlled trials examined the effects of aspirin and heparin (IST only) started within 48 hours of acute ischaemic stroke. The results from IST showed that treatment with low-dose heparin reduced the risk of further ischaemic stroke within the first 14 days, but this benefit was offset by a similar-sized increase in haemorrhagic stroke. At 6 months mortality was identical in both heparin and non-heparin groups. Patients given higher-dose heparin had a worse outcome.*

*Both studies showed that early treatment with aspirin reduces the risk of recurrent stroke in the first 2 weeks (without increasing the risk of haemorrhagic stroke) and reduces mortality or dependency at 6 months.*

## Diener H, Cunha L, Forbes C, Sivenius J, Smets P, Lowenthal A
European stroke prevention study. Dypyridamole and acetylsalicylic acid in the secondary prevention of stroke
*Neurol Sci* 1996;143:1–13

*This large randomised controlled trial studied the effects of dypyridamole Retard and aspirin in patients following acute ischaemic stroke. The results showed that dypyridamole alone led to a 16% reduction in the risk of stroke, com-*

*pared to an 18% reduction with aspirin. However, combination therapy with both drugs reduced the risk of stroke by 37%, equating to the need to treat 18 patients to prevent one stroke over 2 years.*

# Antithrombotic treatment in atrial fibrillation

**Petersen P, Boyson G, Godtfredsen J, Andersen E, Andersen B**
Placebo controlled, randomised trial of warfarin and aspirin for prevention of thromboembolic complications in chronic atrial fibrillation: the AFASAK study.
*Lancet 1989; i:175–9*
**The Boston Area Anticoagulation Trial of Atrial Fibrillation Investigators (BAATAF)**
The effect of low dose warfarin on the risk of stroke in patients with non rheumatic atrial fibrillation.
*New Engl J Med 1990;323:1505–11*
**EAFT (European Atrial Fibrillation Trial) Study Group**
Secondary prevention in non rheumatic atrial fibrillation after transient ischaemic attack or minor stroke.
*Lancet 1993;342:1255–62*
**Connoly SJ, Laupacis A, Gent M et al**
Canadian Atrial Fibrillation Anticoagulation (CAFA) Study
*J Am Coll Cardiol 1991;18:349–55*
**Stroke Prevention in Atrial Fibrillation Investigators (SPAF)**

Warfarin versus aspirin for prevention of thromboembolism in atrial fibrillation: Stroke Prevention in Atrial Fibrillation II study.
*Lancet 1994;343:687–91*

*In recent times the use of anticoagulation and aspirin as prophylaxis against cerebrovascular thromboembolism has been the focus of attention for several large trials. Results from these trials have suggested that, in patients with chronic non-rheumatic atrial fibrillation, warfarin leads to a 69% reduction in the risk of ischaemic stroke compared to only a 25% reduction in the risk with aspirin treatment.*

# Alzheimer's disease

**Roger SL, Farlow MR, Doody RS, Mohs R, Friedhoff LT and the Donepezil Study Group**
A 24 week double blind placebo controlled trial of donepezil in patients with Alzheimer's disease.
*Neurology 1998;50:136–45*

*This study examined the effects of the anticholinesterase inhibitor, donepezil (Aricept) in patients with mild to moderate Alzheimer's disease. The results showed small but significant improvements in cognitive function as measured by the ADAS cog score. It showed that six patients need to be treated with 10 mg/day for one patient to improve by 7 points on the ADAS cog score.*